DATE DUE

Psychological Aspects of Women's Reproductive Health

Michael W. O'Hara, PhD, is Professor and Chair of Psychology at the University of Iowa. He received his doctoral degree from the University of Pittsburgh and is currently Vice-President and President-Elect of the Marcé Society, which is an international society for the understanding, prevention, and treatment of mental illness related to childbearing. He has authored or co-authored over 60 papers and chapters related to depression and postpartum depression. He is also the author of a book, *Postpartum Depression: Causes and Consequences*. Dr. O'Hara has received several grants from the National Institute of Mental Health to study depression, particularly in childbearing women. His current research and clinical interests are in developing specific psychotherapies for postpartum depression.

Robert C. Reiter, MD, is Associate Professor, and Director, Division of Ambulatory Care and Co-Director, Chronic Pelvic Pain Clinic, Department of Obstetrics and Gynecology, University of Iowa College of Medicine. He graduated from the Baylor College of Medicine in Houston, Texas in 1981 and completed residency training in obstetrics and gynecology at the Naval Regional Medical Center in San Diego. Dr. Reiter is a leading investigator in the fields of clinical outcomes research, medical decision-making, and chronic pain management. Over the past 12 years he has co-edited five medical textbooks, authored over 75 published chapters and scientific articles, and received numerous research and teaching awards. He has been recently appointed as the Director of the Office of Outcomes Evaluation and Management at the University of Iowa Hospitals and Clinics.

Susan R. Johnson MD, MS, is Professor of Obstetrics and Gynecology and Acting Associate Dean, College of Medicine, University of Iowa, and is the Director of the Premenstrual Syndrome Clinic and the Menopause Clinic at the University of Iowa Hospitals and Clinics. She graduated from the University of Iowa College of Medicine and completed residency training in obstetrics and gynecology at the University of Iowa. Dr. Johnson has authored or co-authored over 50 papers and chapters on topics related to women's reproductive health. In particular, Dr. Johnson has been an active researcher in the areas of premenstrual syndrome and menopause. She is an investigator in several randomized clinical trials of hormone replacement therapy, including the Postmenopausal Estrogen/Progestin Interventions Trial (PEPI), and the Women's Health Initiative (WHI).

Alison Milburn, PhD, is currently in private practice in Iowa City, Iowa. She worked from 1990 to 1994 as a health psychologist in the Department of Obstetrics and Gynecology at the University of Iowa, where she was Co-Director of the Chronic Pelvic Pain Clinic and the Premenstrual Syndrome Clinic. She received her doctoral degree from The Ohio State University in Columbus. Her clinical and research interests include chronic gynecologic complaints such as chronic pelvic pain, premenstrual syndrome, incontinence, and vulvar symptoms, as well as weight control in women, gynecologic cancer, and sexual functioning in women. She has published several papers and chapters on the topic of chronic pelvic pain and sexual dysfunction in women.

Jane Engeldinger, MD, is an Associate in the Department of Obstetrics and Gynecology, where she is involved in primary patient care and teaching medical students and residents. She is the obstetrics and gynecology liaison for the "Introduction to Clinical Medicine" course for medical students and serves as medical director for the Gynecology Teaching Associates program. She graduated from the University of Iowa College of Medicine and completed her residency in obstetrics and gynecology at the University of Iowa. She has co-authored papers on postpartum depression, and is the author of a chapter on contraception.

PSYCHOLOGICAL ASPECTS *of* WOMEN'S REPRODUCTIVE HEALTH

Michael W. O'Hara, PhD

Robert C. Reiter, MD

Susan R. Johnson, MD

Alison Milburn, PhD

Jane Engeldinger, MD

Editors

 Springer Publishing Company

Springer Publishing Company, Inc.
536 Broadway
New York, NY 10012-3955

Cover Design by Tom Yabut
Production Editor: Joyce Noulas

95 96 97 98 99 / 5 4 3 2 1

RG
103.5
. P7724
1995

Library of Congress Cataloging-in-Publication Data

Psychological aspects of women's reproductive health / Michael W.
    O'Hara . . . [et al.], editors.
        p.   cm
    Includes bibliographical references and index.
    ISBN 0-8261-8660-2
    1. Gynecology—Psychosomatic aspects.   2. Obstetrics—
Psychosomatic aspects.   3. Gynecology—Psychological aspects.
4. Obstetrics—Psychological aspects.   5. Women—Mental health.
I. O'Hara, Michael W.
    [DNLM: 1. Reproduction.   2. Women—psychology.   3. Genital
Diseases, Female—psychology.   4. Decision Making. WQ 205 P9745
1994]
RG103.5.P7724 1994
618'.019—dc20
DNLM/DLC
for Library of Congress   94-36163
                                                                      CIP

Printed in the United States of America

Contents

Contributors

Kristen K. Brewer, MA, received her master's degree in clinical psychology at the University of Iowa, where she is a doctoral candidate. Her research and clinical interests in health psychology include high-risk sexual behavior of college students and the prevention of sexually transmitted diseases.

Kerrie L. Cole, MA, received her master's degree in clinical psychology from Wake Forest University. She is a doctoral candidate at the University of Iowa and is currently doing her clinical internship at the Department of Psychiatry and Behavioral Sciences at the University of Washington in Seattle. Her research interests include chronic pain and neuropsychology. She is planning on a research and clinical career in neuropsychological rehabilitation.

Robin L. Davisson, PhD, received her doctoral degree in physiology from the University of Iowa. She is currently a Fellow in the Cardiovascular Center at the University of Iowa. Her primary interests are in understanding basic mechanisms of cardiovascular functioning. She is currently utilizing transgenic animal models to study abnormalities in the renin-angiotensin system that contribute to the development and maintenance of hypertension.

Laura L. Gorman, MA, received her master's degree in clinical psychology from the University of Iowa, where she is a doctoral candidate. She is currently doing her clinical internship at the St. Louis Psychology Internship Consortium. Her current research and clinical interests include development and evaluation of preventive interventions for postpartum psychological disturbances. She also has interests in cognitive-behavioral and interpersonal interventions with patients who have depressive, anxiety, personality, or eating disorders.

Carol J. Hodne, MA, received her master's degree in social psychology from the University of Iowa, where she is a doctoral candidate. Her research interests include health psychology, with an emphasis on women's health, personal relationships, and empowerment models of social change. She has worked as a health advocate and community organizer among the elderly, poor, rural residents, and women.

Robin M. MacFarlane, MA, received her master's degree in clinical psychology from the University of Iowa, where she is a doctoral candidate. Her research interests are in personality and personality disorders, schizophrenia, and the schizophrenia spectrum.

Lynette A. Menefee, PhD, received her doctoral degree in counseling psychology from the University of Iowa. Her research and clinical interests include adaptation to chronic illness, behavioral medicine, and women's health.

Gail L. Rose, MA, received her master's degree in clinical psychology from the University of Iowa, where she is a doctoral candidate. Her research interests are within the area of women's health. She has conducted research on gender differences in physical and psychological adaptation to myocardial infarction. Her clinical interests are in the area of adaptation to lifestyle change and major life events among health populations, particularly women.

Amy Fuller Stockman, PhD, received her doctoral degree in counseling psychology from the University of Iowa, with a minor in women's health psychology. She is currently a health psychologist in the Department of Obstetrics and Gynecology at the University of Iowa. Her clinical and research interests include psychological issues in women's reproductive health and rural mental health practice.

Elizabeth F. Swanson-Hyland, MA, received her master's degree in clinical psychology from the University of Iowa, where she is a doctoral candidate. She is currently doing her clinical internship at the Kansas City, Missouri Veteran's Administration Medical Center. Her research interests are in the area of social support and health, and her clinical interests are in the area of health psychology.

Mary K. Walling, PhD, received her doctoral degree in clinical psychology at the University of Iowa. She is currently a clinician at the Des Moines Pastoral Counseling Center in Des Moines, Iowa. Her research and clinical interests are in the area of women's health, particularly chronic pelvic pain.

Elizabeth A. Weerts Whitmore, PhD, received her doctoral degree in clinical psychology at the University of Iowa. She is currently an Instructor in the Department of Psychiatry, University of Colorado Health Sciences Center in Denver. Her research and clinical interests are in the areas of women's health issues, personality, and the interaction between psychological and medical factors in problem pregnancies, chronic pelvic pain, and other gynecological problems.

Introduction

Michael W. O'Hara

It has been long recognized that psychological factors play an important role in the health status of both men and women. Originally, recognition of the links between psychological functioning and health was formalized in the discipline of psychosomatic medicine. The research and clinical literature often addressed issues regarding the association between personality traits, psychopathologic states, environmental stressors (e.g., depression, anxiety) and risk for health problems (heart disease, chronic pain, infertility). Within the domain of reproduction, this field became known as psychosomatic obstetrics and gynecology.

The term psychosomatics no longer is adequate to convey the increasing interface between psychology and medicine. Within the domain of women's reproductive health, psychological factors have several roles. In some cases, psychologic factors play a causal role in a health problem. For example, a negative cognitive style will increase the likelihood of depression after childbirth. A low tolerance for the physical discomfort of a normal menstrual flow may put a woman at risk for a hysterectomy. A poor marital relationship may impair adjustment to gynecological cancer. In other cases, psychological factors may be consequences of reproductive health problems. For example, infertility is recognized as a major contributor to psychological distress. Finally, psychological factors may represent part of the complex expression of reproductive health and illness. Examples would include premenstrual syndrome and postpartum depression.

The purpose of the present volume is to explore the interrelationships among psychological and health factors as they relate to women's reproduction. This volume is organized into four parts, *reproductive transitions, gynecology, obstetrics*, and *decision making*. The chapters that make up this volume, with a few exceptions, have a similar organizational structure. The first section of each chapter will provide a brief introduction to and description of the problem that is the focus of the chapter. The second section will provide a critical review of the relevant psychological literature. Finally, the third section will discuss the implications of the psychological literature for the clinical care of the patient. Important issues raised by each chapter are highlighted briefly below.

REPRODUCTIVE TRANSITIONS

With the exception of the menarche, the major reproductive transitions are covered in this part of the book. The menstrual cycle is the transition with which women have the most experience. While for most women discomfort associated with ovulation and impending menstrual flow is a no more than a nuisance, for some women these monthly events cause significant pain and emotional distress. In the chapter on menstruation (Chapter 1) Johnson describes the various menstrually related disorders. Her major focus, however, is on the premenstrual syndrome. In addition to reviewing the etiologic and treatment research, Johnson presents an important model for the clinical evaluation and management of women presenting with premenstrual complaints.

Childbearing (Chapter 2) represents a second reproductive transition that is much more visible and public than menstruation. It is as much of a social event as it is a biological event. O'Hara's focus in this chapter on childbearing is primarily concerned with dysfunctional psychological and social adjustment, particularly postpartum depression. Two important messages of this chapter are 1) that psychological disturbance after childbirth occurs following about 10% of deliveries and deserves prompt recognition and treatment, and 2) that postpartum psychiatric disorders that are not successfully treated may put a woman and her family at risk for future adjustment disorders.

The last major reproductive transition is menopause (Chapter 3) which marks the end of a woman's fertility. Although it was common in the past to view this transition very negatively, associated with loss of social function and high risk for so-called involutional melancholy, psychologists and gynecologists increasingly recognize the generally very good adjustment of menopausal women. Walling does point out the psychological risks associated with surgical menopause, particularly in young women who have not completed their family. Medical management of menopause must recognize that a woman's psychological functioning prior to menopause will in large part determine a woman's adaptation to menopause.

GYNECOLOGY

Many gynecological problems have significant psychological sequelae. Chronic pelvic pain (Chapter 4) has for many years frustrated the best efforts of gynecologists to provide effective pain relief. Patients with pain who did not respond to standard therapies were often given pejorative labels, the belief being that there was no organic basis for their pain. As the pain management field has become more sophisticated, it is now recognized that pain is a complex phenomenon, and that pain sensations reflect both peripheral and central processes. As Walling and Reiter make clear, chronic pelvic pain is best managed by an interdisciplinary team that is sensitive to the physical, emotional, and social features of chronic pain. Another major contribution of Walling and Reiter's chapter is the observation that many women with chronic pain have not only experienced sexual abuse (during childhood or adulthood), but many women have also been physically abused as children or adults. The clinical implications of these observations are discussed as well.

Hysterectomy (discussed in Chapter 5) is among the most common surgical procedures. A very large percentage of American women will undergo a hysterectomy at some time in their lives. Much in the way that menopause was thought to occasion psychological maladjustment, hysterectomy was at one time thought to be associated with an increased risk for psychological disturbance. Prospective research made clear that psychological distress is to some degree relieved by hysterectomy. Rather than being a consequence of hysterectomy, psychological distress also would appear to be a risk factor for hysterectomy. Psychological distress may increase the likelihood that women will seek hysterectomy or the likelihood that women will complain about normal menstrual function and, as a consequence, receive a hysterectomy. However, psychological distress may be a consequence of the medical problems that indicate the need for hysterectomy. As Stockman discusses, careful psychological assessment is often (though not invariably) indicated when a woman presents with questionable indications for a hysterectomy. Stockman also points out the importance of psychological preparation of patients for hysterectomy and other types of gynecological surgery. There is a growing literature pointing to both the psychological and medical consequences of providing both accurate information to patients about their surgery and teaching patients skills (e.g., relaxation, relevant exercises) to manage the consequences.

Gynecological cancer (Chapter 6) may be associated with considerable morbidity and mortality. Menefee argues that patients often benefit from psychological interventions aimed at helping them cope with many of the deleterious consequences of the cancer. Patients can learn to accept and adapt to changes in body shape and function. For example, sexual function is often compromised in patients with gynecological cancer. Psychological interventions can help a couple

adapt to changes in the woman's sexual function and help couples develop
strategies to enhance sexual functioning even when intercourse is difficult or
impossible. Finally, for patients who are terminally ill, psychological interventions can be invaluable in helping patients prepare for their death and in helping
families effectively cope with the loss of a mother or wife.

Managing fertility (covered in Chapter 7) is very important to women, yet
failure to consistently use effective contraceptives is common, particularly among
younger women. In her chapter, Brewer addresses several possible reasons for
this phenomenon. Adolescent women may be exposed to inaccurate information
regarding the likelihood of pregnancy following intercourse, particularly that
which occurs soon after the woman has become sexually active. Brewer discusses the consequences of the difficulty that parents and other sources of
authority have in encouraging abstinence on one hand and encouraging the use
of contraceptives on the other hand. Young people who are not supposed to be
sexually active may feel quite guilty and consequently not plan for sex. Moreover, portrayals in the media of the romantic elements of spontaneous sex are a
further barrier to the proper use of contraceptives. Finally, Brewer reviews several considerations in advising women about contraception at each stage of their
reproductive lives.

In Chapter 8 Milburn and Brewer describe the extent to which sexually
transmitted diseases are a significant public health problem. In addition to AIDS,
sexually transmitted diseases such as herpes and human papillomavirus cause
significant physical and psychological morbidity. The psychological consequences
for the patient with sexually transmitted disease can range from depression and
anxiety to relationship disturbances. Psychological interventions not only play a
role in helping patients adjust to a sexually transmitted disease but, more importantly, they may also be instrumental in helping individuals reduce their risk for
contracting a sexually transmitted disease. Milburn and Brewer conclude their
chapter by outlining preventive strategies that can be implemented with sexually
active young adults.

OBSTETRICS

Although the consequences of unintended pregnancies are of significant concern
to health professionals, infertility (Chapter 9) has become a serious physical and
psychological health problem. Davisson discusses how the inability to conceive
is profoundly discomforting to many couples and challenges their identities as
women and men. Moreover, the expectations of family members and friends
regarding the importance of children to a family may rob the couple of important sources of support. It is unlikely that psychological factors account for
many of the cases of infertility; however, depression, anger, and anxiety are

common consequences of prolonged infertility. These problems are often compounded by difficulties and failures associated with attempts to have a child through medical intervention or adoption.

In Chapter 10 Rose argues that, as couples have waited longer to start families and as technologies have evolved to detect many chromosomal and non-chromosomal abnormalities in the fetus, the psychological burdens associated with prenatal diagnosis have increased. Women over the age of 35 are routinely advised to undergo an amniocentesis because of the risk of Down's Syndrome. The anticipation of procedures such as amniocentesis causes anxiety, and the period of waiting for the results of screening can be very difficult as well. Moreover, maternal serum alphafetoprotein (MSAFP) sampling has a relatively high rate of false positives, requiring further testing to confirm or rule out the original results. Finally, the relatively small subgroup of couples who receive news of a fetal abnormality may be devastated and are immediately faced with the decision to abort the pregnancy or carry to term a defective fetus. All of these facts point to the importance of carefully considering the psychological consequences of prenatal diagnostic testing and the importance of integrating psychological and medical services for couples who undergo these procedures.

Prepared childbirth (discussed in Chapter 11) has become increasingly common for American women. The Lamaze approach, although not the only method, is almost synonymous with childbirth preparation in the minds of most women. As Swanson-Hyland discusses, the central purpose of childbirth preparation is to reduce pain during labor and delivery. Of course, there are other potential benefits of childbirth preparation, including more accurate expectations on the part of the couple regarding the medical elements of childbirth, increased ability to cooperate with the obstetrician and nurses, increased involvement of the spouse during labor and delivery, and less uncertainty and fear regarding the labor, delivery, and the postpartum period. Given the widespread use of childbirth preparation, it is sobering to note that outcome literature regarding the efficacy of prepared childbirth is fraught with methodological problems and, as a consequence, is rather weak.

Pregnancy loss (Chapter 12) is relatively common; however, as Cole argues in her chapter, it is important for the clinician to be sensitive to the grief that couples will experience even when the loss occurs early in pregnancy. Pathological grief may occur in up to 1 in 5 pregnancy losses. Many couples try to repair their loss by trying to conceive again as soon as possible although there as been significant debate about the wisdom of early conception following pregnancy loss. In the final section of her chapter Cole discusses several interventions such as validating the loss and education about grief that may help couples successfully adjust to their loss.

Abortion (Chapter 13) is a complex topic that has significant medical, social, legal, moral, and psychological dimensions. Whitmore briefly reviews the legal status of abortion and argues that much of the psychological knowledge about the consequences of abortion are based on studies conducted when legal abortions were largely unavailable. Whitmore describes the various methods of abortion and the type of follow-up care that is typically provided. She argues that, based on the literature, there is very little evidence that there are pervasive negative psychological consequences of abortion and that in fact, relief is the most common experience after an abortion. Nevertheless, for some women there are negative psychological consequences and some of the risk factors for poor adjustment to abortion are described. In the final section of her chapter, Whitmore provides an overview of counseling interventions that may help some women make a decision regarding abortion and to manage or cope with the consequences of that decision.

High-risk pregnancies (Chapter 14) have important psychological and behavioral causes and consequences. Gorman examines, for example, the extent to which high levels of prenatal anxiety can serve as a risk factor for adverse outcomes. Perhaps more important are health behaviors such as smoking, drinking, and the use of illegal substances, that can put a pregnancy at risk. Psychological and behavioral interventions certainly have a role to play in helping women reduce or eliminate behaviors that put their pregnancy at risk (stopping smoking) and increase behaviors that can facilitate a healthy pregnancy (e.g., proper nutrition).

As MacFarlane makes clear, the United States has one of the highest rates of births to adolescents (Chapter 15) of developed countries. She argues that as a society we give very mixed messages to young people about sexuality—promoting sexual behavior on the one hand and giving adolescents very negative messages about it on the other hand. Several issues are discussed in this chapter including the prevention of adolescent pregnancy, the decision to abort the pregnancy or carry it to term, the decision to keep or adopt out the infant, and the consequences of motherhood for the economic, physical, and social health of the mother. Finally, MacFarlane outlines the various roles that professionals have in intervening with the adolescent woman at each of these points in the childbearing process.

DECISION MAKING

The volume concludes with a thoughtful discussion of psychosocial factors affecting women's medical decision making (Chapter 16). In this chapter, Hodne argues for the active involvement of women in making decisions about their health care and for the benefits to the patient of active involvement. Importantly, she discusses at length some of the judgment biases (e.g., availability bias and framing effects) that can affect medical decision making. Hodne also discusses social influences (e.g., family and friends) on medical decision making. Many more important topics are also considered in this chapter, including sexual and psychosocial issues, competency to grant informed consent, and cultural factors.

In conclusion, we hope that this volume will sensitize the medical and non-medical women's health care professional to the psychological dimensions of the provision of women's reproductive health care. Somatic and psychological causes and consequences of disease are inextricably intertwined. The effective clinician will respect both dimensions in his or her medical care of women.

PART I

Reproductive Transitions

Menstruation

Susan R. Johnson

The menstrual cycle is a common source of minor, and an occasional source of major, symptomatology among reproductive-age women. Knowledge of the basic hormonal events during the normal menstrual cycle helps in understanding these symptoms. The menstrual cycle can be divided into follicular and luteal phases, each defined according to the primary site of hormone secretion by the ovary. During the follicular (or postmenstrual) phase, estrogen is produced by ovarian follicles. One of these follicles becomes the dominant follicle from which an ovum will be released at ovulation. The follicular phase lasts, on average, about two weeks. Ovulation is preceded by a surge of the gonadotropin, luteinizing hormone (LH). Under the influence of LH, the dominant follicle is transformed into the corpus luteum which secretes progesterone. During this phase, called the "luteal phase," both estrogen and progesterone are secreted. After about two weeks, if pregnancy does not occur, the corpus luteum degenerates, and progesterone production ceases. In response to this progesterone "withdrawal," the endometrium (lining of the uterus) is sloughed—that is, the menstrual period.

Each of these phases of the menstrual cycle is commonly accompanied by specific symptoms. Ovulation is often marked by mild, one-sided lower abdominal discomfort (so-called "mittle schmerz") that lasts for a few hours, an increase in clear thin cervical mucous, and occasionally by slight vaginal spotting. A few days before menses, many women experience "moliminal" symptoms, which consist of the same type of complaints that accompany premenstrual syndrome, such as irritability, breast tenderness, appetite cravings, bloating, and so on.

Finally, the menstrual flow itself may be associated with lower midline cramping pain that lasts for a day or two. In severe form these "cramps" are called dysmenorrhea, and often require medical therapy.

The focus of this chapter is premenstrual syndrome (PMS), since this is the menstrual cycle problem most often associated with emotional symptoms. Simply defined, PMS refers to a syndrome in which a group of negative emotional, physical, and/or cognitive symptoms recur in the luteal phase of the menstrual cycle, and are absent in the follicular phase.

One barrier to understanding the literature regarding premenstrual phase phenomena is inconsistently used nomenclature. For some authors, premenstrual syndrome (or premenstrual tension) is used to describe any negative symptoms in the luteal phase, regardless of severity. This broad definition includes as many as 90% of reproductive-age women. At the other extreme, the term is used to delineate the small group of women, perhaps 5%, with symptoms that have a very disruptive impact. The introduction of the label Late Luteal Phase Dysphoric Disorder (LLPDD) in the DSM–III–R (American Psychiatric Association, 1987) was, in part, an attempt to provide this latter group a distinctive diagnostic label. The terms "premenstrual changes" and "molimina" are used to refer to the mild symptoms which are a normal consequence of ovulation in about 50% of women.

In this chapter, the more commonly used name PMS will be used to denote symptoms with adverse impact across a spectrum of severity that includes between 15 and 20% of women. In this scheme, "severe PMS" is equivalent to the subset who meet criteria for the diagnosis of LLPDD.

DIAGNOSTIC CRITERIA

The typical patient with PMS is in her mid-thirties, with symptoms that have been present for several years, but are now more intense and of longer duration. The symptoms begin abruptly, but predictably, between 8 and 14 days before her period is expected. Others, especially family members, often recognize this change. Both physical and emotional symptoms are usually present. Irritability (or sometimes depression) is the most common reason for seeking help. Symptoms improve almost immediately with the onset of menses, and resolve no more than two to three days later. The abrupt "onset" and "offset" has resulted in the often-used Jekyll/Hyde analogy.

Two points made in the earlier description of the menstrual cycle are relevant to our discussion of PMS: 1) The menstrual cycle is characterized by a series of precisely timed events. Progesterone is produced only during the phase in which PMS occurs, leading to focus on the possible causal role of this hormone. 2) Ovulation is a prerequisite to the luteal phase and, by extension, to PMS. Therefore, women who are amenorrhic, menopausal, or have had their ovaries re-moved, cannot have PMS (Hammarbäck, Ekholm, & Bäckström, 1991). On the other hand, a woman who has had her uterus, but not her ovaries, removed, can have PMS. The only clinical difference is that there will be no menstrual period to mark the end of the luteal phase.

In the last ten years several sets of diagnostic criteria for PMS have been developed, as exemplified by the DSM–III–R (appendix) criteria for Late Luteal Phase Dysphoric Disorder (LLPDD), or the criteria proposed by Mortola, Girton, Beck, and Yen (1990). While these sets of criteria have had the positive effect of improving the quality of clinical trials, there is still significant variability among criteria. Hurt, Schnurr, Severino, Freeman, Gise, Rivera-Tovar, and Steege (1992) applied the criteria for LLPDD to 650 subjects drawn from a number of clinical trials in which disparate selection criteria had been used. Between 15 and 44% of the subjects met the criteria, suggesting lack of homogeneity among different diagnostic classification methods.

Fortunately, the same level of precision is not necessary for clinical purposes as for research. All diagnostic criteria sets include requirements for 1) the pres-ence of typical symptoms, that are 2) confined to the luteal phase, and are 3) of sufficient severity to impair function. These requirements serve as a guide to clinical decisions.

The assertion that PMS is associated with an extremely diverse set of symp-toms, numbering over 150 (Tucker & Whalen, 1991) is made repeatedly. How-ever, a more consistent albeit limited phenomenology is suggested by studies which have used rigorously defined cases, that is, cases in which symptom timing is established prospectively, and other medical and psychiatric disorders are excluded. The most common emotional symptoms are irritability, mood swings, hostility, and depression. Physical symptoms are more diverse, and include breast pain, bloating, insomnia, fatigue, hot flashes, hyperphagia, clum-siness, pain, and headaches. Cognitive problems, especially difficulty concentrat-ing, have been more recently recognized. The full syndrome is characterized by a cluster of symptoms, typically six or more, cutting across these categories.

The second criterion, confinement to the luteal phase, requires that the tim-ing of symptoms in relation to the menstrual period be established by a *prospec-tive* symptom diary ("charting"). This requirement is unique among mood disor-ders, and often seems unduly burdensome to both the clinician, who is interested in a rapid disposition, and the woman, who wants prompt treatment. However, most studies have found that about half of the women who complain of premen-strual syndrome do not have a luteal phase pattern confirmed with prospective recording (Rubinow, Roy-Byrne, Hoban, Grover, Stambler, & Post, 1986; Schnurr, 1988).

There are no standardized criteria for assessing the severity of premenstrual symptoms. For most women, the major impact is in their personal life, creating difficulties with partner and/or children and, to a lesser extent, at work (Leather, Holland, Andrews, & Studd, 1993). Mortola et al. (1990) suggest assessing relationship discord, difficulties in parenting, work performance, social isolation, legal difficulties, suicidal ideation, and medical attention-seeking. Serious problems, like suicide attempts, divorce, child abuse, and crime are probably uncommon (Johnson, 1987).

The expression and severity of several problems other than PMS, such as an affective disorder, may be affected by the menstrual cycle. A woman may believe such a problem is PMS either because the symptoms of her condition are similar to those of PMS, or because she believes that any problem that worsens premenstrually is "PMS." Between 30–70% of the women who complain of PMS will have another condition (Chandraiah, Levenson, & Collins, 1991; Chang & Hutchinson-Williams, 1991; Nye, Hurt, Severino, & Shangold, 1992). Therefore, the care giver must be aware of these conditions, and know how to distinguish each from PMS.

Molimina. Molimina refers to normal changes that occur in the late luteal phase of the menstrual cycle as a consequence of ovulation. As described earlier, these symptoms are similar to the ones that characterize PMS, but physical symptoms usually predominate. Typically, symptoms are present for only two or three days, have little functional impact, and disappear promptly with the onset of bleeding. It is not known if PMS simply represents a more extreme form of molimina, or if the two conditions are the result of differing pathophysiological events.

Dysmenorrhea. Dysmenorrhea is characterized by acute, midline-low abdominal pain ("cramps") that begins within a few hours of menstrual bleeding, and usually resolves spontaneously within 48 hours (Johnson, 1992a). Systemic symptoms can occur (headache, fatigue, diarrhea, dizziness), and the syndrome can begin a day or two prior to menses, leading to a picture suggestive of PMS. However, PMS begins sooner in the cycle, begins to resolve (rather than worsening) with the onset of bleeding, and does not have a prominent pain component. The age distribution of this problem differs from PMS. Dysmenorrhea begins within a few months of menarche, and is most common in women between the ages of 15 and 25, whereas PMS does not become a significant problem for most women until after age 25.

Like PMS, dysmenorrhea has a spectrum of severity, with only a small proportion of women experiencing disabling pain. Effective therapies for dysmenorrhea include prostaglandin synthetase inhibitors (e.g., ibuprofen) and oral contraceptive pills.

Perimenstrual exacerbation. A variety of disorders, especially affective disorders, may predictably worsen around the time of the menses (Chisholm, Jung, Cummings, Fox, & Cumming, 1990). Unlike PMS, symptoms in these conditions are not confined to the luteal phase, but rather, occur throughout the cycle. Peak severity typically occurs just prior to or during menses rather than during the luteal phase. Physical symptoms are absent or less prominent. Often, depression or anxiety, rather than irritability, is the dominant symptom. Other syndromes can occur in this pattern as well, such as irritable bowel syndrome, chronic fatigue syndrome, or idiopathic cyclic edema.

Perimenstrual occurrence. Disorders that are episodic in occurrence can also be triggered by menstrual cycle events. Here, the disorder manifests itself primarily in the late luteal or menstrual phase, and tends not to occur at other times. The most common example is migraine headache. As many as 30% of women with migraine headaches note increased frequency in the two weeks prior to and including menstruation. Between 5 and 10% of women with migraines meet the stricter criteria for "menstrual migraine," in which the headaches *only* occur in the late luteal or menstrual phase (Digre & Damasio, 1987). Less common examples are asthma (Gibbs, Coutts, Lock, Finnegan, & White, 1984), epilepsy (Newmark & Penry, 1980), porphyria (Herrick, McColl, Wallace, Moore, & Goldberg, 1990); uveitis (Bell, 1989), and Meniere's disease (Andrews, Ator, & Honrubia, 1992). These disorders are usually easy to distinguish from PMS based on the history and physical examination. Therapy specific to the problem is usually adequate. If perimenstrual recurrence persists despite therapy, ovulation suppression may be useful.

Superimposed PMS. PMS may be coincidentally present along with another problem, including the disorders described above. The prevalence of this situation can be calculated by multiplying the prevalence of PMS by that of the other disorder. For example, if severe PMS has a point prevalence of 5% and major depressive disorder a point prevalence of 1% among women aged 35, you would expect that five in ten thousand ($.05 \times .01 = 0.0005$) women that age will have both. However, if moderate PMS, and all severities of affective disorder are included, the combined prevalence will be more common, approximately 5 in 100 women (0.25×0.2).

The joint occurrence of PMS and an affective disorder can be difficult to distinguish from the premenstrual exacerbation of a mood disorder, since the symptoms of mood disorders and PMS overlap (Siegel, Meyers, & Dineen, 1986). However a woman will often recognize that she develops a new set of symptoms during the late luteal phase that differ from her chronic disorder.

Oral contraceptive pill–associated symptoms. Women taking oral contraceptive pills (oc) may have symptoms that mimic PMS. The pattern may also resemble PMS in that the symptoms are most prominent just prior to withdrawal bleeding. When oc's are stopped, the effect on symptoms is unpredictable: some worsen, some stop and some are unaffected. In addition, many women with PMS are intolerant to oc's; when taking them they develop more severe, PMS-like symptoms either through the entire cycle, or sometimes only during the pre-withdrawal week.

Non-cyclic conditions. Many women who complain of PMS are found to have symptoms which have no relationship to the menstrual cycle when charted prospectively. This conclusion should not be based on a single cycle of charting, since external events can result in an unreliable month. It is important to explain that the symptoms of PMS are nonspecific, and that none are unique to the syndrome.

ETIOLOGY

Some authors theorize that PMS is a culturally linked, learned phenomenon (Bernsted, Luggin, & Petersson, 1984; Ruble & Brooks-Gunn, 1979). The evidence for this theory is largely based on studies of women who have mild premenstrual changes rather than PMS (AuBuchon & Calhoun, 1985). Normal women may indeed attribute some negative physical and emotional symptoms to the premenstrual period based on a learned belief that symptoms should occur then. However, women who meet stringent criteria for moderate to severe PMS do not appear to exhibit this phenomenon (Gallant, Popiel, Hoffman, Chakraborty, & Hamilton, 1992). In addition, a number of biological differences between women with and without PMS have been identified. Examples include: markers of serotonergic activity and beta-endorphin levels (Dinan & O'Keane, 1991); elevated nocturnal temperature (Severino, Wagner, Moline, Hurt, Pollak, & Zendell, 1991); atrial natiuretic peptide concentration (Hussain, O'Brien, DeSouza, Okonofua, & Dandona, 1990); and brainstem auditory evoked responses (Howard, Mason, Taghavi, & Spears, 1992). Finally, the persistence of PMS after hysterectomy with retention of the ovaries is difficult to explain by attribution, since there is no menstrual period to mark the time in the cycle (Bäckström, Boyle, & Baird, 1981).

A conceptual model that incorporates current information regarding pathophysiology of PMS is useful in evaluation and treatment of PMS (Johnson, 1992b). This model suggests that PMS is initiated by events occurring at, or as a result of, ovulation (Hammarbäck et al., 1991). Second, as a result of these events, temporary alterations in neurotransmitters (and perhaps some peripheral substances) occur that lead to a range of emotional, somatic, and cognitive symptoms (Dinan & O'Keane, 1991). Third, the impact of these symptoms on women may depend, in part, on individual differences among women in concomitant psychopathology, situational stressors, social support, and/or coping skills.

The potential roles of luteal phase changes in ovarian, pituitary, and other related hormones have been the subject of interest since Frank (1931) originally described PMS. Despite uncertainty about the precise sequence of events in the pathophysiology of PMS, most data support a biological basis for the disorder.

Progesterone has been the primary focus in the past, but until recently no reproducible differences between women with and without PMS have been found. Although absolute levels of progesterone do not appear to differ, Facchinetti, Genazzani, Martignoni, Fioroni, Nappi, and Genazzani (1993) demonstrated that the pulse frequency and amplitude of progesterone secretion did differ between cases and controls. This same group of investigators (Facchinetti, Genazzani, Martignoni, Fioroni, Sances, & Genazzani, 1990) also found differences in LH pulsatile secretion in women with PMS. Schmidt, Nieman, Grover, Muller, Merriam, and Rubinow (1991) demonstrated that the experimental truncation of the luteal phase with the drug mifepristone did not prevent symptoms in a group of 14 women with PMS. Therefore, rather than being a direct cause of symptoms, the perturbations of progesterone secretion that have been observed may represent an effect of some other primary, perhaps hypothalamic alteration that occurs *at* ovulation. There is currently no evidence of a role for prolactin, renin-angiotensin-aldosterone, sex hormone-binding globulin, or androgens in the pathogenesis of PMS.

Brayshaw and Brayshaw (1986) reported that the majority of a small group of women with PMS had evidence of subtle thyroid dysfunction, and that all responded to therapy with levo-thyroxine. Several studies have investigated this possibility, with mixed results. Casper, Patel-Christopher, and Powell (1989) found no differences in thyroid testing between 15 women with PMS and 19 without PMS. Nikolai, Mulligan, Gribble, Harkins, Meier, and Roberts (1990) studied thyroid function in 44 women with PMS and 15 without PMS. Only one woman had abnormal testing, and there was no benefit of thyroxine therapy in 22 of the women studied in a controlled trial. Schmidt, Grover, Roy-Byrne, and Rubinow (1993) studied 30 women with PMS, and found a rate of subclinical elevated thyroid stimulating hormone (TSH) similar to that expected in a group of reproductive-age women. Thirty percent of the women had an abnormal response to thyroid releasing factor (TRF) stimulation. A subset of the sample was enrolled in a controlled trial of thyroxine, and there was no benefit compared with placebo. Based on these three studies, thyroid testing should be done only if clinically indicated, and thyroxine therapy should be given only to women with documented hypothyroidism.

In the last decade, research has focused on neurotransmitters (Bäckström, 1992; Dinan & O'Keane, 1991). Current evidence suggests that serotonin (Rapkin, 1992), beta-endorphin, and melatonin may all be important in the pathogenesis of PMS.

In women without PMS, an increase in *serotonin* receptors occurs in the luteal phase, perhaps induced by the increasing levels of estradiol from the late follicular phase. There is evidence that this "up regulation" might not occur in women with PMS. A deficiency of receptors could presumably lead to increased serotonin re-uptake, resulting in lowered mood.

Uptake of serotonin and imipramine binding in platelets are both similar to uptake in the brain, so these are studied to make inferences about brain serotonin activity. Rapkin and her collegues found that whole blood (Rapkin, Edelmuth, Chang, Reading, McGuire, & Su, 1987) and platelet uptake of serotonin (Rapkin, Reading, Woo, & Goldman, 1991) are decreased in women with PMS, but the ratio of L-tryptophan to the sum of other neural amino acids is not altered. Rojansky, Halbreich, Zander, Barkai, and Goldstein (1991) found no predictable differences in platelet serotonin uptake, but did find reduced imipramine binding in the early luteal phase. Steege, Stout, Knight, and Nemeroff (1992) observed similar results for imipramine binding. Indirect evidence of the role of serotonin is based on clinical trials in which selective serotonin re-uptake inhibitors, such as fluoxetine, clomipramine, and dextro-fenfluoramine, have been shown to significantly reduce premenstrual symptoms .

The involvement of *beta endorphin* in PMS (Reid & Yen, 1981; Yen, Quigley, Reid, Ropert, & Cetel, 1985) is suggested by evidence that the normal luteal-phase rise in beta-endorphin levels may not occur in women with PMS (Chuong, Coulam, Kao, Bergstralh, & Go, 1985; Facchinetti, Martignoni, Petraglia, Sances, Nappi, & Genazzani, 1987). PMS symptoms can be reduced, but not eliminated, with preovulatory administration of the opioid inhibitor naltrexone (Chuong, Coulam, Bergstralh, O'Fallon, & Steinmetz, 1988). Finally, Parry, Berga, Kripke, Klauber, Laughlin, Yen, and Gillin (1990) have shown differences in secretion patterns of *melatonin* in women with PMS, and have demonstrated that both sleep deprivation (Parry & Wehr, 1987) and bright light therapy (Parry, Berga, Kripke, and Gillin, 1990) can reduce luteal phase symptoms.

It is likely that more than one system is involved, making investigation more challenging. While no single hypothesis adequately accounts for the entire clinical picture of PMS, there is now convincing evidence of a biologic basis for the disorder.

EPIDEMIOLOGY

There are numerous studies of the prevalence of individual premenstrual *symptoms,* but none that have directly measured premenstrual syndrome (Johnson, 1987). Despite methodological differences, there is remarkable consistency among studies in the frequency of individual symptoms. The typical distribution among symptomatic women is 40–60% mild, 15–20% moderate, and 5–10% severe (Johnson, 1987). These studies reinforce the idea that most women who ovulate have some symptoms, since the overall prevalence of at least one symptom is approximately 80%.

Estimates of the prevalence of severe PMS can be extrapolated from these studies of individual symptoms. Assuming that symptoms associated with this entity are reported by women as "severe," the maximum prevalence would be no more than 5–10% of menstruating women. Mortola (1992) further estimates that at least one third of these women have a disorder other than PMS that explains their symptoms, so that the prevalence of severe PMS is more likely less than 5%. Ramcharan, Love, Fick, and Goldfien (1992) provide direct evidence of the relatively low prevalence of the full syndrome. Using a unique design that provided menstrual cycle timing of symptoms, they estimated that only 1% of the 2,000 women studied had an affective syndrome attributable to the luteal phase.

Dalton (1984) proposed several risk factors for PMS, including tubal ligation, pregnancy, preeclampsia, absence of dysmenorrhea, and use of oral contraceptive pills. She also suggests that the problem worsens with age, and that there is a familial pattern. Subsequent investigations have supported some of these hypotheses, but not others.

Prospective studies have not documented a significant rate of menstrual cycle disturbance following sterilization (DeStefano, Perlman, Peterson, & Diamond, 1985). Additionally, Johnson, McChesney and Bean (1988) did not find a difference in the rate of tubal ligation between groups of women with and without severe premenstrual symptoms. On the other hand, 30% of women in this survey reported that their premenstrual symptoms worsened or began after a pregnancy. While there may be biological plausibility for an effect of pregnancy, other factors may account for this attribution. For example, the woman has aged about one year over the course of the pregnancy, which would be of importance if age is an independent risk factor. In addition, having a child generally increases overall stress, which may exaggerate the effect of premenstrual symptoms.

Andersch, Svenson, and Hansson (1991) investigated the role of preeclampsia as a risk factor for PMS in a long-term follow up of 237 women with a prior diagnosis of preeclampsia. In comparison to women who had normotensive pregnancies, the women in the case group who had current hypertensive disease complained of more premenstrual sadness. However, the preeclamptic cases who were currently normotensive had fewer symptoms than controls. Contrary to Dalton's hypothesis, dysmenorrhea appears to be directly correlated with risk of PMS (Johnson et al., 1988; Steege, Stout, & Rupp, 1985).

While there is no evidence that oral contraceptive pills cause PMS, Johnson et al. (1988) found that 30% of the women in a survey with current PMS had discontinued oral contraceptives in the past because of PMS-like side effects. There is also evidence of a familial, probably genetic, component. Kendler, Silberg, Neale, Kessler, Heath, and Eaves (1992) found a significantly increased frequency of severe premenstrual symptoms among monozygotic compared with dizygotic twins of women with PMS. Finally, increasing age may be a risk, as the majority of women who seek help for premenstrual complaints are over 30 years of age.

Many societal troubles are ascribed to PMS, including divorce, substance abuse, child abuse, criminal activity, suicide, and employment inefficiency and absenteeism. However, there is little empirical evidence to link most of these events with PMS (Johnson, 1987). For example, data from a cross-sectional cohort study suggest that there is no difference in divorce rates between women with and without PMS (Johnson et al., 1988). Reports of increased risk for criminal activity are anecdotal, and in most of these cases a rigorous diagnosis of PMS has not been made. Job performance has not been directly studied. Two cross-sectional surveys of reproductive-age women have found significant self-reported work problems only among the small group of women with severe symptoms (Andersch, Wendestam, Hahn, & Ohman, 1986; Johnson, et al., 1988.).

RELATIONSHIP TO DEPRESSIVE DISORDER

Several investigators have raised the important theoretical question as to whether PMS is related to affective disorder. This question arises, in part, because of the phenomenological similarities between these two disorders (Endicott, Halbreich, Schacht, & Nee, 1981; Hallman, 1986; Haskett, Steiner, & Carroll, 1984; Warner, Bancroft, Dixon, & Hampson, 1991). Numerous studies have shown that women who seek care for premenstrual complaints are very likely to have either a concomitant affective disorder, or a history of one (DeJong, Rubinow, Roy-Byrne, Hoban, Grover, & Post, 1985; Hart, Coleman, & Russell, 1987b; Stout, Steege, Blazer, & George, 1986).

Graze, Nee, and Endicott (1990) followed 36 women who had a prospectively confirmed diagnosis of PMS. The long-term risk for major depressive disorder in this group was correlated with the score on the depression subscale of the Premenstrual Assessment Form (Halbreich, Endicott, Schact, & Nee, 1982). These results suggest that at least a subset of women with PMS may be at higher risk for depression, but no other longitudinal studies are available. A longitudinal study comparing the occurrence of new onset affective disorder in women with PMS with women without PMS would be more useful.

Despite the observations that suggest similarities between PMS and affective disorder, several differences have been identified. Mortola, Girton, and Yen (1989) found that depressive episodes in women with PMS differed from those in women with endogenous depressive disorder as measured by cortisol secretory parameters and psychological indices. Conflicting data have been found for results of the dexamethasone suppression test (DST). Roy-Byrne, Rubinow, Gwirtsman, Hoban, and Grover (1986) found no suppression on DST among a group women with PMS, whereas Parry et al. (1991) found a 62% rate of non-suppression in a sample of 8 women. In two studies, women with PMS did not show cognitive changes characteristic of depression (McMillan, Ghadirian, & Pihl, 1989; Rapkin, Chang, & Reading, 1989).

Whatever the answer to this question, the clinician should recognize that there is similarity in the presentation of PMS and the affective disorders. Prospective charting will help identify the woman with depressive illness, because her symptoms will not be confined to the luteal phase (Hammarbäck, Bäckström, MacGibbon-Taylor, 1989).

MANAGEMENT

Diagnosis

The diagnostic process can usually be completed over two visits, separated by at least two menstrual cycles (Johnson, 1992b). At the first visit, a detailed history should be obtained.

First, does the woman ovulate? A recent history of regular spontaneous menses will suffice in most cases. Women on birth control pills are, by definition, not ovulating. If periods are very irregular, or if the woman has had a hysterectomy, but retains her ovaries, additional testing may be necessary.

Second, are the symptoms being described typical for PMS, or are they suggestive of another problem? Because the symptoms of PMS are similar to other mood disorders, a distinction usually cannot be made at this point. However, certain symptoms are suggestive of another problem. For example, panic attacks, bizarre thinking, suicidal plans, or phobias suggest a psychiatric disorder, whereas complaints of a single physical symptom such as headaches, or chest pain, suggests a medical problem.

Third, what is the impact of the symptoms? The clinician should assess the affect on daily functioning, relationships with family and other significant persons, and ability to work.

Fourth, what psychiatric and medical problems have been previously diagnosed? Knowledge of these problems will aid in assessing the etiology of the presenting symptoms, in recognizing how concurrent problems may affect any premenstrual symptoms that are present, and in planning appropriate therapy.

The physical examination is used primarily to identify other problems, since there are no characteristic physical findings for PMS. Similarly, laboratory tests should be obtained only to search for other causes of the symptoms suspected on the basis of the history or physical examination. In particular, determining progesterone or estrogen levels is of no value unless a menstrual cycle problem such as menopause, hyperprolactinemia, or anovulation is suspected.

A differential diagnosis can usually be developed at this point. If there is no need for immediate intervention, the woman should be asked to record her symptoms each day, along with the dates of her menstrual periods, over two menstrual cycles.

Standardized instruments are typically used by investigators to document the severity and timing of symptoms. The two most commonly used are the Moos Menstrual Distress Questionnaire (MDQ) and the Premenstrual Assessment Form (PAF). The MDQ (Moos, 1968) was the first instrument developed for the purpose of measuring PMS. Although it has several characteristics that make it less than adequate, it is still used because there are few alternatives, and study results can be readily compared with the many previous studies in which the MDQ has been used.

The PAF, developed by Halbreich, Endicott, Schact, and Nee (1982), includes 95 symptoms, and its subscales allow classification into several syndromal categories. A special scoring program must be used to analyze the results. Recently, Allen, McBride, and Pirie (1991) described a short form of this instrument which may be more practical clinically.

For clinical purposes, a simple calendar system is adequate. We have the woman select the five most prominent symptoms, and then have her record daily on a calendar grid the occurrence and severity (mild, moderate, or severe) of each symptom. If a more formal instrument is desired, the COPE scale, developed by Mortola et al. (1990), or visual analogue scales for a set of standard symptoms (Casper & Powell, 1986) are relatively easy to use.

Differences between the luteal and follicular phase on the Minnesota Multiphasic Personality Inventory (MMPI) in women with PMS have been reported (Chuong, Colligan, Coulam, & Bergstralh, 1988). Palmer, Lambert, and Richards (1991) attempted to replicate this finding in a group of 214 women with prospectively defined PMS, and found wide variability in profile patterns between the best and worst times in the cycle. These authors advise caution in the use of the MMPI as a diagnostic tool for PMS. If a standardized instrument is used to quantify baseline mood symptoms, it should be administered in the follicular (postmenstrual) phase of the cycle.

At the second visit, the symptom charts should be examined. In most cases, the interpretation of the symptom charts is straightforward. A luteal phase pattern can be diagnosed if the symptoms begin within 14 days of the first day of menses, and are completely gone by day two of menses. If the symptoms persist beyond the last day of menstrual flow, another diagnosis is probably present, either alone, or in addition to premenstrual syndrome.

THERAPY

Diet, Exercise, and Nutritional Supplements

The therapeutic approach to the woman with PMS will depend on the severity of her symptoms and the presence of any concomitant psychopathology. For the woman with "pure" premenstrual syndrome, we recommend that most women initially try the so-called "self-help" therapies. These consist of nutritional changes, exercise, and mineral supplements.

Diet appears to have an affect on symptoms. Complex carbohydrates have been shown to reduce depressive symptoms in the luteal phase in one controlled trial (Wurtman, Brzezinski, Wurtman, & Laferrere, 1989). The mechanism of action may be via modification of serotonergic activity. Eating a healthy, balanced diet may also have a nonspecific beneficial effect. Caffeine intake has been shown by Rossignol and Bonnlander (1990) to be greater among women with severe premenstrual symptoms. These same investigators (Rossignol, Bonnlander, Song, & Phillis, 1991) further showed that women with PMS tend to consume more caffeine in the luteal phase, perhaps in a misdirected attempt at self-medication. Finally, Rossignol and Bonnlander (1991) found, among a large group of university students, that foods high in sugar content (chocolate, caffeine-free soda, and fruit juice) as well as alcoholic beverages, were directly associated with the severity of premenstrual symptoms. These observations support the clinical recommendation to decrease caffeine intake and to avoid foods and beverages high in sugar.

The theoretical basis for the hypothesized effect of *exercise* on PMS has to do with alterations of endorphins and, perhaps, other neurotransmitters. There is some direct evidence that premenstrual symptoms are reduced in women who regularly exercise (Prior, Vigna, Sciarretta, Alojado, & Schulzer, 1987), although there has never been a direct trial of vigorous exercise in women with PMS.

Evidence from controlled trials that supplementation with *minerals*, either calcium (Thys-Jacobs, Ceccarelle, & Bierman, 1989) or magnesium (Facchinetti, et al., 1991) are helpful. We therefore recommend a trial of one or both of these mineral supplements prior to considering prescription drug therapy. The dosages are elemental calcium, 1000 mg daily, or magnesium, 400 mg daily.

Vitamin supplements are widely recommended, but the evidence of benefit is limited. Kleijnen, Ter Riet, and Knipschild (1990) reviewed 12 controlled trials of pyridoxine (vitamin B6) therapy, and concluded that the evidence for a benefit is weak. Women who choose to take pyridoxine need to be aware of the potential for peripheral neurotoxicity if doses greater than 200 mg daily are taken regularly (Parry & Bredesen, 1985). We usually recommend limiting the dose to no more than 100 mg daily. Alpha-tocopherol (vitamin E), in a dose of 600 mg daily, is sometimes recommended as well, especially for breast tenderness (London, Sundaram, Murphy, & Goldstein, 1983). Two controlled trials have found improvement with a high-dose multiple vitamin, Optivite® (Chakmakjian, Higgins, & Abraham, 1985; London, Bradley, & Chiamori, 1991). However, this supplement contains magnesium, and so it is not clear that the more expensive multiple vitamin formulation is necessary.

Psychological Therapy

Psychological interventions have been studied in two controlled trials. The "relaxation response" was compared with two comparison interventions, quietly reading a book for 30 minutes per day, and education about premenstrual syndrome (Goodale, Domar, & Bensen, 1990). Women in the group assigned to the relaxation response reported a significant reduction in symptoms over the 3 months. Morse, Dennerstein, Farrell, and Varnavides (1991) compared cognitive–behavioral therapy to both relaxation and hormone therapy. The latter two groups did not demonstrate sustained benefit over 3 months, whereas the cognitive therapy group did.

Pharmacological Therapy

If self-help therapies are ineffective, pharmacological therapy may be considered. Based on controlled trials, the most effective drugs appear to be those that either inhibit ovulation or block serotonin re-uptake.

Diuretics are widely prescribed but most types have not been studied. The exception is spironolactone, which acts as an aldosterone inhibitor *and* as an antagonist of testosterone (O'Brien, Craven, Selby, & Symonds, 1979). Clinical trial results have been inconsistent for effects on mood, but fluid-retention symptoms are usually improved (Hellberg, Claesson, & Nilsson, 1991; Vellacott, Shroff, Pearce, Stratford, & Akbar, 1987). Burnet, Radden, Easterbrook, and McKinnon (1991) found no overall benefit of spironolactone for PMS symptoms, but the subset of women who did respond had higher androgen levels in the luteal as compared with the follicular phase of the cycle. The usual dose of spironolactone is 100 mg daily in the luteal phase.

Progesterone vaginal suppositories are worth specific comment. Dalton has promulgated the use of this therapy for the past 20 years, based on her clinical experience (Dalton, 1984). However, over a dozen controlled trials have failed to find a significant benefit. Freeman, Rickels, Sondheimer, and Plansky (1990) conducted the most definitive study of this question. Doses of either 400 or 800 mg daily were administered in a blinded cross-over fashion to 168 women with rigorously defined PMS, and no significant differences between progesterone and placebo were found.

Three selective serotonin re-uptake inhibitors (SSRI), fluoxetine, clomipramine, and dextro-fenfluoramine, have been shown in controlled trials to be superior to placebo. Fluoxetine is given in a dose of 20 mg daily (Menkes, Taghavi, Mason, Spears, & Howard, 1992; Rickels, Freeman, Sondheimer, & Albert, 1990; Stone, Pearlstein, & Brown, 1991). Wood, Mortola, Chan, Moossazadeh, and Yen (1992) studied the use of fluoxetine in subjects who had no personal history of either current or past affective disorder, to better control for the possibility that fluoxetine merely acts as an antidepressant. Symptoms were reduced nearly to baseline follicular phase levels among the group on active therapy. These results suggest that the effect of fluoxetine is not simply to improve underlying depression. Clomipramine has been effective in doses between 25 and 75 mg daily (Eriksson, Lisjö, Sundblad, Andersson, Andersch, & Modigh, 1989; Stone, Pearlstein, & Brown, 1991; Sundblad, Hedberg, & Eriksson, 1993; Sundblad, Modigh, & Andersch, 1992). The dextro isomer of fenfluoramine is not available in the United States, but its effectiveness further supports the role of SSRI is the therapy of PMS (Brzezinski et al., 1990).

Tricyclic antidepressants have also been studied on a limited basis. Imipramine (Glick, Harrison, Endicott, McGrath, & Quitkin, 1991) and nortryptilline (Harrison, Endicott, & Nee, 1989) given in modest doses (between 25 and 125 mg daily) have been shown in controlled trials to reduce premenstrual depression.

Ovulation inhibition should usually be reserved for women who do not respond to other therapies. In the one controlled trial of oral contraceptive pills, physical symptoms were improved, but psychological symptoms were not (Graham & Sherwin, 1992). Approaches shown to be effective include continuous administration of high-dose estradiol (Watson, Studd, Savvas, Garnett, & Baber, 1989), danazol (Halbreich, Rojansky, & Palter, 1991), or gonadotropin-releasing hormone agonist (Muse, Cetel, Futterman, & Yen, 1984). Although these regimens can be quite effective in reducing symptoms, each has its disadvantages for long-term use.

GnRH agonist therapy appears to be the most effective, but the high price makes it impractical for most patients. Hormone replacement must be given concomitantly to reduce the risks of hypoestrogenemia, primarily osteopenia. Mortola, Girton, and Fischer (1991) demonstrated that PMS symptoms do not return when "add-back" cyclic estrogen-progestin is given along with GnRH agonist therapy. *Danazol* is also costly and has short-term side effects of weight gain and some androgen effects that are unacceptable to many women. In addition, danazol depresses HDL cholesterol, so that long-term (in excess of 1 or 2 years) administration is not advisable because of the potential adverse impact on heart disease risk. *High-dose estradiol* is effective either via an estradiol implant, or the transdermal patch, in a dose of 0.2 mg daily. Cyclic progestin must be given to reduce the risk of endometrial neoplasia (Watson, Studd, Savvas, & Baber, 1990). The long-term effects of this high dose are not known.

Removal of the ovaries appears to be an effective treatment. In two open trials, women with prospectively defined PMS who had responded to a trial of danazol therapy, underwent hysterectomy with oophorectomy (Casper & Hearn, 1990; Casson, Hahn, VanVugt, & Reid, 1990). After two years of follow-up, all continued to have complete resolution of symptoms. However, surgical therapy is expensive, and is accompanied by both intraoperative and long-term risks. Oophorectomy will only eliminate symptoms associated with PMS, so that prospective confirmation of the diagnosis is absolutely essential before considering surgical therapy. Surgical therapy should be reserved for the minority of women with severe premenstrual symptoms, who have not responded to other therapies except either danazol or GnRH, and who have a significant number of menstrual years remaining. In these selected cases, surgical therapy may be offered as an alternative to using expensive, side-effect-producing drugs for prolonged intervals of ten to fifteen years.

In summary, the diagnosis of PMS can generally be made if a rigorous approach is used. Careful evaluation of concomitant pathology will aid in establishing a rational treatment plan. Using this approach, the majority of women with PMS can be helped by the currently available therapies.

REFERENCES

Allen, S. S., McBride, C. M., & Pirie, P. L. (1991). The shortened premenstrual assessment form. *Journal of Reproductive Medicine, 36,* 769–772.

American Psychiatric Association. (1987). *Diagnostic and statistical manual of mental disorders.* 3rd Edition, Revised. (DSM–III-R), p. 367. Washington, DC: American Psychiatric Association.

Andersch, B., Svenson, A., & Hansson, L. (1991). Pre-eclampsia, hypertension and the premenstrual tension syndrome. *International Journal of Gynaecology and Obstetrics, 32,* 123–127.

Andersch, B., Wendestam, C., Hahn, L., & Ohman, R. (1986). Premenstrual complaints. I. Prevalence of premenstrual symptoms in a Swedish urban population. *Journal of Psychosomatic Obstetrics and Gynecology, 5,* 39–49.

Andrews, J.C., Ator, G.A., & Honrubia, V. (1992). The exacerbation of symptoms in Meniere's disease during the premenstrual period. *Archives of Otolaryngology, Head and Neck Surgery, 118,* 74–78.

AuBuchon, P.G., & Calhoun, K. S. (1985). Menstrual cycle symptomatology: The role of social expectancy and experimental demand characteristics. *Psychosomatic Medicine, 47,* 35–45.

Bäckström, T. (1992). Neuroendocrinology of premenstrual syndrome. *Clinical Obstetrics and Gynecology, 35,* 612–628.

Bäckström, C.T., Boyle, H., & Baird, D.T. (1981). Persistence of symptoms of premenstrual tension in hysterectomized women. *British Journal of Obstetrics and Gynaecology, 88,* 530–536.

Bell, J.A. (1989). Danazol, premenstrual tension, and uveitis. *Archives of Ophthalmology*, *107*, 796.

Bernsted, L., Luggin, R., & Petersson, B. (1984). Psychosocial considerations of the premenstrual syndrome. *Acta Psychiatrica Scandinavica*, *69*, 455–460.

Brayshaw, N.D. and Brayshaw, D.D. (1986). Thyroid hypofunction in premenstrual syndrome [letter]. *New England Journal of Medicine*, *315*, 1486–1487.

Brzezinski, A. A., Wurtman, J.J., Wurtman, R.J., Gleason, R., Greenfield, J., & Nader, T. (1990). d-Fenfluramine suppresses the increased calorie and carbohydrate intakes and improves the mood of women with premenstrual depression. *Obstetrics and Gynecology*, *76*, 296–301.

Burnet, R.B., Radden, H.S., Easterbrook, E.G., & McKinnon, R.A. (1991). Premenstrual syndrome and spironolactone. *Australian and New Zealand Journal of Obstetrics and Gynaecology*, *31*, 366–368.

Casper, R.F., & Hearn, M.T. (1990). The effect of hysterectomy and bilateral oophorectomy in women with severe premenstrual syndrome. *Obstetrics and Gynecology*, *162*, 105–109.

Casper, R.F., Patel-Christopher, A., Powell, A.-M. (1989). Thyrotropin and prolactin responses to thyrotropin-releasing hormone in premenstrual syndrome. *Journal of Clinical Endocrinology and Metabolism*, *68*, 608–612.

Casper, R.F., & Powell, A.-M. (1986). Premenstrual syndrome: Documentation by a linear analog scale compared with two descriptive scales. *American Journal of Obstetrics and Gynecology*, *155*, 862–867.

Casson, P., Hahn, P. M., VanVugt, D.A., & Reid, R.L. (1990). Lasting response to ovariectomy in severe intractable premenstrual syndrome. *American Journal of Obstetrics and Gynecology*, *162*, 99–109.

Chakmakjian, Z.H., Higgins, C.E., & Abraham, G.E. (1985). The effect of a nutritional supplement, Optivite, for women, on premenstrual tension *Journal of Applied Nutrition*, *37*, 12–17.

Chandraiah, S., Levenson, J.L., & Collins, J.B. (1991). Sexual dysfunction, social maladjustment, and psychiatric disorders in women seeking treatment in a premenstrual syndrome. *International Journal of Psychiatry and Medicine 21*, 189–204.

Chang, G., & Hutchinson-Williams, K.A. (1991). Lifetime psychiatric illness and premenstrual syndromes. *Connecticut Medicine*, *55*, 683–686.

Chisholm, G., Jung, S.O.J., Cummings, C.E., Fox, E.E., Cumming, D.C. (1990). Premenstrual anxiety and depression: Comparison of objective psychological tests with a retrospective questionaire. *Acta Psychiatrica Scandinavica*, *81*, 52–57.

Chuong, C.J., Colligan, R.C., Coulam, C.B., & Bergstralh, E.J. (1988). The MMPI as an aid in evaluating patients with premenstrual syndrome. *Psychosomatics*, *29*, 197–202.

Chuong, C.J., Coulam, C.B., Bergstralh, E.J., O'Fallon, W.M., & Steinmetz, G.I. (1988). Clinical trial of naltrexone in premenstrual syndrome. *Obstetrics and Gynecology*, *72*, 332–336.

Chuong, C.J., Coulam, C.B., Kao, P.C., Bergstralh, E.J., & Go, V.L. (1985). Neuropeptide levels in premenstrual syndrome. *Fertility and Sterility*, *44*, 760–765.

Dalton K. (1984). *The premenstrual syndrome and progesterone therapy*. London: W.

Heinemann Medical Book, Ltd.; 2nd edition, Chicago: Yearbook Medical Publishers.

DeJong, R., Rubinow, D.R., Roy-Byrne, P., Hoban, M.C., Grover, G.N., & Post, R.M. (1985). Premenstrual mood disorder and psychiatric illness. *American Journal of Psychiatry, 142*, 1359–1361.

DeStefano, F., Perlman, J.A., Peterson, H.B., & Diamond, E.L. (1985). Long-term risk of menstrual disturbances after tubal sterilization. *American Journal of Obstetrics and Gynecology, 152*, 835–841.

Digre, K., & Damasio, H. (1987). Menstrual migraine: Differential diagnosis, evaluation, and treatment. *Clinical Obstetrics and Gynecology, 30*, 417–430.

Dinan, T., O'Keane, V. (1991). The premenstrual syndrome: a psychoneuroendocrine perspective. *Bailliere's Clinical Endocrinology and Metabolism, 5*, 143–165.

Endicott, J., Halbreich, U., Schact, S., & Nee, J. (1981). Premenstrual changes and affective disorders. *Psychosomatic Medicine, 43*, 519–529.

Eriksson, E., Lisjö, E.E., Sundblad, C., Andersson, K., Andersch, B., & Modigh, K. (1989). Effect of clomipramine on premenstrual syndrome. *Acta Psychiatrica Scandinavica, 81*, 87–88.

Facchinetti, F., Borella, P., Sances, G., Fioroni, L., Nappi, R.E., & Genazzani, A.R. (1991). Oral magnesium successfully relieves pre-menstrual mood changes. *Obstetrics and Gynecology, 78*, 177–181.

Facchinetti, F., Genazzani, A.D., Martignoni, E., Fioroni, L.,Nappi, G., & Genazzani, A.R. (1993). Neuroendocrine changes in luteal function in patients with premenstrual syndrome. *Journal of Clinical Endocrinology and Metabolism, 76*, 1123–1127.

Facchinetti, F., Genazzani, A.D., Martignoni, E., Fioroni, L., Sances, G., & Genazzani, A.R. (1990). Neuroendocrine correlates of premenstrual syndrome: Changes in the pulsatile pattern of plasma LH. *Psychoneuroendocrinology, 15*, 269–277.

Facchinetti, F., Martignoni, E., Petraglia, F., Sances, M.G., Nappi, A.R., & Genazzani, A.R. (1987). Premenstrual fall of plasma beta-endorphin in patients with premenstrual syndrome. *Fertility and Steritlity, 47*, 570–573.

Frank, R.T. (1931). The hormonal causes of premenstrual tension. *Archives of Neurology and Psychiatry, 26*, 1053–1057.

Freeman, E.W., Rickels, K, Sondheimer, S.J., & Plansky, M., (1990). Ineffectiveness of progesterone suppository treatment for premenstrual syndrome. *Journal of the American Medical Association, 264*, 349–353.

Gallant, S.J., Popiel, D.A., Hoffman, D.M., Chakraborty, P.K., & Hamilton, J.A. (1992). Using daily ratings to confirm premenstrual syndrom/late luteal phase dysphoric disorder. Part I. Effects of demand characteristics and expectations. *Psychosomatic Medicine, 54*, 149–166.

Gibbs, C.J., Coutts, I.I., Lock, R., Finnegan, O.C., & White, R.J. (1984). Premenstrual exacerbation of asthma. *Thorax, 39*, 833–836.

Glick, R., Harrison, W., Endicott, J., McGrath, P., & Quitkin, F.M. (1991). Treatment of premenstrual dysphoric symptoms in depressed women. *Journal of the American Medical Women's Association, 46*, 182–185.

Goodale, I.L., Domar, A.D., & Bensen, H. (1990). Alleviation of premenstrual syndrome symptoms with the relaxation response. *Obstetrics and Gynecology, 75*, 649–655.

Graham, C.A., & Sherwin, B.B. (1992). A prospective treatment study of premenstrual symptoms using a triphasic oral contraceptive. *Journal of Psychosomatic Research*, *36*, 257–266.

Graze, K.K., Nee, J., & Endicott, J. (1990). Premenstrual depression predicts future major depressive disorder. *Acta Psychiatrica Scandinavica*, *81*, 201–205.

Halbreich, U., Endicott, J., Schact, S., & Nee, J. (1982). The diversity of premenstrual changes as reflected in the Premenstrual Assessment Form. *Acta Psychiatrica Scandinavica*, *65*, 46–65.

Halbreich, U., Rojansky, N., & Palter, S. (1991). Elimination of ovulation and menstrual cyclicity (with danazol) improves dysphoric premenstrual syndrome. *Fertility and Sterility*, *56*, 1066–1069.

Hallman, J. (1986). The premenstrual syndrome: An equivalent of depression. *Acta Psychiatrica Scandinavica*, *73*, 403–411.

Hammarbäck, S., Bäckström, T., & MacGibbon-Taylor, B. (1989). Diagnosis of premenstrual tension syndrome: Description and evaluation of a procedure for diagnosis and differential diagnosis. *Journal of Psychosomatic Obstetrics and Gynaecology*, *10*, 25–42.

Hammarbäck, S., Ekholm, U.-B., & Bäckström, T. (1991). Spontaneous anovulation causing disappearance of cyclical symptoms in women with the premenstrual syndrome. *Acta Endocrinologica (Copenhagen)*, *125*, 132–137.

Harrison, W.M., Endicott, J., & Nee, J. (1989). Treatment of premenstrual depression with nortriptyline: A pilot study. *Journal of Clinical Psychiatry*, *50*, 136–139.

Hart, W.G., Coleman, G.J., & Russel, J.W. (1987a). Assessment of premenstrual symptomatology: A re-evaluation of the predictive validity of self-report. *Journal of Psychosomatic Research*, *31*, 185–190.

Hart, W.G., Coleman, G.J., & Russel, J.W. (1987b). Psychiatric screening in the premenstrual syndrome. *Medical Journal of Australia*, *146*, 518–520.

Haskett, R.F., Steiner, M., & Carroll, B.J. (1984). A psychoendocrine study of premenstrual tension syndrome: A model for endogenous depression? *Journal of Affective Disorders*, *6*, 191–199.

Hellberg, D., Claesson, B., & Nilsson, S. (1991). Premenstrual tension: A placebo-controlled efficacy study with spironolactone and medroxyprogesterone acetate. *International Journal of Gynaecology and Obstetrics*, *34*, 243–248.

Herrick, A.L., McColl, K.E.L., Wallace, A.M., Moore, M.R., & Goldberg, A. (1990). LHRH analogue treatment for the prevention of premenstrual attacks of acute porphyria. *Quarterly Journal of Medicine, New Series 75*, *276*, 355–363.

Howard, R., Mason, P., Taghavi, E., & Spears, G. (1992). Brainstem auditory evoked responses (BAERs) during the menstrual cycle in women with and without premenstrual syndrome. *Biological Psychiatry*, *32*, 682–690.

Hurt, S.W., Schnurr, P.P., Severino, S.K., Freeman, E.W., Gise, L.H., Rivera-Tovar, A., & Steege, J.F. (1992). Late luteal phase dysphoric disorder in 670 women evaluated for premenstrual complaints. *American Journal of Psychiatry*, *149*, 525–530.

Hussain, S.Y., O'Brien, P.M.S., & DeSouza, V., Okonofua, F., & Dandona, P. (1990). Reduced atrial natiuretic peptide concentrations in premenstrual syndrome. *British Journal of Obstetrics and Gynaecology*, *97*, 397–401.

Johnson, S.R. (1987). The epidemiology and social impact of premenstrual symptoms. *Clinical Obstetrics and Gynecology*, 30, 367–376.

Johnson, S.R. (1992a). Premenstrual syndrome and dysmenorrhea. In W.F. Rayburn & F.P. Zuspan (Eds.), *Drug therapy in obstetrics and gynecology, 3rd edition*, pp. 335–374. St. Louis: Mosby Year Book.

Johnson, S.R. (1992b). Clinician's approach to the diagnosis and management of premenstral syndrome. *Clinical Obstetrics and Gynecology*, 35, 637–657.

Johnson, S.R., McChesney C., & Bean, J.A. (1988). Epidemiology of premenstrual symtpoms in a nonclinical sample. I. Prevalence, natural history and help-seeking behavior. *Journal of Reproductive Medicine*, 33, 340–346.

Kendler, K.S., Silberg, J.L., Neale, M.C., Kessler, R.C., Heath, A.C., & Eaves, L.J. (1992). Genetic and environmental factyors in the aetiology of menstrual, premenstrual and neurotic symptoms: A population-based twin study. *Psychological Medicine*, 22, 85–100.

Kleijnen, J., Ter Riet, G., & Knipschild, P. (1990). Vitamin B6 in the treatment of the premenstrual syndrome—a review. *British Journal of Obstetrics and Gynaecology*, 97, 847–852.

Leather, A.T., Holland, E.F.N., Andrews, G.D., & Studd, J.W.W. (1993). A study of the referral patterns and therapeutic experiences of 100 women attending a specialist premenstrual syndrome clinic. *Journal of the Royal Society of Medicine*, 86, 199–201.

London, R.S., Bradley, L., & Chiamori, N.Y. (1991). Effect of a nutritional supplement on premenstrual symptomatology in women with premenstrual syndrome: A double-blind longitudinal study. *Journal of the American College of Nutrition*, 10, 494–499.

London, R.S., Sundaram, G.S., Murphy, L., & Goldstein, P.J. (1983). Evaluation and treatment of breast symptoms in patients with the premenstrual syndrome. *Journal of Reproductive Medicine*, 28, 503–508.

McMillan, M.J., Ghadirian, A.M., & Pihl, R.O. (1989). Premenstrual depression in women with a history of affective disorder: Mood and attentional processes. *Canadian Journal of Psychiatry*, 34, 791–795.

Menkes, D.B., Taghavi, E., Mason, P.A., Spears, G.F.S., & Howard, R.C. (1992). Fluoxetine treatment of severe premenstrual syndrome. *British Medical Journal*, 305, 346–347.

Moos, R.H. (1968). The development of menstrual distress qustionnaire. *Psychosomatic Medicine, 30*, 853–867.

Morse, C.A., Dennerstein, L., Farrell, E., & Varnavides, K. (1991). A comparison of hormone therapy, coping skills training, and relaxation for the relief of premenstrual syndrome. *Journal of Behavioral Medicine*, 14, 469–489.

Mortola, J. F., (1992). Issues in the diagnosis and research of premenstrual syndrome. *Clinical Obstetrics and Gynecology, 35*, 587–598.

Mortola, J. F., Girton, L., Beck L., & Yen, S.S.C. (1990). Diagnosis of premenstrual syndrome by a simple, prospective, and reliable instrument; the Calendar of Premenstrual Experiences. *Obstetrics and Gynecology*, 76, 302–307.

Mortola, J.F., Girton, L., & Fischer, U. (1991). Successful treatment of severe premenstrual syndrome by combined use of gonadotropin-releasing hormone agonist and estrogen/progestin. *Journal of Clinical Endocrinology and Metabolism*, 72, 252A–252F.

Mortola, J.F., Girton, L., & Yen, S.S.C. (1989). Depressive episodes in premenstrual syndrome. *American Journal of Obstetrics and Gynecology*, 161, 1682–1687.

Muse, K.N., Cetel, N.S., Futterman, L.A., & Yen, S.S.C. (1984). The premenstrual syndrome: Effects of "medical ovariectomy." *New England Journal of Medicine, 311*, 1345–1349.

Newmark, M.E., & Penry, J.K. (1980). Catamenial epilepsy: A review. *Epilepsia, 21*, 281–300.

Nikolai, T.F., Mulligan, G.M., Gribble, R.K., Harkins, P.G., Meier, P.R., & Roberts, R.C. (1990). Thyroid function and treatment in premenstrual syndrome. *Journal of Clinical Endocrinology and Metabolism, 70*, 1108–1113.

Nye, S.S., Hurt, S.W., Severino, S. K., & Shangold, G.A. (1992). Characterizing women who seek treatment for late luteal phase dysphoric disorder (LLPDD). *Journal of Women's Health, 1*, 301–305.

O'Brien, P.M.S., Craven, D., Selby, C., & Symonds, E.M. (1979). Treatment of premenstrual syndrome by spironolactone. *British Journal of Obstetrics and Gynaecology, 86*, 142–147.

Palmer, S.A., Lambert, M.J., & Richards, R.L. (1991). The MMPI and premenstrual syndrome: Profile fluctuations between best and worst times during the menstrual cycle. *Journal of Clinical Psychology, 47*, 215–221.

Parry, B.L., Berga, S.L., Kripke, D.F., & Gillin, J.C. (1990). Melatonin and phototherapy in premenstrual depression. *Progress in Clinical and Biological Research, 341B*, 35–43.

Parry, B.L., Berga, S.L., Kripke, D.F., Klauber, M.R., Laughlin, G.A., Yen, S.S.C., & Gillin, J.C. (1990). Altered waveform of plasma nocturnal melatonin secretion in premenstrual depression. *Archives of General Psychiatry, 47*, 1139–1146.

Parry, G.J., & Bredesen, D.E. (1985). Sensory neuropathy with low-dose pyridoxine. *Neurology, 35*, 1466–1468.

Parry, B.L., Gerner, R.H., Wilkins, J.N., Halaris, A.E., Carlson, H.E., Hershman, J.M., Linnoila, M. Merrill, J., Gold, P.W., Gracely, R., Aloi, J., & Newton, R. (1991). CSF and endocrine studies of premenstrual syndrome. *Neuropsychopharmacology, 5*, 127–137.

Parry, B.L., & Wehr, T.A. (1987). Therapeutic effect of sleep deprivation in patients with premenstrual syndrome. *American Journal of Psychiatry, 144*, 808–810.

Prior, J.C., Vigna, Y., Sciarretta, D., Alojado, N., & Schulzer, M. (1987). Conditioning exercise decreases premenstrual symptoms: A prospective, controlled 6–month trial. *Fertility and Sterility, 47*, 423–428.

Ramcharan, S., Love, E.J., Fick, G.H., & Goldfien, A. (1992). The epidemiology of premenstrual symptoms in a population-based sample of 2650 urban women: Attributable risk and risk factors. *Journal of Clinical Epidemiology, 45*, 377–392.

Rapkin, A.J. (1992). The role of serotonin in premenstrual syndrome. *Clinical Obstetrics and Gynecology, 35*, 629–636.

Rapkin, A.J., Chang, L.C., & Reading, A.E. (1989). Mood and cognitive style in premenstrual syndrome. *Obstetrics and Gynecology, 74*, 644–649.

Rapkin, A.J., Edelmuth, E., Chang, L.C., Reading, A.E., McGuire, M.T., & Su, T.-P. (1987). Whole-blood serotonin in premenstrual syndrome. *Obstetrics and Gynecology, 70*, 533–537.

Rapkin, A.J., Reading, A.E., Woo, S., & Goldman, L.M. (1991). Tryptophan and neutral amino acids in premenstrual syndrome. *American Journal of Obstetrics and Gynecology, 165*, 1830–1833.

Reid, R.L., & Yen, S.S.C. (1981). Premenstrual syndrome. *American Journal of Obstetrics and Gynecology, 139*, 85–104.

Rickels, K., Freeman, E.W., Sondheimer, S, & Albert, J. (1990). Fluoxetine in the treatment of premenstrual syndrome. *Current Therapeutic Research, 48*, 161–166.

Rojansky, N., Halbreich, U., Zander, K., Barkai, A., & Goldstein, S. (1991). Imipramine receptor binding and serotonin uptake in platelets of women with premenstrual changes. *Gynecologic and Obstetric Investigation, 31*, 146–152.

Rossignol, A.M., & Bonnlander, H., (1990). Caffeine-containing beverages, total fluid consumption, and premenstrual syndrome. *American Journal of Public Health, 80*, 1106–1110.

Rossignol, A.M., & Bonnlander, H. (1991). Prevalence and severity of the premenstrual syndrome. Effects of foods and beverages that are sweet or high in sugar content. *Journal of Reproductive Medicine, 36*, 131–136.

Rossignol, A.M., Bonnlander, H., Song, L., & Phillis, J.W. (1991). Do women with premenstrual symptoms self-medicate with caffeine? *Epidemiology, 2*, 403–408.

Roy-Byrne, P.P., Rubinow, D.R., Gwirtsman, H, Hoban, M.C., & Grover, G.N. (1986). Cortisol response to dexamethasone in women with premenstrual syndrome. *Neuropsychobiology, 16*, 61–63.

Rubinow, D.R., Roy-Byrne, R., Hoban, M.C., Grover, G.N., Stambler, N., & Post, R.M. (1986). Premenstrual mood changes: Characteristic patterns in women with and without premenstrual syndrome. *Journal of Affective Disorders, 10*, 85–90.

Rubinow, D.R., & Schmidt, P.J. (1992). Premenstrual syndrome: A review of endocrine studies. *Endocrinologist, 2*, 47–54.

Ruble, D.N., & Brooks-Gunn, J. (1979). Menstrual symptoms: A social cognition analysis. *Journal of Behavioral Medicine, 2*, 171–194.

Schmidt, P.J., Nieman, L.K., Grover, G.N., Muller, K.L., Merriam, G.R., & Rubinow, D.R. (1991). Lack of effect of induced menses on symptoms in women with premenstrual syndrome. *New England Journal of Medicine, 324*, 1174–1179.

Schmidt, P.J., Grover, G.N., Roy-Byrne, P.P., & Rubinow, D.R. (1993). Thyroid function in women with premenstrual syndrome. *Journal of Clinical Endocrinology and Metabolism, 76*, 671–674.

Schnurr, P.P. (1988). Some correlates of prospectively defined premenstrual syndrome. *American Journal of Psychiatry, 1988*, 491–494.

Severino, S.K., Wagner, D.R., Moline, M.L., Hurt, S.W., Pollak, C.P., & Zendell, S. (1991). High nocturnal body temperature in premenstrual syndrome and late luteal phase dysphoric disorder. *American Journal of Psychiatry, 148*, 1329–1335.

Siegel, J.P., Meyers, B., & Dineen, M.K. (1986). Comparison of depressed and nondepressed women with severe premenstrual tension syndrome. *Psychotherapy & Psychosomatics, 45*, 113–117.

Steege, J.F., Stout, A.L., & Rupp, S.L. (1985). Relationships among premenstrual symptoms and menstrual cycle characteristics. *Obstetrics and Gynecology, 65*, 389–402.

Steege, J.F., Stout, A.L., Knight, D.L., & Nemeroff, C.B. (1992). Reduced platelet tritium-labeled imipramine binding sites in women with premenstrual syndrome. *American Journal of Obstetrics and Gynecology, 167*, 168–172.

Stone, A.B., Pearlstein, T.B., & Brown, W.A. (1991). Fluoxetine in the treatment of premenstrual syndrome. *Journal of Clinical Psychiatry*, 52, 290–293.

Stout, A.L., Steege, J.F., Blazer, D.G., & George, L.K. (1986). Comparison of lifetime psychiatric diagnoses in premenstrual syndrome clinic and community samples. *Journal of Nervous and Mental Disease*, 174, 517–529.

Sundblad, C., Hedberg, M.A., & Eriksson, E. (1993). Clomipramine administered during the luteal phase reduces the symptoms of premenstrual syndrome: A placebo-controlled trial. *Neuropsychopharmacology*, 9, 133–145.

Sundblad, C., Modigh, K., & Andersch, B. (1992). Clomipramine effectively reduces premenstrual irritability and dysphoria: A placebo-controlled trial. *Acta Psychiatrica Scandinavica*, 85, 39–47.

Thys-Jacobs, S., Ceccarelle, S., & Bierman, A. (1989). Calcium supplementation in premenstrual syndrome: A randomized crossover trial. *Journal of General Internal Medicine*, 4, 183–189.

Tucker, J.S., & Whalen, R.E. (1991). Premenstrual syndrome. *International Journal of Psychiatry in Medicine*, 21, 311–341.

Vellacott, I.D., Shroff, N.E., Pearce, M.Y., Stratford, M.E., & Akbar, F.A. (1987). A double-blind, placebo-controlled evaluation of spironolactone in the premenstrual syndrome. *Current Medical Research and Opinion*, 10, 450–456.

Warner, P., Bancroft, J., Dixon, A., & Hampson, M. (1991). The relationship between perimenstrual depressive mood and depressive illness. *Journal of Affective Disorders*, 23, 9–23.

Watson, N.R., Studd, J.W.W., Savvas, M., Garnett, T., & Baber, R.J. (1989). Treatment of severe premenstrual syndrome with oestradiol patches and cyclical oral norethisterone. *Lancet*, 2, 730–732.

Watson, N.R., Studd, J.W., Savvas, M., & Baber, R.J. (1990). The long-term effects of estradiol implant therapy for the treatment of premenstrual syndrome. *Gynecologic Endocrinology*, 4, 99–107.

Wood, S.H., Mortola, J.F., Chan, Y.F., Moossazadeh, F., & Yen, S.S.C. (1992). Treatment of premenstrual sydrome with fluoxetine: A double-blind, placebo-controlled, cross-over study. *Obstetrics and Gynecology*, 80, 339–344.

Wurtman, J.J., Brzezinski, A., Wurtman, R.J., & Laferrere, B. (1989). Effect of nutrient intake on premenstrual depression. *American Journal of Obstetrics and Gynecology*, 161, 1228–1234.

Yen, S.S.C., Quigley, M.E., Reid, R.L., Ropert, J.F., & Cetel, N.S. (1985). Neuroendocrinology of opioid peptides and their role in the control of gonadotropin and prolactin secretion. *American Journal of Obstetrics and Gynecology*, 152, 485–493.

2

Childbearing

Michael W. O'Hara

Pregnancy and the puerperium represent a major period of transition for women and their families. Ordinarily, this transition to parenthood is made without major difficulty; however, for some women the transition is a difficult one. Frequently, pregnant women may experience nausea and fatigue, lose interest in sex, have problems sleeping, or experience difficulty in keeping up with their usual activities. These problems are usually taken in stride and few significant problems with adjustment occur. However, some women experience significant adjustment problems that affect mood and social functioning during pregnancy or after delivery. Such difficulties may be relatively short-lived and mild in the degree to which they cause impairment, or they may be relatively long-lived and cause serious disruption in the woman's ability to function. These types of problems are often called pregnancy-related and postpartum psychiatric disorders.

Postpartum blues, postpartum depression, and postpartum psychosis have garnered the most attention as psychiatric complications of childbearing (O'Hara, 1991). Women, however, may experience psychiatric disturbances during pregnancy. Also, forms of psychopathology other than depression (e.g., panic and obsessive–compulsive disorder) do emerge during pregnancy and the puerperium (Cohen, Heller, & Rosenbaum, 1989; Watson, Elliott, Rugg, & Brough, 1984). Because much of the clinical and research literature has been concerned with depression, it will receive the most attention in this chapter. In the first section of this chapter normal adjustment during pregnancy and after delivery will be discussed, followed by a brief characterization of postpartum blues,

26

depression, and psychosis. Third, current knowledge regarding the causes and consequences of these conditions will be outlined. Finally, a strategy for identifying and managing women who develop psychiatric disorders during pregnancy or after delivery will be presented.

SYMPTOMS AND NORMAL ADJUSTMENT

An influential early study suggested that women may experience relatively high levels of anxiety in the first and third trimesters of pregnancy relative to the second trimester (Lubin, Gardener, & Roth, 1975). However, as Elliott (1984) has pointed out, these findings have not been widely replicated. For example, Elliott, Rugg, Watson, and Brough (1983) followed 128 women from the end of the first trimester of pregnancy until one year postpartum. They performed regular assessments during pregnancy and after delivery, obtaining measures of depression, anxiety, somatic symptoms, personality, marital relationship, interest in sex, and a number of other psychological variables. Elliott et al. (1983) found that during pregnancy and after delivery women were within the normal ranges on these measures. Moreover, they observed little change during pregnancy or during the puerperium, and pregnancy to postpartum changes were in the direction of improved physical and psychological health. The psychological variables which did show significant change included interest, satisfaction, and frequency of sex and the perception of decreased "understanding" by the husband from pregnancy to three months postpartum. Based on these findings, Elliott et al. (1983) argued that, except for some obvious physical consequences of pregnancy, childbearing women show little evidence of disturbed psychological functioning and show good evidence of a high degree of stability in symptoms that are present during pregnancy and the puerperium.

In a more recent study, O'Hara, Zekoski, Philipps, and Wright (1990) followed a large sample ($N = 182$) of childbearing women and a matched sample of nonchildbearing women ($N = 179$) from the second trimester of pregnancy until nine weeks postpartum (based on the deliveries of the childbearing women). Each nonchildbearing woman was assessed with the same measures and at the same times as the childbearing woman with whom she was matched. This strategy allowed the determination of the extent to which women during pregnancy and after delivery experienced changes in levels of symptoms of depression or changes in the quality of their social adjustment. O'Hara et al. (1990) found that for some variables the findings were consistent with Elliott et al. (1983) and for other variables the findings were not consistent.

Somatic complaints associated with depression, such as difficulty sleeping and fatigue, distinguished childbearing and nonchildbearing women from the second trimester of pregnancy until nine weeks postpartum, when those differences disappeared. Childbearing women also reported higher levels of cognitive and affective symptoms of depression than nonchildbearing women (such as feeling guilty or worthless) during pregnancy and the early puerperium. These differences were especially apparent late in pregnancy and toward the end of the first week postpartum (this latter period, a time when the postpartum blues are often observed) and began to diminish by about six weeks postpartum. Finally, there was evidence that overall social adjustment was poorer in childbearing women during the first six weeks postpartum. Marital adjustment among the childbearing women was as good as that among the nonchildbearing women during the second trimester of pregnancy. However, by the third trimester and through nine weeks postpartum childbearing women were reporting poorer marital adjustment than nonchildbearing women. These differences may have been explained in part, but not completely, by decreased libido among the childbearing women.

There are several points of similarity between the findings of Elliott et al. (1983) and O'Hara et al. (1990). First, it would appear that, overall, women do show improvement in symptoms and social adjustment after delivery compared with pregnancy. Somatic symptoms are greatly increased during pregnancy and diminish within a few weeks of delivery. Sexual interest is diminished; however, there are difficulties in social adjustment of childbearing women that go beyond simple loss of libido. The findings of O'Hara et al. (1990) also point to the possibility that cognitive and affective symptoms are elevated in childbearing women, particularly during late pregnancy and the early puerperium.

In summary, pregnancy and the puerperium is not a time of particularly poor adjustment for women. Problems associated with the physical demands of pregnancy, childbirth, and child care do occur and do impact on mood and social adjustment. However, the general trend is for women to feel and function better after delivery. As will be discussed in the next section, about 10% to 15% of women have symptoms of sufficient severity and duration to be considered a psychiatric disorder. These are the women who must be identified and treated.

PSYCHOLOGICAL DISTURBANCE DURING PREGNANCY AND AFTER DELIVERY

Women with major and minor mental disorders *do* become mothers and must be managed with sensitivity during pregnancy and after delivery by the obstetrician and the rest of the health care team. All types of psychiatric disorder may be present in the pregnant woman, including schizophrenia, bipolar and unipolar depression, anxiety disorders, personality disorders and, of course, substance abuse disorders. Many of these women have already been in treatment, and coordination of care with the treating psychiatrist, psychologist, or other mental health professional is essential. The major issues involved in managing the psychiatric patient during pregnancy have been well described elsewhere (American Academy of Pediatrics, 1989; Cohen et al., 1989; Oates, 1989; Robinson, Schou, 1990; Spielvogel & Wile, 1986; Stewart & Flak, 1986; Wisner & Perel, 1988). Later in this chapter some of the issues involved in managing the patient who is at high risk for psychiatric disorder after delivery will be discussed. The rest of this section will be concerned with the three phenomena that are most often encountered as psychological disturbance in the puerperium—*postpartum blues*, *postpartum depression*, and *postpartum psychosis*.

Postpartum Blues

Many women within the first week after delivery (and sometimes later) will experience periods of tearfulness and crying, mood lability, anxious or sad mood, sleep and appetite disturbances, and irritability (Kennerley & Gath, 1989; O'Hara, 1991; O'Hara, Schlechte, Lewis, & Wright, 1991). One or more of these symptoms occurring together is called the postpartum blues. Reported prevalence rates are variable, ranging from 26% to 85% (O'Hara, 1991) The symptoms most characteristic of the postpartum blues, based on work by Kennerley and Gath (1989), are detailed in Table 2.1 Although these symptoms are usually mild in their intensity and brief in their duration, they are often experienced as unpleasant and may be atypically severe or persistent. Symptoms of the blues often peak between the fifth and seventh day postpartum (Kendell, McGuire, Connor, & Cox, 1981; Kennerley & Gath, 1989; O'Hara, Schlechte, Lewis, & Wright, 1991). This late onset pattern distinguishes the postpartum blues from the psychological consequences of other stressful medical events such as surgery. Several studies have demonstrated that postsurgical symptoms are high immediately after surgery and diminish over time (Iles, Gath, & Kennerley, 1989; Kendell, MacKenzie, West, McGuire, & Cox, 1984; Levy, 1987).

Postpartum Depression

Much less common than the blues is depression. Approximately 10% to 15% of childbearing women experience a major or minor depression during the puerperium (O'Hara, 1991; O'Hara, Zekoski, Philipps, & Wright, 1990; Watson, Elliott, Rugg, & Brough, 1984). Rates may be much higher for childbearing adolescents (Troutman & Cutrona, 1990). Some of these episodes begin during pregnancy; however, most begin after delivery (Kumar & Robson, 1984; O'Hara et al., 1990; Watson et al., 1984). Episodes are variable in duration, lasting anywhere from a few weeks to many months. For example, Watson et al. (1984) found that 50% of their postpartum depressed subjects had episodes lasting 3 months or more. Kumar and Robson (1984) reported that 50% of their postpartum

TABLE 2.1   Symptoms of the Postpartum Blues

1. Tearful	15. Emotionally numb
2. Mentally tense	16. Depressed
3. Able to concentrate	17. Over-emotional
4. Low-spirited	18. Happy
5. Elated	19. Confident
6. Helpless	20. Changeable in your spirits
7. Difficulty showing feelings	21. Tired
8. Alert	22. Irritable
9. Forgetful, muddled	23. Crying without being able to stop
10. Anxious	24. Lively
11. Wishing you were alone	25. Over-sensitive
12. Mentally relaxed	26. Up and down in your mood
13. Brooding on things	27. Restless
14. Feeling sorry for yourself	28. Calm, tranquil

Note: For the positive symptoms (e.g., 3, 5, 8, 12, etc.), it is their absence that reflects a symptom of the blues. These symptoms are included in a measure of the postpartum blues (Kennerley & Gath, 1989).

depressed subjects had episodes lasting 6 months or more. These findings suggest that depressions that occur after childbirth have serious consequences and often require the attention of the health professional.

The symptoms used to define postpartum depression are the same as for depressions that occur at other times. The Research Diagnostic Criteria (RDC; Spitzer, Endicott, & Robins, 1978) or the DSM–III–R criteria (American Psychiatric Association, 1987), which are commonly used in clinical practice and have often been used in research on postpartum depression (especially the RDC), are appropriate for defining clinically significant depression during the puerperium. Symptoms reflecting the DSM–III–R criteria for major depression, which are similar to the RDC for depression, are presented in Table 2.2. The one feature not captured by the DSM–III–R criteria that is worth noting is that some women will experience what is called a minor depression (in the RDC), a depression that has fewer symptoms (e.g., three rather than the necessary five for major depression) than a major depression, but one that still causes distress for the woman and, possibly, her family. These minor depressions, while not requiring psychiatric treatment, should not be ignored because they can persist for a very long period of time and may evolve into a major depression.

There has been a great deal of debate about the extent to which the puerperium represents a high-risk time for depression (O'Hara & Zekoski, 1988). There is little question that within the first 90 days after delivery women are at greatly increased risk to be hospitalized for a psychiatric disorder, particularly a psychotic one (Kendell, Chalmers, & Platz, 1987). However, recent studies have called into question whether nonpsychotic depressions actually occur more fre-

TABLE 2.2 Symptoms Characteristic of Major Depression (Based on DSM–III–R)

Depressed mood
Loss of interest in pleasurable activities
Appetite disturbance
Sleep disturbance
Excessive fatigue
Excessive guilt
Difficulties in thinking and concentration
Thoughts of suicide
Psychomotor disturbance

quently after childbirth (Cooper, Campbell, Day, Kennerley, & Bond, 1988; Cox, Murray, & Chapman, 1993; O'Hara, Zekoski, Philipps, & Wright, 1990; Troutman & Cutrona, 1990). These studies have demonstrated that although depression is common after childbirth, it is just as common in nonchildbearing women. Depression is a frequently occurring disorder and recent epidemiological studies confirm that young women of childbearing age are most at risk (Myers et al., 1984).

Postpartum Psychosis

Psychosis represents the most severe form of postpartum psychiatric disorder (Kendell, 1985; O'Hara, 1991). Fortunately, postpartum psychoses are relatively rare, occurring subsequent to 1 in 1000 deliveries (Kendell, 1985; Kendell, Chalmers, & Platz, 1987). Despite the low incidence of postpartum psychosis, the postpartum period conveys a high relative risk for psychosis over nonchildbearing times, on the order of a thirteenfold increase in risk (Kendell et al., 1987). The first 30 to 90 days after delivery represent the period of highest risk.

Women experiencing postpartum psychosis are grossly impaired in their ability to function, usually because of delusions and hallucinations (O'Hara, 1991). Affective psychoses will present as depression or mania. Schizophrenia will also present in the puerperium (Brockington & Cox-Roper, 1988). The fact that these severe disorders seem to be relatively more common in the puerperium and follow in time close to childbirth has engendered a great deal of debate over the years about whether psychotic disorders occurring in the puerperium are distinct (Hamilton, 1992). The current diagnostic nomenclatures (i.e., DSM–IV; American Psychiatric Association, 1994, and ICD–9, World Health Organization, 1978) do not include postpartum psychiatric disorders as separate entities. The consensus is that postpartum disorders are best understood within the framework of disorders they resemble (i.e., depression, etc.).

CAUSAL FACTORS

Most of the research reviewed in this section will bear on our understanding of the causes of postpartum depression. There are several reasons for this emphasis. First, the blues, though relatively common, are rather transient and do not appear to have serious consequences for women. Second, depression is the most common postpartum psychiatric disorder that the health care professional will encounter. Finally, psychosis is very uncommon and is rarely encountered in normal clinical practice. Nevertheless, potential causal factors for the blues and psychosis will be discussed in each of the sections on depression.

Postpartum depression has been variously defined and those definitions affect interpretation of research on causal factors. At the most general level, postpartum depression has been defined categorically and dimensionally. Categorical definitions are those that define depression in terms of presence or absence. The woman is afflicted or not. In defining depression categorically, many investigators will use standard diagnostic criteria such as the DSM–III–R (APA, 1987). Measures that reflect depression severity such as the Beck Depression Inventory (Beck, Ward, Mendelson, Mock, & Erbaugh, 1961) are used to define depression dimensionally. There are at least two practical consequences of using different methods to define postpartum depression. First, who gets identified as "depressed" will often be different when different measures are used. Second, potential causal factors associated with depression may be different depending upon the methods used to define depression. In this section, risk factors that seem most pertinent to depression when defined categorically (i.e., by its presence or absence) will be reviewed.

Background Factors

There is little evidence that demographic variables (e.g., age, education, social and marital status) are associated with risk for the postpartum blues or depression (Kennerley & Gath, 1986; O'Hara, 1991). This observation is surprising for at least two reasons. Social disadvantage (low socio-economic status [SES]) should make the postpartum period more stressful and, in fact, there is evidence that in other contexts severe social disadvantage is related to depression (Brown & Harris, 1978). Also, primiparity is related to increased risk for postpartum psychosis (Kendell, 1985). However, it should be noted that the rate of depression is very high among childbearing adolescents (Troutman & Cutrona, 1990) and that methodological difficulties in previous research (e.g., the use of demographically homogeneous samples) may have contributed to the absence of an observed relation between background factors and postpartum blues and depression.

Hormonal Factors

The timing of the postpartum blues and psychosis and, to a lesser extent, depression, have led to intense speculation regarding the etiologic/causal role of reproductive hormones such as progesterone, estrogens, and prolactin in the genesis of postpartum mood disorders (George & Sandler, 1988; Hamilton & Harberger, 1992). Hormonal hypotheses have also come from the more general biological models of depression (Schlesser, 1986). In general, the findings from a great deal of research have been weak and inconsistent at best. For example, progesterone withdrawal as a cause of postpartum mood disorders has been a prominent hypothesis. However, no evidence of lowered levels of progesterone in postpartum blues or depression was found in a recent study (O'Hara, Schlechte, Lewis, & Varner, 1991; O'Hara, Schlechte, Lewis, & Wright, 1991). Interestingly, Harris, Johns, Fung, Thomas, Walker, Read, and Riad-Fahmy (1989) observed lowered levels of progesterone in depressed breastfeeding women but higher levels of progesterone among depressed bottlefeeding women. The findings for estrogens have been similarly mixed. For example, O'Hara, Schlechte, Lewis, and Wright (1991) observed higher levels of free and total estriol during pregnancy and immediately after delivery and a greater change in free estriol levels from late pregnancy to day 1 postpartum in women experiencing the blues. The higher late pregnancy levels and the greater change were in accord with estrogen hypotheses for the blues. Lower levels of estradiol were also observed for postpartum depressed women at week 36 gestation and day 2 postpartum (O'Hara, Schlechte, Lewis, & Varner, 1991). Few other significant findings for estrogens have been observed (see George & Sandler, 1988; Hamilton & Harberger, 1992).

In nonchildbearing women there is some evidence that very high levels of prolactin (hyperprolactinemia) are associated with depression, anxiety, and hostility (Campbell & Winokur, 1985). The findings in the literature have been mixed with some studies finding a positive relation between prolactin levels and depressed mood (George, Copeland, & Wilson, 1980), other studies finding a negative relation (Harris et al., 1989), and still other studies finding no relation (O'Hara, Schlechte, Lewis, & Varner, 1991; O'Hara, Schlechte, Lewis, & Wright, 1991).

Because of its potential importance in nonpuerperal major depression, the role of cortisol in the blues and depression has been investigated in a number of studies. There have been no consistent findings for cortisol. Some studies have found higher levels of cortisol during late pregnancy in women who later experienced the blues (Handley, Dunn, Waldron, & Baker, 1980); however, these findings were not replicated in two later studies (Gard, Handley, Parsons, & Waldron, 1986; O'Hara, Schlechte, Lewis, & Wright, 1991). Moreover, there is little evidence that any aspects of cortisol dynamics, such as dexamethasone nonsuppression, are related to postpartum depression (Greenwood & Parker, 1984; O'Hara, Schlechte, Lewis, & Varner, 1991).

Many other biological variables have been investigated for a relation with postpartum blues or depression, including beta-endorphin, electrolytes, vitamins, tryptophan, and thyroid dysfunction (George & Sandler, 1988; Hamilton & Harberger, 1992; O'Hara, 1991). Of these variables, a potential role for thyroid dysfunction in postpartum depression has shown the most promise in recent studies. Two investigations have documented evidence of an association between thyroid dysfunction (either hyper- or hypothyroidism) assessed at various times in the postpartum period and depression defined by DSM–III or RDC criteria (Harris et al., 1989; Pop et al., 1991).

Gynecological and Obstetrical Factors

Several investigators have posited links between menstrual problems and postpartum mood disturbances (e.g., Steiner, 1979). The underlying assumption is that a similar hormonal dysfunction may underlie both premenstrual and postpartum mood disorders. One recent study, for example, compared women with prospectively determined premenstrual syndrome with women who had no premenstrual problems and found a marginally higher rate of past postpartum depression among the women with premenstrual syndrome (Dennerstein, Morse, & Varnavides, 1988). We found that past history of premenstrual major depression (Endicott, Halbriech, Schacht, & Nee, 1981) was related to the postpartum blues, but not to depression (O'Hara, 1995). A number of other studies have found associations between premenstrual tension (defined in various ways) and postpartum mood disturbance (e.g., Nott, Franklin, Armitage, & Gelder, 1976).

The findings for obstetrical stress have been inconsistent. Several studies have found that women experiencing higher levels of obstetrical complications have reported lower levels of postpartum mood disturbance (O'Hara, Rehm, & Campbell, 1982; Paykel, Emms, Fletcher, & Rassaby, 1980). Other studies have found higher levels of obstetrical stress associated with higher levels of postpartum mood disturbance (Campbell & Cohn, 1991; O'Hara, Neunaber, & Zekoski, 1984). One problem in this area is the variability in the way obstetrical stressors are defined. The measures tend not to be comparable across studies, which might explain some of the inconsistent findings. Also, certain types of obstetrical stressors, such as having a cesarean section, may cue the social environment (e.g., the spouse) to provide high levels of postpartum support that more than compensates for the stressful obstetric event. This perspective emphasizes the importance of considering social support as a buffer against the effects of peripartum stress.

Stressful Life Events

Obstetrical stressors are not the only negative life events that occur during pregnancy and the early postpartum period. The full range of psychosocial stressors may occur, including events such as loss of a loved one (including neonatal illness or death), moving the household, loss of employment, marital disruption or divorce, and illness in spouse or parent. Events which have implications for the woman's ability to properly care for her infant (e.g., severe financial reversal, abandonment by spouse) might be especially potent in bringing on a depressive episode. In fact, the literature is relatively consistent in suggesting that there is a clear link between negative life events, which occur during pregnancy or in the early postpartum period, and postpartum depression (O'Hara, 1986; 1991; O'Hara, Schlechte, Lewis, & Varner, 1991; Paykel et al., 1980).

Marital Relationship and Social Support

The quality of the marital relationship is obviously important to childbearing women. A poor marital relationship negatively impacts on a childbearing woman in a number of ways. The satisfaction associated with having a baby may be greatly attentuated by poor marital adjustment. The conflict associated with marital discord may interfere with the woman's ability to care for her child. Practical help and emotional support that might ordinarily be provided by a husband may be absent. All of these potential consequences of a poor marital relationship should increase the likelihood of depression. A number of studies have confirmed this hypothesis. Women who report lower marital satisfaction during pregnancy are at increased risk for depression after delivery (Gotlib, Whiffen, Wallace, & Mount, 1991; Kumar & Robson, 1984; O'Hara, 1986). Not surprisingly, many studies have also found lower levels of marital satisfaction in postpartum depressed women (O'Hara, Rehm, & Campbell, 1983; Paykel et al., 1980; Cox, Connor, & Kendell, 1982). Finally, several studies have assessed social support received by women during pregnancy and after delivery and have found that lack of support from the social network, particularly the spouse, is associated with increased risk for postpartum depression (Blair, Playfair, Tisdall, & O'Shea, 1970; Feggetter & Gath, 1981; O'Hara, 1986).

Personal and Family Psychopathology

Although postpartum depressions sometimes do afflict women who have been psychologically healthy all of their lives, many women who experience postpartum depression have been depressed in the past (O'Hara, 1991; O'Hara Schlechte, Lewis & Varner, 1991; Paykel et al., 1980; Watson et al., 1984). Also, these women frequently have family members who have experienced depression (O'Hara, et al., 1984; Watson et al., 1984). Interestingly, depression during pregnancy is not necessarily a good predictor of postpartum depression. In one recent study, women who were depressed during pregnancy were found to be at increased risk for postpartum depression (O'Hara Schlechte, Lewis, & Varner, 1991). Most studies have not documented this association (Kumar & Robson, 1984; O'Hara et al., 1984). Nevertheless, studies of risk for postpartum depression do suggest that women who are prone to depression before becoming pregnant are at elevated risk for depression after delivery. Finally, it should be noted that personal and family history of psychosis are also associated with increased risk for postpartum psychosis (Kendell, 1985; O'Hara, 1991).

Psychological Variables

Depression theorists have developed models to account for psychological processes that lead individuals to become depressed (Abramson, Seligman, & Teasdale, 1978; Beck, Rush, Shaw & Emery, 1979; Lewinsohn, Youngren, & Grosscup, 1979; Rehm, 1977). In general, these models suggest that individuals prone to depression perceive themselves and their environment in particularly negative and dysfunctional ways. For example, the depression-prone individual may be especially likely to blame herself for a failure, but not take credit for a success, or set very high or stringent standards for personal success, or misinterpret the meaning of situations. All of these cognitive behaviors lead the individual to experience herself and life in general as much more negative and unrewarding than would someone with a more adaptive cognitive style. A number of prospective studies of postpartum depression have tested these hypotheses. In general, the findings suggest that these negative cognitive styles are associated with increased likelihood of negative affect after delivery (i.e., high levels of depressive symptomatology) but not with increased risk for clinical postpartum depression (O'Hara et al., 1984; O'Hara, Schlechte, Lewis, & Varner, 1991; Whiffen, 1988).

Summary of Causal Factors

Although no potential causal factor for postpartum depression (or the blues or psychosis for that matter) has received unambiguous support in the literature, a "composite sketch" of the woman who is most likely to be at risk can be developed. The vulnerable pregnant woman is one who has had a past episode of depression (or other serious psychiatric disorder). During pregnancy or after delivery she may experience some significant negative life events such as loss of housing or loss of employment for herself or her partner. She may be in an unsatisfying relationship with her partner or she may have no partner to provide support and assistance to her. Finally, during the early postpartum period she may experience the blues which may persist longer than usual. All of these features will increase the woman's risk for a postpartum depression. Hormonal factors may ultimately be understood as playing a causal role in postpartum depression, but as yet specific hormonal events during the puerperium that would put a woman at risk for postpartum depression have not been identified.

CONSEQUENCES

For the Child

In recent years a rather large literature has emerged suggesting that parental psychopathology may have negative consequences for children (Downey & Coyne, 1990; Gelfand & Teti, 1990). These studies have examined the effects of both paternal and maternal psychopathology; however, most of the work has been done with mothers. The most consistent findings have been that children (of all ages) of depressed mothers are at increased risk both for problems in social adjustment and depression. Most of this research has been done with depressed mothers of older children and adolescents. However, in recent years several studies have followed childbearing women and their children on a prospective basis over a period of 3 to 5 years. The other strategy has been to identify depressed women after delivery and assess the functioning of their infants.

Studies of infants of depressed mothers have found that depressed mothers are more negative in their interactions with their infants (Cohn, Campbell, Matias, & Hopkins, 1990; Field, Healy, Goldstein, Perry, Bendell, Schanberg, Zimmerman, & Kuhn, 1988). For example, Cohn et al. (1990) observed 24 depressed and 22 nondepressed mother–infant dyads at 2 months postpartum in structured and unstructured interactions. Depressed mothers showed higher levels of negative affect, especially irritation and intrusiveness, during face-to-face interactions. Interestingly, the only effect on infant observable behavior was that babies of nonworking depressed mothers showed a lower proportion of positive affect than babies of nondepressed mothers and depressed mothers who worked.

Representative of long-term follow-up studies of childbearing women and the children was one conducted by Kumar and Robson (1984). They found that at age 4½ the children of postpartum depressed mothers performed significantly worse on a standard measure of cognitive abilities than did children of postpartum nondepressed mothers (Cogill, Caplan, Alexandra, Robson, & Kumar, 1986). They did not, however, observe differences in the social or emotional development in these two groups of children (Caplan, Cogill, Alexandra, Robson, Katz, & Kumar, 1989). Despite these findings, other studies have found evidence of long-term social and emotional consequences of maternal postpartum depression (Philipps & O'Hara, 1991; Wrate, Rooney, Thomas, & Cox, 1985).

For the Mother

The major consequence to the mother of having experienced a postpartum depression is risk for future depression. The findings of these studies have been relatively consistent. Women who experience a postpartum depression are at increased risk for future depressions over a 5-year period (Ghodsian, Zajicek, & Wolkind, 1984; Kumar & Robson, 1984; Philipps & O'Hara, 1991). This increased risk for future depressions is not necessarily due to the postpartum depression per se. As discussed earlier, women who experienced a postpartum depression frequently have had earlier episodes of depression. The postpartum depression may simply be an index of an enduring vulnerability to depressive episodes that extends into the future following a postpartum depression. Nevertheless, these future episodes of depression that build on top of the postpartum depression have serious implications for the woman's ability to function effectively in all of her social roles (e.g., mother, spouse, worker).

The consequences for children and women who have experienced a postpartum psychosis are similar to what has been described for postpartum depression. The children are at risk for social and cognitive deficits (O'Hara, 1991). Mothers are at risk for future psychotic episodes, particularly following the birth of another child (Brockington, Winokur, & Dean, 1982).

TREATMENT

In general, postpartum depressed women receive the same treatments that other depressed patients would receive in clinical settings. However, because of the timing of postpartum depression, the possible role of reproductive hormones, and the special significance that many women and clinicians attach to depression during the postpartum period, some specific treatments for postpartum depression have been developed. These treatments have been of two general sorts, treatments given during pregnancy or early in the puerperium, often to at-risk women, designed to prevent the development of a postpartum depression, and treatments that are given after delivery to a woman who is already depressed.

Several prevention studies have been conducted and each of them involved a series of group sessions (two or more) that helped women (and sometimes their partners) prepare for the postpartum responsibilities (Elliott, Sanjack, & Leverton, 1988; Gordon & Gordon, 1960; Halonen & Passman, 1985). The targets of these preventive interventions varied from the very practical, such as advice-giving regarding the necessity of getting help during the postpartum period and identifying a pediatrician prior to delivery, to more therapeutic activities such as learning to relax or simply discussing common concerns in a group setting. Overall, women receiving each of these interventions had better postpartum emotional adjustment than women receiving a control intervention. In another study, women with a history of postpartum depression were given progesterone regularly after delivery for about two months (Dalton, 1985). No cases of postpartum depression were observed; however, the lack of a control group and the self-selection of these women make these findings difficult to interpret.

Few well-designed treatment studies of postpartum depressed women have been undertaken. The most adequate study was conducted in Scotland with women who met the RDC for major depression (Holden, Sagovsky, & Cox, 1989). Women who received eight brief client-centered counseling sessions that were conducted in their homes by health visitors experienced significantly lower levels of depressive symptomatology following treatment than a control group of nontreated women. One other treatment study of postpartum depression is currently under way in which the treated group is receiving transdermal estrogen (Gregoire, Henderson, Studd, & Kumar, 1992). Preliminary results suggest some benefit for the estrogen therapy.

Too little treatment research has been conducted to draw confident conclusions regarding the efficacy of various treatments for postpartum depression. Conventional treatments for depression appear to be effective for women experiencing a postpartum depression. However, caution is advised. For example, little is known about the extent to which women experiencing postpartum depression have been represented in therapy outcome studies. Given concerns about the effects of antidepressants in breast milk it is unlikely that childbearing women have been included in general trials of antidepressants. The childbearing status of women in therapy outcome studies is rarely mentioned so it is unclear whether depression in the puerperium is responsive to conventional pharmacotherapies and psychotherapies. Also, the clinician must remain sensitive to these women's needs as new mothers during the postpartum period. Medical centers are increasingly developing specialized units to treat women with postpartum mood disorders. In Great Britain special mother–baby units have been developed to care for women who require hospitalization for depression or other psychiatric disorder after delivery (Sneddon, 1992). These units allow the baby to stay with the mother so that development of the mother–infant relationship and the mother's parenting skills are disrupted as little as possible.

CLINICAL MANAGEMENT

Little additional time is required by the obstetrician and the obstetrical care staff to accommodate the psychological needs of women during pregnancy and after delivery. It is time well spent when the obstetrician has been able to identify the high-risk patient during pregnancy, provide reassurance to the low-risk patient where appropriate, or validate the feelings of a depressed postpartum patient and facilitate her entry into treatment. Both nurses and physicians have a role to play in this domain.

Prenatal Screening

As part of a general health history, patients should be asked to provide information regarding any past episodes of psychiatric disorder. The obstetrician should be sensitive to past hospitalizations or formal treatment for depression or other disorders. However, many individuals do not obtain treatment when they are depressed (or suffer from an anxiety disorder) and so relying on past treatment as the sole index of past psychopathology is inadequate. Obstetricians should inquire about times when the patient might have been out of her normal mood state for more than two weeks at a time. If the patient is able to identify such a period, the obstetrician should follow-up with questions regarding depressive symptoms for DSM–III–R mood disorders (American Psychiatric Association, 1987). Of course, the obstetrician should be alert for the presence of any current mood disorder. In sum, the obstetrician should have a good understanding of the patient's psychiatric history.

A second element of prenatal screening involves what might be called a psychosocial screening. The obstetrician should inquire about psychosocial difficulties that would make adjustment during pregnancy or after delivery more difficult, including adequacy of financial resources and housing; employment and the potentiality of work hazards; the quality of the marital relationship; the availability of support from family or friends; and the occurrence of any recent negative events that may have long-term implications (e.g., announcement of future layoffs at spouse's place of employment). Information gained from this sort of psychosocial interview will alert the obstetrician to the potential of significant present and future stress in the patient's life and provide the opportunity for an informed referral for the patient (e.g., to hospital social services).

Prenatal Preparation

The type of preparation that the obstetrician does with the patient will depend in part upon the results of the prenatal screening. It should also be recognized that although prenatal classes (e.g., Lamaze) play an important role in preparing women for childbirth and beyond, it is often (though not necessarily) the case that relatively little emphasis is placed on emotional adjustment. Perhaps more importantly, prenatal preparation is disconnected from obstetrical care such that no information flows between the obstetrician and the individuals doing the prenatal preparation. Ideally, these services should be integrated in order to best serve the patient. Wherever prenatal preparation occurs, it should be emphasized to the pregnant woman that although mild mood disturbances (i.e., the blues) are common after delivery, they are not very severe and are usually short-lived. The more serious disorders such as postpartum depression and particularly postpartum psychosis are much less common.

Although there is not a large research base for recommendations that an obstetrician might make to a patient, there are some suggestions that can be made that reflect common sense and have some objective support (Gordon & Gordon, 1960; O'Hara & Engeldinger, 1989). Examples would include: a) reassurance that the blues are normal and may reflect the effects of exhaustion or relief of built-up tension after delivery; b) emphasizing to the couple that having a baby is a shared responsibility (i.e., encouraging provision of help by partner); c) encouraging primiparas, in particular, to seek help and advice from women more experienced in child care to reduce excessive or unnecessary worrying; and d) suggesting that couples avoid major life changes such as moving or changing jobs during the puerperium. Finally, a woman should know who to contact if she experiences emotional problems after delivery (e.g., symptoms in Table 2.2 that persist for two weeks or more).

Women who have a history of previous psychiatric illness, and particularly women who are currently depressed (or are experiencing some other disorder), should be monitored more closely than the low-risk patient. In the case of women who have had a prior serious disorder (e.g., psychotic depression, manic–depressive disorder) arrangements should be made during pregnancy for the woman to consult with a psychiatrist (preferably one that she knows and trusts). The risk of recurrence of psychiatric illness is high after delivery for these women and they should be intensively monitored for at least 30 days after delivery and less intensively monitored for another 60 days. Because of the potential teratogenic effects of most psychotropic medications, psychiatrists are usually reluctant to undertake drug treatment during pregnancy (Cohen et al., 1989).

Postnatal Assessment

Obstetricians usually have contact with patients during the period that they are in the hospital after delivery and then at about six weeks after delivery. The obstetrician should inquire about the patient's mood prior to sending her home from the hospital. Patients who are doing well can be advised to call if problems develop. Patients who are experiencing some mood disturbance can be reassured regarding the likelihood that it will be short-lived. Also, based on the prenatal screening, the obstetrician may be aware of various psychosocial stressors that may impair the patient's ability to function. Referral to hospital social work, clinical psychologic, or psychiatric resources may be indicated in these cases. Follow-up is important because women may find it difficult to follow through on a referral because of overwhelming responsibilities at home and lack of help.

At the time of the postnatal visit it is useful to ask the patient to complete a depression screening measure like the Beck Depression Inventory (BDI; Beck et al., 1961) or the Edinburgh Postnatal Depression Scale (EPDS; Cox, Holden, & Sagovsky, 1987). These questionnaires allow the patient to rate the severity of a number of depression symptoms (e.g., dysphoric mood, guilt, problems in concentration, appetite and sleep disturbance, fatigue). Measures such as the BDI and the EPDS cannot yield diagnoses but they can alert the obstetrician to those women who need more intensive assessment.

Postnatal Treatment

Ordinarily, the obstetrician is not going to undertake the treatment of depression. In most cases, a referral should be made to a clinical psychologist or psychiatrist for psychotherapy or, possibly, pharmacotherapy. In most cases, the treating clinician will use whatever methods, he/she has typically used to treat a depressed female patient. A large number of antidepressant medications are available for use, including newer ones such as fluoxetine (Prozac®), which have relatively mild side effects. One consideration for breastfeeding women taking medication during the puerperium is the presence of the drug in breast milk. The conservative clinical view is that women should bottle feed if they are taking psychotropic medications (Cohen et al., 1989; Robinson et al., 1986). However, there is growing evidence that some antidepressants (e.g., nortriptyline) are present in very low levels in breast milk and at almost undetectable levels in infants' blood (Wisner & Perel, 1988). Of course, many women will not want to take medication because of their desire to breast-feed, their general reluctance to take medication, or their previous nonresponse to medication. Fortunately, there are several psychological interventions that have the same efficacy as antidepressant treatment (Elkin et al., 1989).

The two major psychotherapies that have been validated as effective treatments for patients experiencing major depression are cognitive therapy (Beck et al., 1979) and interpersonal psychotherapy (IPT; Klerman, Weissman, Rounsaville, & Chevron, 1984). Both of these therapies have undergone rigorous evaluations and have been found to be as effective as antidepressant medication (Elkin et al., 1989). Cognitive therapy is based on Aaron Beck's cognitive model of depression (Beck et al., 1979) and assumes that by identifying, challenging, and changing dysfunctional negative cognitions, depression can be effectively managed. Details of cognitive therapy procedures are outlined in the treatment manual developed by Beck and his colleagues (Beck et al., 1979). Interpersonal psychotherapy was originally developed as an adjunct to antidepressant medication treatment (Klerman et al., 1984). It has also been used as a continuation and maintenance treatment to prevent depression relapse or recurrence (Frank et al., 1990). As might be understood from the name of the therapy, IPT is concerned with interpersonal aspects of depression and, in particular, problems that depressed patients have in their various social roles (e.g., mother, spouse, daughter, employee, friend). A distinct advantage of IPT and cognitive therapy, as well, is that they are both designed to be administered as relatively short-term therapies (16 to 24 sessions). Finally, they both are problem focused and appeal to the common sense of the patient and either can be confidently recommended to a depressed patient.

SUMMARY

Most women make a healthy psychological adjustment to pregnancy and the postpartum period. However, because psychiatric disorders, especially depression, are common in childbearing-aged women, obstetrical staff must be sensitive to the needs of women who are at high risk for depression during pregnancy and after delivery. The obstetrical staff members, as the providers of primary health care for childbearing women, are in the best position to educate women about how to lessen their risk for difficulties after delivery and to identify women who are experiencing the early stages of a psychiatric disorder during pregnancy or after delivery. Hopefully, these roles will be increasingly taken on by physicians and nurses in the field of health care for women.

REFERENCES

Abramson, L. Y., Seligman, M.E.P., & Teasdale, J. D. (1978). Learned helplessness in humans: Critique and reformulation. *Journal of Abnormal Psychology, 87*, 49–74.

American Academy of Pediatrics, Committee on Drugs. (1989). The transfer of drugs and other chemicals into human breast milk. *Pediatrics, 84*, 924–936.

American Psychiatric Association (1987). *Diagnostic and statistical manual of mental disorders*. 3rd Edition, Revised. (DSM–III–R). Washington, DC: American Psychiatric Association.

American Psychiatric Association (1994). *Diagnostic and statistical manual of mental disorders*. (4th Edition, DSM–IV). Washington, DC: American Psychiatric Association.

Beck, A. T., Rush, A. J., Shaw, B. F., & Emery, G. (1979). *Cognitive therapy of depression*. New York: Guilford Press.

Beck, A. T., Ward, C. H., Mendelson, M., Mock, J., & Erbaugh, J. (1961). An inventory for measuring depression. *Archives of General Psychiatry, 4*, 561–569.

Blair, R. A., Gilmore, J. S., Playfair, H. R., Tisdall, M. W., & O'Shea, M. W. (1970). Puerperal depression: A study of predictive factors. *Journal of the Royal College of General Practitioners, 19*, 22–25.

Brockington, I. F., & Cox-Roper, A. (1988). In R. Kumar & I. F. Brockington (Eds.), *Motherhood and mental illness 2 Causes and consequences* (pp. 1–16). London: Wright.

Brockington, I. F., Winokur, G., & Dean, C. (1982). Puerperal psychosis. In I. F. Brockington & R. Kumar (Eds.), *Motherhood and mental illness* (pp. 37–69). New York: Grune and Stratton.

Brown, G. W., & Harris, T. (1978). *Social origins of depression: A study of psychiatric disorder in women*. New York: Free Press.

Campbell, J. L., & Winokur, G. (1985). Post-partum affective disorders: Selected biological aspects. In D. G. Inwood (Ed.), *Recent advances in post-partum psychiatric disorders* (pp. 19–40). Washington, DC: American Psychiatric Press.

Campbell, S. B., & Cohn, J. F. (1991). Prevalence and correlates of postpartum depression in first-time mothers. *Journal of Abnormal Psychology, 100*, 594–599.

Caplan, H. L., Cogill, S. R., Alexandra, H., Robson, K. M., Katz, R., & Kumar, R. (1989). Maternal depression and the emotional development of the child. *British Journal of Psychiatry, 154*, 818–822.

Cogill, S. R., Caplan, H. L., Alexandra, H., Robson, K. M., & Kumar, R. (1986). Impact of maternal postnatal depression on cognitive development of young children. *British Medical Journal, 292*, 1165–1167.

Cohen, L. S., Heller, V. L., & Rosenbaum, J. F. (1989). Treatment guidelines for psychotropic drug use in pregnancy. *Psychosomatics, 30*, 25–33.

Cohn, J. F., Campbell, S. B., Matias, R., & Hopkins, J. (1990). Face-to-face interactions of postpartum depressed and nondepressed mother–infant pairs at 2 months. *Developmental Psychology, 26*, 15–23.

Cooper, P. J., Campbell, E. A., Day, A., Kennerley, H., & Bond, A. (1988). Non-psychotic psychiatric disorder after childbirth: A prospective study of prevalence, incidence, course and nature. *British Journal of Psychiatry, 152*, 799–806.

Cox, J. L., Connor, Y., & Kendell, R. E. (1982). Prospective study of the psychiatric disorders of childbirth. *British Journal of Psychiatry, 140*, 111–117.

Cox, J. L., Holden, J. M., & Sagovsky, R. (1987). Detection of postnatal depression: Development of the 10-item Edinburgh Postnatal Depression Scale. *British Journal of Psychiatry, 150*, 782–786.

Cox, J. L., Murray, D., & Chapman, G. (1993). A controlled study of the onset, duration, and prevalence of postnatal depression. *British Journal of Psychiatry, 163*, 27–31.

Dalton, K. (1985). Progesterone prophylaxis used successfully in postnatal depression. *The Practitioner, 229*, 507–508.

Dennerstein, L., Morse, C. A., & Varnavides, K. (1988). Premenstrual tension and depression—is there a relationship? *Journal of Psychosomatic Obstetrics and Gynecology, 8*, 45–52.

Downey, G., & Coyne, J. C. (1990). Children of depressed parents: An integrative review. *Psychological Bulletin, 108*, 50–76.

Elkin, I., Shea, M. T., Watkins, J. T., Imber, S. D., Sotsky, S. M., Collins, J. F., Glass, D. R., Pilkonis, P. A., Leber, W. R., Docherty, J. P., Fiester, S. J., & Parloff, M. B. (1989). National Institute of Mental Health Treatment of Depression Collaborative Research Program: General effectiveness of treatments. *Archives of General Psychiatry, 46*, 971–982.

Elliott, S. A. (1984). Pregnancy and after. In S. Rachman (Ed.), *Contributions to medical psychology*, Vol. 3, (pp. 93–116). Oxford: Pergamon.

Elliott, S. A., Rugg, A. J., Watson, J. P., & Brough, D. I. (1983). Mood changes during pregnancy and after the birth of a child. *British Journal of Clinical Psychology, 22*, 295–308.

Elliott, S. A., Sanjack, M., & Leverton, T. J. (1988). Parents groups in pregnancy: A preventive intervention for postnatal depression? (pp. 87–110). In B. H. Gottlieb (Ed.), *Marshaling social support: Formats, processes, and effects*. Newbury Park, CA: Sage.

Endicott, J., Halbreich, U., Schacht, S., & Nee, J. (1981). Premenstrual changes and affective disorder. *Psychosomatic Medicine, 43*, 519–529.

Feggetter, P., & Gath, D. (1981). Non-psychotic psychiatric disorders in women one year after childbirth. *Journal of Psychosomatic Research, 25*, 369–372.

Field, T., Healy, B., Goldstein, S., Perry, S., Bendell, D., Schanberg, S., Zimmerman, E. A., & Kuhn, C. (1988). Infants of depressed mothers show "depressed" behavior even with nondepressed adults. *Child Development, 59*, 1569–1579.

Frank, E., Kupfer, D. J., Perel, J. M., Cornes, C., Jarrett, D. B., Mallinger, A. G., Thase, M. E., McEachran, A. B., & Grochocinski, V. J. (1990). Three-year outcomes for maintenance therapies in recurrent depression. *Archives of General Psychiatry, 47*, 1093–1099.

Gard, P. R., Handley, S. L., Parsons, A. D., & Waldron, G. (1986). A multivariate investigation of postpartum mood disturbance. *British Journal of Psychiatry, 148*, 567–575.

Gelfand, D. M., & Teti, D. M. (1990). The effects of maternal depression on children. *Clinical Psychology Review, 10*, 329–353.

George, A., & Sandler, M. (1988). Endocrine and biochemical studies in puerperal mental disorders. In R. Kumar & I. F. Brockington (Eds.), *Motherhood and mental illness 2 Causes and consequences* (pp. 78–112). London: Wright.

George, A. J., Copeland, J.R.M., & Wilson, K.C.M. (1980). Serum prolactin and the postpartum blues syndrome. *British Journal of Pharmacology, 70*, 102–103.

Ghodsian, M., Zajicek, E., & Wolkind, S. (1984). A longitudinal study of maternal depression and child behavior problems. *Journal of Child Psychology and Psychiatry and Allied Disciplines, 25*, 91–109.

Gordon, R. E., & Gordon, K. K. (1960). Social factors in the prevention of postpartum emotional problems. *Obstetrics and Gynecology, 15*, 433–438.

Gotlib, I. H., Whiffen, V. E., Wallace, P. M., & Mount, J. H. (1991). Prospective investigation of postpartum depression: Factors involved in onset and recovery. *Journal of Abnormal Psychology, 100*, 122–132.

Greenwood, J., & Parker, G. (1984). The dexamethasone suppression test in the puerperium. *Australian and New Zealand Journal of Psychiatry, 18*, 282–284.

Gregoire, A., Henderson, A., Studd, J., & Kumar, R. (1992 June). *Percutaneous oestrogens in the treatment of postnatal depression*. Paper presented at the 10th International Congress of Psychosomatic Obstetrics and Gynaecology, Stockholm.

Halonen, J. S., & Passman, R. H. (1985). Relaxation training and expectation in the treatment of postpartum distress. *Journal of Clinical and Consulting Psychology, 53*, 839–845.

Hamilton, J. A. (1992). The issue of unique qualities. In J. A. Hamilton & P. N. Harberger (Eds.), *Postpartum psychiatric illness: A picture puzzle* (pp. 15–32). Philadelphia: University of Pennsylvania Press.

Hamilton, J. A., & Harberger, P. N. (Eds.). (1992). *Postpartum psychiatric illness: A picture puzzle*. Philadelphia: University of Pennsylvania Press.

Handley, S. L., Dunn, T. L., Waldron, G., & Baker, J. M. (1980). Tryptophan, cortisol and puerperal mood. *British Journal of Psychiatry, 136*, 498–508.

Harris, B., Johns, S., Fung, H., Thomas, R., Walker, R., Read, G., & Riad-Fahmy, D. (1989). The hormonal environment of post-natal depression. *British Journal of Psychiatry, 154*, 660–667.

Holden, J. M., Sagovsky, R., & Cox, J. L. (1989). Counselling in a general practice setting: Controlled study of health visitor intervention in treatment of postnatal depression. *British Medical Journal, 298*, 223–226.

Iles, S., Gath, D., & Kennerley, H. (1989). Maternity blues II. A comparison between post-operative women and post-natal women. *British Journal of Psychiatry. 155*, 363–366.

Kendell, R. E. (1985). Emotional and physical factors in the genesis of puerperal mental disorders. *Journal of Psychosomatic Research, 29*, 3–11.

Kendell, R. E., Chalmers, J. C., & Platz, C. (1987). Epidemiology of puerperal psychoses. *British Journal of Psychiatry, 150*, 662–673.

Kendell R. E., Mackenzie W. E, West C., McGuire R. J., & Cox J. L. (1984). Day-to-day mood changes after childbirth: Further data. *British Journal of Psychiatry, 145*, 620–625.

Kendell, R. E., McGuire, R. J., Conner, Y., & Cox, J. L. (1981). Mood changes in the first three weeks after childbirth. *Journal of Affective Disorders, 3*, 317–326.

Kennerley, H., & Gath, D. (1986). Maternity blues reassessed. *Psychiatric Developments, 4*, 1–17.

Kennerley, H., & Gath, D. (1989). Maternity blues I. Detection and measurement by questionnaire. *British Journal of Psychiatry, 155*, 356–362.

Klerman, G. L., Weissman, M. M., Rounsaville, B. J., & Chevron, E. S. (1984). *Interpersonal psychotherapy of depression*. New York: Basic Books.

Kumar, R., & Robson, K. M. (1984). A prospective study of emotional disorders in childbearing women. *British Journal of Psychiatry, 144*, 35–47.

Levy, V. (1987). The maternity blues in post-partum and post-operative women. *British Journal of Psychiatry, 151*, 368–372.

Lewinsohn, P. M., Youngren, M. A., & Grosscup, S. J. (1979). Reinforcement and depression. In R. A. Depue (Ed.), *The psychobiology of depressive disorders: Implications for the effects of stress* (pp. 291–316). New York: Academic Press.

Lubin, B., Gardener, S. H., & Roth, A. (1975). Mood and somatic symptoms during pregnancy. *Psychosomatic Medicine, 37*, 136–146.

Myers, J. K., Weissman, M. M., Tischler, G. L., Holzer, C. E., Leaf, P. J., Orvaschel, H., Anthony, J. C., Boyd, J. H., Burke, J. D., Jr., Kramer, M., & Stoltzman, R. (1984). Six-month prevalence of psychiatric disorders in three communities. *Archives of General Psychiatry, 41*, 959–967.

Nott, P. N., Franklin, M. Armitage, C., & Gelder, M. G. (1976). Hormonal changes in mood in the puerperium. *British Journal of Psychiatry, 128*, 379–383.

Oates, M. (1989). Management of major mental illness in pregnancy and the puerperium. In M. R. Oates (Ed.), *Baillière's clinical obstetrics and gynaecology: International practice and research*, Volume 3, Number 4, (pp. 905–920). London: Baillière Tindall.

O'Hara, M. W. (1986). Social support, life events, and depression during pregnancy and the puerperium. *Archives of General Psychiatry, 43*, 569–573.

O'Hara, M. W. (1991). Postpartum mental disorders. In J. J. Sciarra (Ed.), *Gynecology and obstetrics*. Volume 6, Chapter 84. Philadelphia: Harper & Row.

O'Hara, M. W. (1995). *Postpartum depression: Causes and consequences*. New York: Springer-Verlag.

O'Hara, M. W., & Engeldinger, J. (1989). Postpartum mood disorders: Detection and prevention. *The Female Patient, 14*, 19–27.

O'Hara, M. W., Neunaber, D. J., & Zekoski, E. M. (1984). A prospective study of postpartum depression: Prevalence, course, and predictive factors. *Journal of Abnormal Psychology, 93*, 158–171.

O'Hara, M. W., Rehm, L. P., & Campbell, S. B. (1982). Predicting depressive symptomatology: Cognitive-behavioral models and postpartum depression. *Journal of Abnormal Psychology, 91*, 457–461.

O'Hara, M. W., Rehm, L. P., & Campbell, S. B. (1983). Postpartum depression: A role for social network and life stress variables. *Journal of Nervous and Mental Disease, 171*, 336–341.

O'Hara, M. W., Schlechte, J. A., Lewis, D. A., & Varner, M. W. (1991). A controlled prospective study of postpartum mood disorders: Psychological, environmental, and hormonal variables. *Journal of Abnormal Psychology, 100*, 63–73.

O'Hara, M. W., Schlechte, J. A., Lewis, D. A., & Wright, E. J. (1991). Prospective study of postpartum blues: Biologic and psychosocial factors. *Archives of General Psychiatry, 48*, 801–806.

O'Hara, M. W., & Zekoski, E. M. (1988). Postpartum depression: A comprehensive review. In R. Kumar & I. F. Brockington (Eds.), *Motherhood and mental illness 2 Causes and consequences* (pp. 17–63). London: Wright.

O'Hara, M. W., Zekoski, E. M., Philipps, L. H., & Wright, E. J. (1990). A controlled prospective study of postpartum mood disorders: Comparison of childbearing and nonchildbearing women. *Journal of Abnormal Psychology, 99*, 3–15.

Paykel, E. S., Emms, E. M., Fletcher, J., & Rassaby, E. S. (1980). Life events and social support in puerperal depression. *British Journal of Psychiatry, 136*, 339–346.

Philipps, L.H.C. & O'Hara, M. W. (1991). Prospective study of postpartum depression: 4 1/2-year follow-up of women and children. *Journal of Abnormal Psychology, 100*, 151–155.

Pop, V.J.M., de Rooy, H.A.M., Vader, H. L., van der Heide, D., van Son, M., Komproe, I. H., Essed, G.G.M., & de Geus, C. A. (1991). Postpartum thyroid dysfunction and depression in an unselected population. *New England Journal of Medicine. 324*, 1815–1816.

Rehm, L. P. (1977). A self-control model of depression. *Behavior Therapy, 8*, 787–804.

Robinson, G. E., Stewart, D. E., & Flak, E. (1986). The rational use of psychotropic drugs in pregnancy and postpartum. *Canadian Journal of Psychiatry, 31*, 183–190.

Schlesser, M. A. (1986). Neuroendocrine abnormalities in affective disorder. In A. J. Rush & K. Z. Altshuler (Eds.), *Depression: Basic mechanisms, diagnosis, and treatment* (pp. 45–71). New York: Guilford Press.

Schou, M. (1990). Lithium treatment during pregnancy delivery, and lactation: An update. *Journal of Clinical Psychiatry, 51*, 410–413.

Sneddon, J. (1992). The mother and baby unit: An important approach to treatment. (pp. 102–114). In J. A. Hamilton & P. N. Harberger (Eds.), *Postpartum psychiatric illness: A picture puzzle*. Philadelphia: University of Pennsylvania Press.

Spielvogel, A., & Wile, J. (1986). Treatment of psychotic pregnant patient. *Psychosomatics, 27*, 487–492.

Spitzer, R. L., Endicott, J., & Robins, E. (1978). Research diagnostic criteria: Rationale and reliability. *Archives of General Psychiatry, 36*, 773–782.

Steiner, M. (1979). Psychobiology of mental disorders associated with childbearing. *Acta Psychiatrica Scandinavica, 60*, 449–464.

Troutman, B. R., & Cutrona, C. E. (1990). Nonpsychotic postpartum depression among adolescent mothers. *Journal of Abnormal Psychology, 99*, 69–78.

Watson, J. P., Elliott, S. A., Rugg, A. J., & Brough, D. I. (1984). Psychiatric disorder in pregnancy and the first postnatal year. *British Journal of Psychiatry, 144*, 453–462.

Whiffen, V. E. (1988). Vulnerability to postpartum depression: A prospective multivariate study. *Journal of Abnormal Psychology, 97*, 467–474.

Wisner, K. L., & Perel, J. M. (1988). Psychopharmacologic agents and electroconvulsive therapy during pregnancy and the puerperium. In R. L. Cohen (Ed.), *Psychiatric consultation in childbirth settings: Parent- and child-oriented approaches* (pp. 165–206). New York: Plenum.

World Health Organization. (1978). Mental disorders: Glossary and guide to their classification in accordance with the ninth revision of the *International Classification of Diseases*. Geneva: Author.

Wrate, R. M., Rooney, A. C., Thomas, P. F., & Cox, J. L. (1985). Postnatal depression and child development: A three-year follow-up study. *British Journal of Psychiatry, 146*, 622–627.

3

Menopause

Mary K. Walling

Menopause will be experienced by every woman who lives long enough. For many centuries various physical and psychological problems have been attributed to the experience of menopause. Early studies employing menopause clinic samples seemed to support these attributions while more recent cross-sectional and longitudinal studies of non-patients are not as supportive of psychological effects. It is the purpose of this chapter to examine the empirical research bearing on the impact that menopause may (or may not) have on a woman's psychological well-being and to discuss the clinical implications of these findings.

First, the various phases that occur in the transition from the reproductive to the nonreproductive years of a woman's life will be presented. Next will be a brief discussion of the physiological basis of this transition and the physical effects of the hormonal deficiency resulting from ovarian failure. This will be followed by a discussion of methodological issues to consider when examining this body of literature. A summary of the literature employing clinical samples and a more extensive review of the literature employing non-patients will then be offered. Finally, the practical implications of this research will be discussed.

Various terms have been used to describe the menstrual status of women. Although there are no universally accepted definitions, those offered by the World Health Organization (1981) will be used in the remainder of this chapter: 1) *premenopause* refers to the reproductive years before menopause; 2) *perimenopause* (or "climacteric") begins when signs of the approaching menopause (e.g., irregular periods, hot flushes) appear and lasts until approximately one year after the menopause; 3) *menopause* is the permanent cessation of menstruation and occurs with the conclusion of a woman's final menstrual period; 4) *postmenopause* begins one year after the last menstrual period.

PHYSIOLOGICAL BASIS OF MENOPAUSE

Menopause occurs following decades of age-related changes in ovarian functioning. In order better to understand the changes that occur with ovarian atresia, it is helpful to examine the normal menstrual cycle. Briefly, a newborn girl carries within her ovaries her lifetime supply of eggs (ova). Each egg and its surrounding cells constitute a *follicle*. After puberty, many follicles begin to mature each month under the influence of follicular stimulating hormone (FSH), a hormone released by the pituitary gland and regulated by the hypothalamus. FSH causes the cells surrounding the egg to multiply and fill with fluid, which has a high concentration of cholesterol. The cholesterol is converted into estradiol, a potent estrogen, which eventually finds its way into the blood stream. All but one of the maturing follicles usually regress and the surviving ("dominant") follicle continues to grow as it is prepared for ovulation.

The estrogen circulating in the blood stream not only acts upon the uterus, fallopian tubes, and cervix, it also influences tissues throughout the body, either directly (e.g., the skin, vagina, and breasts) or indirectly (e.g., the heart and blood vessels). The estrogen, or follicular, phase of the cycle lasts about 10 days. When the level of estrogen in the blood peaks, the hypothalamus signals the pituitary gland to decrease secretion of FSH and to start secreting luteinizing hormone (LH). A surge of LH precedes ovulation by 24–48 hours and stimulates the follicle further, causing ovulation to occur (i.e., the egg is released through the surface of the ovary).

The cells of the ruptured follicle remain behind to multiply and swell under the influence of LH, taking on a yellowish appearance and hence the name *corpus luteum* or "yellow body". The corpus luteum continues to secrete some estrogen, but secretes predominantly progesterone, which governs the luteal phase of the cycle. Progesterone controls the effects of estrogen, halting multiplication of the endometrial cells lining the uterus. The endometrial cells mature under the influence of progesterone, which also quiets the muscle of the uterus and inhibits secretion of FSH to prevent the start of another cycle. If conception does not occur, LH declines and the corpus luteum begins to degenerate, leading to a drop in production of progesterone. As progesterone levels fall, the endometrium is sloughed from the uterine wall and flows out through the cervix and vagina as the menstrual period. The hypothalamus is no longer inhibited by progesterone and can once again signal the pituitary to secrete FSH, initiating another cycle.

It is important to note that estrogen and progesterone are not the only sex steroids produced by the female. The central region of the ovary also produces small quantities of two androgens—testosterone and androstenedione (which is converted by the fat cells to estrone, an estrogen that is less potent than estradiol), and secretes them into the blood stream (Abraham, Lobotsky, & Lloyd, 1969; Korenman, Sherman, & Korenman, 1978). The adrenal cortex, however, serves as the primary source of androgens in the female (about 5% of the amount found in males).

At about age 25, a woman's ovaries begin a slight but steady decline in estrogen production. As the ovaries age further, there is a decrease in the number of follicles responsive to FSH, resulting in a decrease in the luteal phase levels of estrogen and progesterone. Levels of these hormones will eventually decline drastically as ovulation becomes more and more erratic and finally ceases. Additionally, there is a significant rise in the amounts of FSH and LH secreted by the pituitary to spur maturation of follicles which no longer respond.

The postmenopausal ovary does not cease hormonal production with the end of ovulation. The androgens continue to be produced for many years, sometimes in higher amounts than in the ovaries of younger women. Eventually all ovarian function fails, leaving the adrenal cortex as the only source of estrogen precursors. These are converted into estrone in fat cells and continue to be produced in the postmenopausal years.

PHYSICAL EFFECTS OF ESTROGEN DEFICIENCY

Ovarian hormones, particularly estrogen, have direct effects on genital tissue. Decreased hormone production is associated with the following: thinning of the genital epithelium (the lining of the vagina); loss of subcutaneous fat; flattening of the labia majora; decrease in the size of the introitus and labia minora; and vaginal atrophy (i.e., a decrease in vaginal lubrication along with a decrease in vaginal length and width) (Lang & Aponte, 1967; Utian, 1987). Some of these effects, particularly vaginal atrophy, may be less severe in women who remain sexually active after menopause (Utian, 1987).

The direct effects of estrogen deficiency are not limited to the genital structures. "Hot flushes" are experienced by roughly 50%–80% of women, although there are individual differences in frequency and intensity (Kletzky & Borenstein, 1987; Walsh & Schiff, 1989). Typically, a hot flush is preceded by a vague aura which is then followed within a minute or two by a sudden onset of warmth in the face and neck which spreads to the chest. The wave of heat is accompanied by dilation of the superficial blood vessels, leading to a noticeable redness of the skin. While not a health threat, these sensations may be extremely uncomfortable and may also be accompanied by palpitations, dizziness, headache, and a drenching sweat. Night sweats, in which a woman awakens one or more times in the night with profuse sweating, are also associated with estrogen deficiency. These vasomotor symptoms, along with vaginal atrophy, are known as the hall-marks of the estrogen deficiency syndrome. Vasomotor symptoms decline in severity, although they can continue for as long as ten years following the end of menses, but genital symptoms such as vaginal atrophy worsen with time (Bar-ber, 1988; Perlmutter, 1977).

While vasomotor symptoms and vaginal atrophy can be quite annoying and cause significant alterations in life-style, they are not associated with increased morbidity or mortality. In contrast, the more "silent" effects of estrogen defi-ciency, osteoporosis and cardiovascular disease, increase both morbidity and mortality (e.g., Bengtsson & Lindquist, 1978; Gordon, Kannel, & Hjortland, 1978; Lindsay, 1989). Although Albright, Bloomberg, and Smith (1940) high-lighted the importance of ovarian failure in the pathogenesis of osteoporotic fracture, noting the unusually high proportion of oophorectomized women who presented with osteoporosis, this relationship remained controversial until the publication of carefully controlled clinical studies demonstrating that the admin-istration of estrogen prevents bone loss and fractures in both surgically and naturally menopausal women (Horsman, Gallagher, Simpson, & Nordin, 1977; Hutchinson, Polansky, & Feinstein, 1979; Lindsay et al., 1980). Other factors which appear to be important in bone loss are poor calcium intake, physical inactivity, heredity, smoking, and alcohol use (Barber, 1988).

A relationship between menopause and cardiovascular disease has also been established, but important questions remain. Perlman et al. (1989), conclude that, although it appears clear that surgically induced early menopause is a risk factor for heart disease, the role of natural menopause remains less obvious. Findings from numerous prospective studies of the relation between estrogen use and cardiovascular disease in both surgically and naturally postmenopausal women suggest that a significant reduction in risk of cardiovascular mortality can be achieved with estrogen use (e.g., Colditz et al., 1987; Cornoni-Huntley et al., 1983; Petitti, Perlman, & Sydney, 1987). Surgically menopausal women appear to be at greatest risk and benefit the most from estrogen use.

METHODOLOGICAL CONSIDERATIONS

Before reviewing the literature concerning psychological symptoms traditionally attributed to the climacteric, a discussion of important methodological issues will be presented. These issues include the use of clinical samples, failure to distinguish between women undergoing surgical versus natural menopause, vari-ability in the determination of menopausal status, and failure to assess poten-tially important psychosocial variables.

The use of clinical samples is by no means unique to the menopause literature. Although the ready availability of a pool of subjects enhances the desirability of sampling from those who present to a clinic for treatment of the condition of interest, threats to the external validity of results are formidable when such samples are used. Not the least of these threats is seen in the literature on illness behavior. This literature suggests strongly that individuals who report more life stress tend to report more symptoms (both physical and psychological) and to seek medical help for their symptoms (e.g., Ilfeld, 1977). Thus there may be differences between those who present for medical treatment and those who do not that are of sufficient magnitude to raise questions about the validity of generalizations from one group to the other.

The second methodological consideration is the failure to distinguish between women undergoing surgical menopause and those undergoing natural menopause. Natural menopause occurs gradually after many years of declining ovarian function. Additionally, the ovaries do not cease production of all estrogen precursors at the point of the final menses. With surgical menopause, however, the loss of ovarian function is immediate and complete. Additionally, there is some evidence that women who undergo surgical menopause may differ in important ways from those undergoing natural menopause in terms of symptom reporting and use of medical services (e.g., McKinlay & McKinlay, 1989; Roos, 1983). Therefore, employing "mixed" samples that include both women who have undergone surgical menopause and those who have undergone natural menopause may yield results of questionable value. When samples are restricted to those undergoing surgical menopause, generalizations to the population of women undergoing natural menopause may not be valid.

A third methodological difficulty is the establishment of menopausal status. Some studies have sorted subjects into pre-, peri-, and postmenopausal groups on the basis of age, deducing a relation between chronological age and endocrine status that may not exist for any given subject (Dennerstein, 1987). Other studies rely on the woman's self-report of symptom onset and/or cessation of menses to establish group membership. This method suffers from the problems associated with self-report, retrospective reporting, and effort-after-meaning in the case of women who may be attributing new or worrisome symptoms to the approach of menopause whether or not such attributions are warranted. The most accurate method of determining group membership is the use of hormonal assays. Although this method is invasive and more expensive than employing age or self-report to establish menopausal status, the use of rigorous methodology in determining group membership is vital to both internal and external validity. If questionable criteria are employed at this step, any inferences drawn from the results will be equally questionable.

The final methodological issue to be considered is the failure to assess potentially important variables such as life events, socioeconomic status, and marital and job satisfaction. For example, it now appears that although socioeconomic status (SES) is unrelated to the experience of vasomotor symptoms, women from the lower social classes may experience more psychological symptoms during the perimenopausal years than women from higher social classes (Hunter, Battersby, & Whitehead, 1986). Also, several investigators have found that psychosocial factors such as stressful life events are more predictive of psychological distress than is menopausal status (Cooke, 1985; Greene, 1980).

PSYCHOLOGICAL SYMPTOMS

Although many psychological symptoms have been attributed to the climacteric and postmenopausal years, there is little agreement as to which symptoms, if any, are directly related to hormonal insufficiency. Many early studies were based on clinical samples and, not surprisingly, a wide variety of frequently reported psychological symptoms emerged from these studies (Dennerstein & Burrows, 1978). These symptoms included diminished energy and drive, depression, anxiety, irritability, reduced concentration, aggressiveness, mood lability, tension, worry, and sleep difficulties. When the relation between these symptoms and estrogen deficiency was tested in several double-blind cross-over studies of hormone replacement therapy (HRT), results generally revealed no differences between treated and untreated groups (e.g., Coope, 1981; Coope, Thompson, & Poller, 1975; George, Beaumont, & Beardwood, 1973). A strong placebo effect was frequently demonstrated. When significant differences have been found, improvements in psychological symptoms could be interpreted as secondary to relief of vasomotor symptoms and/or vaginal atrophy and normalization of sleep patterns (e.g., Aylward, Holly, & Parker, 1974; Bakke, 1965; Judd, 1987). For example, decreases in irritability, fatigue, and sleep disturbances have been shown to be associated with a reduction in the night sweats that occur during the climacteric, allowing the woman to have adequate sleep (Judd, 1987).

In summary, early studies of clinical samples seemed to indicate that an increase in psychological symptoms occurred in the climacteric years but results of HRT studies were somewhat equivocal in determining the nature of the relation between these symptoms and estrogen deficiency. This is not surprising when one considers the previously mentioned problems associated with the use of clinical samples. The obvious approach to circumventing these difficulties is to study non-clinical samples of women undergoing natural menopause. Cross-sectional and longitudinal studies employing non-clinical samples will be described next.

Neugarten and Kraines (1965) conducted a cross-sectional study of 460 women aged 13–54. Women with major illnesses or surgical menopause were excluded. Subjects were divided into five groups on the basis of age and menopausal status, which was determined by self-report. A 28-item checklist composed of somatic (e.g., hot flushes; cold sweats; weight gain), psychosomatic (e.g., headaches; pounding heart; dizzy spells), and psychological (e.g., irritable and nervous; blue and depressed; crying spells) symptoms was administered to subjects. Perimenopausal women reported more somatic and psychosomatic symptoms than women in the other groups, but were not differentiated from the others on the basis of psychological symptoms. This study served as something of a landmark, as it was the first well-designed study to suggest that the perimenopausal years were not associated with a higher incidence of psychological symptoms.

Ballinger (1985) employed a cross-sectional comparative design to examine the relation between psychosocial stress and symptoms (psychologic, hypothalamic, and metabolic) in menopause clinic patients and non-patients. One hundred and twenty-three patients were compared to 164 non-patients. All women were postmenopausal (i.e., between 12 months and 5 years past the date of their last menses). The Hamilton Rating Scale for Depression (Hamilton, 1960) and a life events questionnaire designed for middle-aged women were used to measure depression, anxiety, and life events. A semi-structured interview was used to determine clinical impressions of the vulnerability and coping skills of each subject in the face of stressors in her life. Other symptoms were assessed by open-ended questions and symptom scales. These included hypothalamic (e.g., hot flushes; sweating; palpitations), metabolic (e.g., dry vagina; dyspareunia; dry skin), and psychological (e.g., anxiety, depression, irritability) symptoms. There were no significant differences between groups in the incidence of either hot flushes or vaginal atrophy. However, the patient group reported that their hot flushes were significantly more severe than the non-patient group. Additionally, patients reported significantly more life stress, psychological symptoms, and clinician-rated depression than did the non-patients. It should also be noted that significantly more patients reported experiencing depression during their premenopausal years than did the non-patients.

On the basis of the consistency of her results with the literature on illness behavior (i.e., a relation appears to exist between perceived life stress, psychological symptoms such as depression and anxiety, and help-seeking behavior in the medical setting), Ballinger suggests that a fundamental difference exists between patients presenting to menopause clinics and non-patients with respect to coping style in the face of stressful life events. That is, symptoms of women who present to menopause clinics may be driven more by their individual responses to life stress than by hormonal insufficiency per se.

Hunter, Battersby, and Whitehead (1986) conducted a carefully designed cross-sectional study of 850 pre-, peri-, and postmenopausal women, aged 45–65 years. These subjects were not drawn from a menopause clinic but were recruited from women presenting for routine ovarian screening. The assessment battery included measures of general health, psychosocial factors (SES, employment and marital status), and psychological, somatic, and vasomotor symptoms. Menopausal history was used to divide the subjects into pre-, peri-, and post-menopausal groups. As expected, vasomotor symptoms increased significantly across groups (i.e., *pre < peri < post*), as did sleep difficulties. Vaginal dryness was reported significantly more frequently by the postmenopausal group than the pre- or perimenopausal groups, while sexual interest declined across groups. However, sexual satisfaction showed no significant differences across groups. Depressed mood was significantly higher in the peri- and postmenopausal groups than in the premenopausal group. Importantly, however, psychosocial factors (e.g., SES; employment status) were better predictors of both somatic and psychological symptoms than was menopausal status. These authors concluded that changes in menopausal status are probably not directly related to psychological symptoms occurring during this time and they caution that symptoms should not be attributed too quickly to menopausal status when assessing women in this age range.

McKinlay and McKinlay (1989) conducted a study of 2,300 women who were randomly sampled from a general population and who were premeno-pausal at the start of the survey. The study was designed to identify physical and mental health changes that were clearly related to the physiological changes of the climacteric and those that could be attributed to other psychosocial factors. During a 4.5-year follow-up, 55% of these women experienced menopause. These investigators used extensive telephone interviews that covered current menstrual status, health status, health history, psychosocial factors (e.g., marital and family status, job status, income, persons causing worry [children, parents], social networks, and help-seeking behavior). Each instrument was administered twice, 27 months apart. The most consistent message from this study was that menopause has almost no impact on subsequent perceived physical or mental health. The one exception was surgical menopause. Not surprisingly, women who underwent surgical menopause had both poorer health and higher use of medical services prior to surgery and reported poorer health following surgery. This finding is consistent with a Canadian study (Roos, 1983) which identified a distinct subgroup of women who are at higher risk for surgical menopause. Most women in the McKinlays' study reported positive or neutral feelings about meno-pause, consistent with its failure to produce adverse health outcomes.

Cross-sectional data on the effects of multiple social roles (e.g., wife, daugh-ter, mother) and the stress associated with them indicate that these factors may have a negative effect on the woman's health, particularly if she is not employed outside the home. McKinlay and McKinlay argued that their findings indicated that there may be an identifiable group of women who respond to certain events or circumstances in predictable ways and that increases in symptoms are more closely related to the social circumstances in which these women find them-selves in middle-age rather than to menopause. This finding is consistent with the findings of other studies suggesting that psychological symptom-reporting peaks in adolescence or the premenopausal years and that increases during the climacteric years are more strongly associated with psychosocial factors (Greene & Cooke, 1980; Neugarten & Kraines, 1965).

Finally, Matthews et al. (1990) conducted a longitudinal study of psychological and physical symptom outcomes in a sample of 541 initially premenopausal healthy women. At the three-year follow-up, 69 women had experienced natural menopause at least 12 months previously and were not on hormone replacement therapy. At this time, the postmenopausal group was compared to a group (*n* = 101) who had not yet experienced menopause and a group (*n* = 32) of women who had been on hormone replacement therapy within 2 months of reevaluation. The assessment battery included self-report measures of depression, anxiety, anger, perceived stress, and self-consciousness. Results showed no significant differences in psychological symptoms with the exceptions that postmenopausal women who were not taking hormone replacement therapy had lower private self-consciousness scores than at baseline and the hormone-user group increased significantly in depression level from baseline to follow-up while the other two groups did not. The authors concluded that, with respect to psychological outcomes, natural menopause is a relatively innocuous event for the majority of healthy women and suggest that assessment and treatment of such women should focus more on their individual life situations and risk factors than menopausal status.

In summary, it appears that, with respect to psychological symptoms, natural menopause alone is a fairly benign event for the majority of women. For those women who do experience an increase in psychological symptoms such as depression, anxiety, and irritability, it appears that psychosocial factors such as stressful life events, role demands, inadequate coping skills, and past history of psychiatric disorder may be more important than the experience of menopause, per se.

CLINICAL IMPLICATIONS

Assessment

The importance of thorough assessment of a peri- or postmenopausal woman presenting with complaints of psychological distress cannot be overstated in light of the literature to date. Patients are not the only ones who fall into the trap of seizing the most salient of the possible explanations for their symptoms. Clinicians, too, may misattribute psychological distress in a middle-aged woman to the hormonal changes associated with the climacteric (Hunter, 1988). Failure to assess the total person who has presented, under the assumption that her symptoms are due to "the change of life," may result in an inappropriate choice of treatment.

Assessment should begin with a careful evaluation of current symptoms. This should include both the presenting complaints and those symptoms that might not be mentioned by the woman initially. For example, a woman may present complaining of irritability, fatigue, and sleep disturbance. Upon further questioning the clinician may learn that the woman has been experiencing frequent hot flushes and night sweats that regularly interrupt her sleep. In such a case, it would be reasonable to hypothesize that the psychological symptoms were the result of inadequate sleep caused by vasomotor symptoms. If no vasomotor symptoms are reported even upon further questioning, that possibility is ruled out. Similarly, sexual complaints may (or may not) be a function of dyspareunia resulting from vaginal dryness.

In addition to current symptoms, important areas of assessment include medical and psychiatric history, marital status and satisfaction, sexual functioning, "motherhood" status and satisfaction, health status of parents and in-laws and the role of the patient in their care, employment status and satisfaction, stressful life events not covered by the preceding areas of assessment (e.g., loss events), availability and use of social support, and coping abilities. "Red flags" that may emerge from such an assessment include an extensive history of help-seeking behavior that pre-dates menopause, history of psychiatric disorder, and the presence of major life stressors. In addition to the woman herself, if she is married, it may be important to assess her husband's adjustment to this stage of life and his health (both physical and psychological) as well, because his well-being may impact that of the patient. If possible, an interview with him would be the optimal choice.

Therapy

Estrogen replacement will often improve psychological functioning if the mood symptoms are secondary to symptoms of estrogen deficiency such as hot flushes. However, psychological distress in the peri- or postmenopausal woman is not necessarily driven by her hormonal state. A variety of psychosocial factors may be playing an important role as well. For that reason, a multi-modal approach to treatment that is tailored to the woman's individual needs may be needed if hormone therapy does not significantly improve the symptoms. In addition to estrogen replacement, components of such treatment might include education and reassurance (Whitehead, 1983), behavioral interventions such as relaxation training or "prescribed" physical exercise, cognitive therapy directed at the woman's perceptions of her life circumstances and relationships with others, or even assertiveness training if she is faced with unreasonable demands from her parents, spouse, and children.

The potential for a multi-modal treatment approach with these patients can be seen in a study by Greene and Hart (1987). These investigators conducted an evaluation of a psychological treatment program for climacteric women whose vasomotor symptoms had responded to hormone replacement therapy but who continued to experience symptoms and complaints thought to be psychogenic in origin. At the first appointment, a detailed history of their complaints was obtained, as well as information about personal and family circumstances, ongoing or new sources of stress or worry, and threatening life experiences within the past year. Psychological and somatic symptoms were assessed, as was subjective adaptation. The treatment model assumed that certain women become more vulnerable to the effects of psychosocial stressors during the climacteric years. The treatment program included education, counseling about current problems and concerns, exploration of feelings and attitudes, behavioral techniques such as anxiety management, and cognitive–behavioral therapy for depressive symptoms. Patients were seen at 3–4 week intervals. Results showed a highly significant decrease in the mean severity rating of the main presenting complaint. There was also a significant reduction in other symptoms and subjective adaptation. In subjective overall improvement ratings, 7 subjects said they were "considerably improved", 9 were "much improved", 4 were "slightly to moderately improved", 3 rated "no change", and 1 was "worse". However, there was clear evidence that response depended on the nature of the presenting complaint. Those presenting with anxiety as their main complaint improved most, followed by those with complaints of depression. Those with psychosomatic complaints or loss of libido as their main presenting complaint showed little or no response to treatment.

Evidence to date clearly highlights the importance of viewing each peri- or postmenopausal woman as a complex and unique individual rather than the simple biological product of her hormonal status. This is true for both assessment and the formulation of treatment plans. Thorough physical examination and assessment of psychosocial factors provide the information necessary for offering treatment designed to optimize the outcome for each woman.

REFERENCES

Abraham, G. E., Lobotsky, J., & Lloyd, W. (1969). Metabolism of testosterone and androstenedione in normal and ovariectomized women. *Journal of Clinical Investigation, 48,* 696–703.

Albright, F., Bloomberg, F., & Smith, P. H. (1940). Postmenopausal osteoporosis. *Transactions of the Association of American Physicians, 55,* 298–305.

Aylward, M., Holly, F., & Parker, R. J. (1974). An evaluation of clinical responses to piperazine oestrone sulphate ("Harmogen") in menopausal patients. *Current Medical Research Opinion, 2,* 417–423.

Bakke, J. L. (1965). A double-blind study of a progestin-estrogen combination in the management of the menopause. *Pacific Medicine and Surgery, 73*, 200–205.

Barber, H.R.K. (1988). *Perimenopausal and geriatric gynecology*. New York: Macmillan.

Bengtsson, C., & Lindquist, O. (1978). Coronary heart disease during the menopause. In M. G. Oliver (Ed.), *Coronary heart disease in young women* (pp. 234–239). Edinburgh: Churchill Livingstone.

Colditz, G.A., Willett, W.C., Stampher, M.J., Rosner, B., Speizer, F.E., & Hennekens, C.H. (1987). Menopause and the risk of coronary heart disease in women. *New England Journal of Medicine, 316*, 1105–1110.

Cooke, D. J. (1985). Psychosocial vulnerability to life events during the climacteric. *British Journal of Psychiatry, 147*, 71–75.

Coope, J. (1981). Is oestrogen therapy effective in the treatment of menopausal depression? *Journal of the Royal College of General Practitioners, 31*, 134–140.

Coope, J., Thompson, J. M., & Poller, L. (1975). The effects of natural oestrogen therapy on menopausal symptoms and blood clotting. *British Medical Journal, 4*, 139–143.

Cornoni-Huntley, J., Barbano, H.E., Brody, J.A., Cohen, B., Feldman, J.J., Kleinman, J.C., & Madans, J. (1983). National Health and Nutrition Examination I—Epidemiologic Follow-up Survey. *Public Health Reports, 98*, 245–261.

Dennerstein, L. (1987). Psychologic changes. In D. Mishell (Ed.), *Menopause: Physiology and pharmacology* (pp. 115–126). Chicago: Year Book Medical Publishers.

Dennerstein, L., & Burrows, G. D. (1978). A review of studies of the psychological symptoms found at the menopause. *Maturitas, 1*, 55–64.

George, G.C.W., Beaumont, P.J.V., & Beardwood, C. J. (1973). Effects of exogenous oestrogens on minor psychiatric symptoms in postmenopausal women. *South African Medical Journal, 47*, 2387–2394.

Gordon, T., Kannel, B., & Hjortland, M. (1978). Menopause and coronary disease. The Framingham Study. *Annals of Internal Medicine, 89*, 157–161.

Greene, J. G. (1980). Stress at the climacterium: The assessment of symptomatology. In I. G. Sarason & C. D. Spielberger (Eds.), *Stress and anxiety* (Vol. 7) (pp. 127–138). Washington, DC: Hemisphere.

Greene, J. G., & Cooke, D. J. (1980). Life stress and symptoms at the climacterium. *British Journal of Psychiatry, 136*, 486–491.

Greene, J. G., & Hart, D. M. (1987). Evaluation of a psychological treatment programme for climacteric women. *Maturitas, 9*, 41–48.

Hamilton, M. (1960). A rating scale for depression. *Journal of Neurology, Neurosurgery, and Psychiatry, 23*, 56–62.

Horsman, A., Gallagher, J. C., Simpson, M., & Nordin, B.E.C. (1977). Prospective trial of oestrogen and calcium in postmenopausal women. *British Medical Journal, 2*, 789–792.

Hunter, M. S. (1988). Psychological aspects of the climacteric and postmenopause. In J. W. W. Studd & M. I. Whitehead (Eds.), *The menopause* (pp. 55–64). Oxford: Blackwell Scientific Publications.

Hunter, M., Battersby, R., & Whitehead, M. (1986). Relationships between psychological symptoms, somatic complaints, and menopausal status. *Maturitas, 8*, 217–228.

Hutchinson, T. A., Polansky, S. M., & Feinstein, A. R. (1979). Post-menopausal oestrogens protect against fractures of hip and distal radius: A case-control study. *Lancet, 2*, 705–709.

Ilfeld, F. W. (1977). Current social stressors and symptoms of depression. *American Journal of Psychiatry, 134*, 161–166.

Judd, H. L. (1987). Oestrogen replacementtherapy: Physiological considerations and new applications. *Baillieres Clinical Endocrinology and Metabolism, 1*, 177–206.

Kletzky, O. A., & Borenstein, R. (1987). Vasomotor instability of the menopause. In D. Mishell (Ed.), *Menopause: Physiology and pharmacology* (pp 53–66). Chicago: Year Book Medical Publishers.

Korenman, S. G., Sherman, B. M., & Korenman, J. C. (1978). Reproductive hormone function: The perimenopausal period and beyond. *Clinics in Endocrinology and Metabolism, 7*, 625–643.

Lang, W. R., & Aponte, G. F. (1967). Gross and microscopic anatomy of the aged female reproductive organs. *Clinics in Obstetrics and Gynecology, 10*, 454–465.

Lindsay, R. (1989). Postmenopausal osteoporosis. In C. B. Hammond, F. P. Haseltine, & I. Schiff (Eds.), *Menopause: Evaluation, treatment, and health concerns* (pp. 253–262). New York: Alan R. Liss.

Lindsay, R., Aitken, J. M., Anderson, J. B., Hart, D. M., MacDonald, E. B., & Clarke, A. C. (1980). Long-term prevention of postmenopausal osteoporosis by oestrogen. *Lancet, 2*, 1038–1041.

Matthews, K. A., Wing, R. R., Kuller, L. H., Meilahn, E. N., Kelsey, S. F., Costello, E. J., & Caggiula, A. W. (1990). Influences of natural menopause on psychological characteristics and symptoms of middle-aged healthy women. *Journal of Consulting and Clinical Psychology, 58*, 345–351.

McKinlay, S. M., & McKinlay, J. B. (1989). The impact of menopause and social factors on health. In C. B. Hammond, F. P. Haseltine, & I. Schiff (Eds.), *Menopause: Evaluation, treatment, and health concerns* (pp. 137–162). New York: Alan R. Liss.

Neugarten, B. L., & Kraines, R. J. (1965). Menopausal symptoms in women of various ages. *Psychosomatic Medicine, 27*, 266–273.

Perlman, J., Wolf, P., Finucane, F., & Madans, J. (1989). Menopause and the epidemiology of cardiovascular disease in women. In C. B. Hammond, F. P. Haseltine, & I. Schiff (Eds.), *Menopause: Evaluation, treatment, and health concerns* (pp. 283–312). New York: Alan R. Liss.

Perlmutter, J. (1977). Temporary symptoms and permanent changes. In L. Rose (Ed.), *The menopause book* (pp. 18–34). New York: Hawthorn Books.

Petitti, D., Perlman, J., & Sydney, S. (1987). Non-contraceptive estrogens and mortality: A long-term followup of women in the Walnut Creek Study. *Obstetrics and Gynecology, 70*, 289–293.

Utian, W. H. (1987). The fate of the untreated menopause. *Obstetrics and Gynecology Clinics of North America, 14*, 1–11.

Walsh, B., & Schiff, I (1989). Vasomotor flushes. In C. B. Hammond, F. P. Haseltine, & I. Schiff (Eds.), *Menopause: Evaluation, treatment, and health concerns* (pp. 71–88). New York: Alan R. Liss.

Whitehead, M. I. (1983). The menopause: Part A: Hormone "replacement" therapy—the controversies. In L. Dennerstein & G. Burrows (Eds.), *Handbook of psychosomatic obstetrics and gynaecology* (pp. 445–481). Amsterdam: Elsevier.

World Health Organization (1981). Research on the menopause. W. H. O. Tech. Rep. Ser. No. 670. Geneva: Author.

PART II
Gynecology

4

Chronic Pelvic Pain

Mary K. Walling and Robert C. Reiter

Chronic pelvic pain, defined as noncyclic pelvic pain of greater than 6 months duration, is a major health concern in women of childbearing age. In spite of an impressive array of proposed somatic contributors to chronic pelvic pain (Reiter, 1990a; Stenchever, 1990), no significant pathology can be found in many women seeking relief from chronic pelvic pain. For many others, pain remains or recurs following treatment of presumed somatic "causes." Further, many women who present with the symptom of chronic pelvic pain are also experiencing psychological distress (e.g., depression, anxiety) and behavioral changes typically associated with the chronic pain syndrome seen in many chronic pain populations (Merskey, 1978). Taken together, evidence to date strongly suggests that, in addition to biological factors, psychological and environmental factors contribute significantly to the etiology and maintenance of chronic pelvic pain and must be taken into consideration in assessment and case management.

The importance of achieving a clearer understanding of the phenomenon of chronic pelvic pain and its treatment can be seen in an examination of its costs, both fiscal and personal. This enigmatic symptom accounts for up to 10% of all gynecology outpatient visits and is the indication for up to 25% of laparoscopies performed annually in the U.S. (Reiter, Shakerin, Gambone, & Milburn, 1991). Of even greater consequence, it is the third leading indication for hysterectomy in the U.S., accounting for approximately 80,000 hysterectomies annually (Reiter & Gambone, 1990a). While total direct and indirect costs in the United States have been estimated to exceed one billion dollars (Reiter, 1990b), the personal costs to women with chronic pelvic pain in terms of unrelieved suffering and its associated consequences cannot be measured.

This chapter will examine the phenomenon of chronic pelvic pain from a multidimensional perspective. First, the distinction between acute and chronic pain will be discussed. This will be followed by a brief summary of several theories of chronic pain. Next, the literature concerning psychosocial aspects of chronic pelvic pain will be reviewed. Finally, a multidisciplinary approach to the assessment and treatment of chronic pelvic pain will be presented.

ACUTE VERSUS CHRONIC PAIN

An appreciation of the distinction between acute and chronic pain is crucial to an understanding of the phenomenon of chronic pain. Acute pain is usually associated with tissue damage (actual or impending) or disease. It is fairly abrupt in onset, of relatively short duration, and there is generally (but not always) a strong correlation between the site and extent of injury and the location and intensity of pain experienced (France, Krishnan, & Houpt, 1988). Acute pain serves as a signal that something is wrong and is accompanied by the physiological and neuroendocrine responses of sympathetic arousal and the psychological experience of acute anxiety (Bonica, 1985). These responses prompt the individual to engage in behaviors (e.g., rest the injured body part; self-treat with analgesics; seek medical care) that will correct the cause of pain, eliminate the symptom of pain, or both. Patients with acute pain usually obtain relief with the use of appropriate analgesics (Crue, 1988). When resulting from injury or disease, acute pain and its associated responses usually diminish and finally disappear as healing occurs. Although psychological factors influence the experience of acute pain, these factors are rarely implicated in the etiology of the pain (Bonica, 1985). In general, the traditional medical model (i.e., an underlying biological substrate is "causing" the disorder) fits the phenomenon of acute pain fairly well.

In its broadest definition, chronic pain is typically defined as pain that has occurred without substantial relief for a period of at least 6 months. It may be caused by chronic disease processes (e.g., rheumatoid arthritis; cancer) or dysfunction of the peripheral or central nervous system (e.g., trigeminal neuralgia; causalgia). Chronic pain may also occur in the absence of an identifiable somatic cause or it may evolve when acute pain due to illness or injury persists beyond an expected healing time. While acute pain serves as a warning that something is physically wrong, pain in its chronic, persistent form rarely has such a function. In contrast to acute pain patients, chronic pain patients seldom display autonomic hyperactivity and acute anxiety. Rather, they often suffer from neurovegetative symptoms frequently associated with depression (France, Krishnan, & Houpt, 1988).

Another difference between acute and chronic pain is seen in response to pharmacotherapy. Analgesics and narcotic agents are effective for only a short time, at best, in providing relief from chronic pain (Crue, 1988). Also, while the expected duration of acute pain is predictable once the underlying cause is determined, the time course of chronic pain remains unknown since physical examination and diagnostic tests rarely yield satisfactory explanations for the pain. For these reasons, chronic pain is not well explained by the medical model. More complex models are required to explain this perplexing and frequently frustrating phenomenon.

THEORIES OF PAIN PERCEPTION

Several models which suggest mechanisms involved in the evolution of a chronic pain syndrome have been proposed. As has already been mentioned, the *traditional* medical model, based on the Cartesian notion of pain perception, proposes a direct relationship between tissue damage or other stimulation of nociceptors and pain. Traditionally, this has led to an "either–or" attitude with respect to chronic pain—chronic pain is either physical (i.e., "real") or it is psychological (i.e., "not real"). In spite of the fact that this model is of little value in explaining chronic pain, it is the model that has most influenced the diagnosis and treatment of chronic pain until the fairly recent past and continues to exert a powerful influence in both medical and popular thinking about chronic pain.

The *gate control* theory of pain perception (Melzack & Wall, 1965) acknowledges the importance of both peripheral and central influences on the experience of pain. Pain is postulated to be the result of an interaction of sensory, cognitive–evaluative, and emotional–affective factors. This model proposes that stimulation of nociceptors is not the starting point of the pain experience. Rather, the sensory input of nociceptors enters an active nervous system that is already busily processing sensory input from both internal and external sources. Additionally, the nervous system bears the influence of past experience, culture, and a variety of other psychosocial factors. In sum, the experience of pain is not a linear function of the sensory transmission system but is a dynamic process consisting of continuous interactions among both ascending and descending systems (Dennis & Melzack, 1977). Although some of the physiological bases of the original theory have since been challenged (Nathan, 1976), its multidimensional view of pain continues to have a major influence on chronic pain research and treatment.

A third model, the model of *operant conditioning* (Fordyce, 1976), proposes that, since pain is not directly observable, all that can be known about it is based on pain behaviors, either verbal (e.g., self-reports of pain) or nonverbal (e.g., grimacing; lying down). These behaviors are capable of producing desired outcomes (e.g., attention from significant others; relief from household chores) and are thus subject to the laws of operant conditioning. As a consequence, pain behaviors may be maintained by the reinforcing properties of these outcomes. Fordyce proposes that pain behaviors, rather than the subjective experience of pain, should be the targets of treatment. The operant conditioning perspective departs from the traditional medical model by asserting that tissue damage is neither a necessary nor sufficient condition for pain, or at least pain behaviors. In a more recent version of his model, Fordyce (1989) adopts a more cognitive–behavioral perspective, but the focus is still on the effects of learning and conditioning and he asserts that chronic pain is best conceptualized as "something people *do*, not something they *have*" (p. 63).

More recently, the biopsychosocial model of chronic pain has been proposed by Turk (1986). This model is an extended version of the cognitive–behavioral transaction model proposed by Turk, Meichenbaum, and Genest (1983). This model proposes that the gate control model and the operant conditioning model are complementary rather than mutually exclusive and emphasizes the importance of cognitive, affective, sensory, and behavioral factors in the experience of pain. According to this model, it is the patient's interpretation of her situation that reciprocally interacts with emotional responses, sensory input, and pain behaviors. The biopsychosocial model proposes that chronic pain results from the synergistic relationship found among the components of sensory stimulation, psychological factors (i.e., cognitive, affective, and behavioral), and socioenvironmental factors, with each component capable of influencing each of the other components and being influenced by them in return (Turk & Rudy, 1987).

A MULTIDIMENSIONAL MODEL OF CHRONIC PELVIC PAIN

Steege, Stout, and Somkuti (1991) have proposed an integrative model of chronic pelvic pain that parallels the biopsychosocial model of chronic pain. The integrative model proposes that the interaction of psychological and neurological mechanisms may explain the evolution of chronic pelvic pain, regardless of the degree of tissue damage present or the functional disorder that might have provided the initial nociceptive stimulation. This theory takes into consideration the interaction of 1) biological events which initiate nociception, 2) the alteration of life-styles and relationships with time, and 3) anxiety and affective disorders.

These three components interact in a circular fashion resulting in a vicious cycle. Sexually transmitted diseases, endometriosis, recurrent bladder and/or vaginal infections, alterations of bowel motility, and abdominal wall pain are examples of physiological factors that may contribute individually, or in combination, to providing a chronic sensory stimulus. Initially this may result in alteration of physical activity, with rest providing relief of acute pain. Interaction with family members is altered because the individual is perceived as being "sick." In time, interaction and communication with the patient is focused on her pain. Depression, which is observed in a significant number of chronic pelvic pain patients (Magni, Salmi, de Leo, & Ceola, 1984; Walker et al., 1988), may occur as a cumulative result of disability, altered attentional focus, and feelings of despair that she will ever return to "normal."

The integrative model of chronic pelvic pain also proposes that pre-existing factors may predispose an individual to become caught in the "vicious cycle" that results in the syndrome of chronic pelvic pain. These include being reared in a severely dysfunctional home environment and a genetic predisposition to depression. This may, in part, explain the observation that individuals with a family history of depression appear to benefit more from treatment of chronic pain with tricyclic antidepressants than patients with no family history of depression (Steege et al., 1991).

With respect to treatment, this model postulates that the longer the chronic pelvic pain has been a part of a woman's life, the less effective treatment of tissue pathology or "organicity" alone will be in relieving her pain and restoring her physical and emotional well-being.

On the basis of the preceding discussion, it is clear that the theoretical model of chronic pain adopted carries important implications for the diagnosis and management of chronic pelvic pain. For example, in this population it is essential that the traditional medical model of assignment of cause and effect be identified and changed in both patients and health care providers. This model encourages continued inappropriate health care utilization and diverts efforts away from investigating underlying psychosocial variables, symptom management, and recovery in all areas of dysfunction (i.e., physical, affective, behavioral). Furthermore, the correlation between medical diagnoses—such as endometriosis, adhesions, uterine fibroids, and ovarian cysts—and the presence or severity of symptoms is notoriously poor (Rapkin, 1986; Walker et al., 1988), with many of the patients with these findings reporting no symptoms whatsoever (Reiter & Gambone, 1990b). For these reasons, assignment of somatic causality of symptoms in the majority of women presenting with chronic pelvic pain is of little practical value, except to the extent that the stimulus is amenable to a specific therapeutic intervention. Further, the absence of identifiable medical pathology does not obviate the need for treatment, nor does it substantially change the general format of diagnosis and treatment.

PSYCHOSOCIAL FACTORS IN CHRONIC PELVIC PAIN

Available data regarding psychological characteristics of women with chronic pelvic pain will be reviewed in three parts. First, reports without comparison data will be summarized. This will be followed by a more extensive review of studies that included comparison groups and a summary of these study results. Finally, a discussion of methodological shortcomings of the literature to date will be presented.

A number of published reports of psychological characteristics of chronic pelvic pain patients have failed to provide comparison data. However, several characteristics and patterns of behavior have been described with regularity in these reports. Depression, somatization, and hypochondriacal concerns are frequent findings (Benson, Hanson, & Matarazzo, 1959; Duncan & Taylor, 1952; Locke & Donnelly, 1947; Wood, Wiesner, & Reiter, 1990), as are traumatic childhoods and stressful interpersonal relationships (Benson et al., 1959; Duncan & Taylor, 1952; Gross et al., 1980/1981).

Although the data obtained in the studies summarized above are useful for identifying areas for further study, their failure to provide comparison data precludes drawing inferences about psychosocial factors that may be important in the etiology and maintenance of chronic pelvic pain or important ways in which women with chronic pelvic pain differ from other groups of women. Following is a selective review of studies that have included a comparison group of women.

Gidro-Frank, Gordon, and Taylor (1960) studied 40 patients referred from a gynecological pain clinic and a comparison group of 25 pregnant women. Results of semistructured psychiatric interviews indicated that women in the pelvic pain group were more likely to report traumatic childhoods, unhappy marriages, and more nongynecologic symptoms than the pregnant subjects.

Beard, Belsey, Lieberman, and Wilkinson (1977) studied 35 women with chronic pelvic pain who were divided into a negative laparoscopy group ($N = 18$) and a positive laparoscopy group ($N = 17$). A comparison group of women with no gynecologic complaint was included ($N = 9$). Measures of interest included the Eysenck Personality Inventory (EPI; Eysenck & Eysenck, 1964). Neuroticism scores on the EPI were significantly higher for the negative laparoscopy group than for the pain-free women. No significant differences were found for the subjects' ratings of their relationships with their families. Significantly fewer women in both pain groups reported experiencing orgasm during sexual intercourse than women in the pain-free group.

Renaer, Vertommen, Nijs, Wagemans, and Van Hemelrijck (1979) compared chronic pelvic pain patients with negative laparoscopy ($N = 15$) to those with positive laparoscopy ($N = 22$) and pain-free gynecology patients ($N = 23$). The Dutch version of the MMPI was administered to all groups. Mean scores for both pain groups were significantly elevated on the hypochondriasis, depression, hysteria, psychasthenia, social inversion, and anxiety scales, and were lower than the controls on the ego strength scale.

Magni, Salmi, de Leo, and Ceola (1984) conducted a study of 29 women with chronic pelvic pain, 18 with positive laparoscopy (Group A) and 11 with negative laparoscopy (Group B). A comparison group of 11 women with chronic perianal pain (Group C) was included. The Zung Self-Rating Depression Scale (SDS; Zung, 1965) was completed by all groups and semistructured interviews were conducted with women in Groups A and B. Scores on the SDS were significantly higher for Groups B and C than for Group A, with no significant difference between Groups B and C. Women in Group B endorsed significantly more physical symptoms in addition to pain than women in Group A. Further, significantly more women in Group B reported a history of depressive disorder as well as depression spectrum disorders in first-degree relatives. Five women in Group B and none in Group A met DSM–III criteria for major depression.

Walker et al. (1988) conducted structured psychiatric and sexual abuse interviews with 25 women undergoing laparoscopy for chronic pelvic pain and 30 pain-free women undergoing laparoscopy for bilateral tubal ligation or evaluation of infertility problems. No significant group differences were found at laparoscopy with respect to type or severity of pathology. The women in the chronic pelvic pain group endorsed significantly more somatic symptoms than the pain-free group and had a significantly higher prevalence of both lifetime and current major depressive disorder, history of drug abuse or dependence, functional dyspareunia, inhibited orgasm, and inhibited sexual desire. Women in the pelvic pain group also had significantly higher prevalences of both childhood and adulthood sexual abuse. When sexual abuse was categorized as mild or severe, all of the women who reported severe sexual abuse as children ($n = 4$) had chronic pelvic pain.

Reiter (1990c) reported on a study of demographic, medical, and psychosexual variables in 106 women referred to a chronic pelvic pain clinic and 92 consecutive age-matched women presenting for routine gynecologic examination. Women in the chronic pelvic pain group reported significantly more symptoms for which they had sought treatment or self-medicated, reported taking significantly more prescription medications, and had undergone significantly more nongynecologic surgical procedures than the controls. Significantly more women in the chronic pelvic pain group reported a history of sexual abuse.

Rapkin, Kames, Darke, Stampler, and Naliboff (1990) studied the sexual and physical abuse histories of 31 women with chronic pelvic pain, 142 women with "other" chronic pain complaints, and 32 pain-free women presenting for routine gynecologic care. The chronic pelvic pain group was further differentiated in those with and without somatic pathology. Results of standardized interviews revealed no significant differences in either childhood or adulthood sexual abuse.

However, no attempt was made to differentiate between abuse involving direct contact with the genitals, and other forms of sexual abuse and isolated instances of adulthood sexual assault (including rape) were not included. The chronic pelvic pain group was found to have significantly higher prevalences of childhood physical abuse as well as any (i.e., sexual or physical) childhood abuse than the other two groups. They also had a higher lifetime prevalence of physical abuse and any abuse than the pain-free group but not the "other" pain group.

Finally, Walker, Katon, Neraas, Jemelka, and Massoth (1992) conducted a study of 43 women who attended a women's health clinic, 22 who reported a prior history of chronic pelvic pain and 21 of whom did not. Structured sexual abuse interviews and various self-report measures of psychological functioning were employed. Results revealed that women with a history of chronic pelvic pain were significantly more likely to amplify physical symptoms, see themselves as medically disabled, report psychological distress and impaired vocational and social functioning, use dissociation as a coping mechanism, and report childhood sexual abuse.

In summary, a number of characteristics of women with chronic pelvic pain have emerged from this literature. Depression, somatization, anxiety, and hypochondriacal concerns are frequent findings. When structured psychiatric interviews have been conducted, depressive disorders and sexual dysfunction are frequently diagnosed. Additionally, it appears that a significant number of women with chronic pelvic pain have been both sexually and physically abused.

Many inferences have been drawn about the etiology and maintenance of chronic pelvic pain on the basis of the literature to date, particularly concerning the specific role that childhood sexual abuse may play (e.g., Walker et al., 1988). However, studies to date have been plagued with methodological shortcomings. Among these have been small sample sizes, the failure to include appropriate comparison groups, and the failure to include an assessment of physical abuse as well as sexual abuse.

With respect to the inclusion of appropriate comparison groups, in many studies, women determined to have pelvic pathology sufficient to account for their pain have been used as a comparison group for those found not to have sufficient pathology. This is a carryover effect from the traditional medical model's assertion that pain must be either somatic or psychogenic. Evidence to date, however, suggests that the role of pelvic pathology in the experience of chronic pelvic pain is uncertain, at best, since women who are pain-free have been found to have equivalent "amounts" of pathology at laparoscopy as those who have pain (Rapkin, 1986; Walker et al., 1988). Furthermore, when the determination of "sufficiency" is made by individuals who are not blind to the specifics of each case (e.g., medical history; psychological distress; history of abuse), this knowledge may lead to selection bias. For example, a woman with minimal pathology but a very dramatic description of her pain, evidence of depressive symptomatology, and a history of sexual abuse might be assigned to the "nonsomatic" group while a woman with equally minimal pathology but who describes her pain calmly and has no evidence of depression or history of sexual abuse might be assigned to the "somatic" group. This leads to a circularity of reasoning when variables influencing group assignment (e.g., depression; sexual abuse) are also used as outcome variables.

The failure to include specific assessment of both childhood and adulthood sexual abuse precludes inferences about the specificity of the relation between childhood sexual abuse and chronic pelvic pain, or the nature of the association between childhood sexual abuse and psychological morbidity. Results of a study by Walling (1992) indicate that, while a specific relation appears to exist between major sexual abuse (i.e., that involving penetration or other direct contact with the genitals) and chronic pelvic pain, women with chronic pelvic pain also had a higher prevalence of physical abuse than pain-free women, but not women with chronic headache. Further, significantly more women in the chronic pelvic pain group had experienced both major sexual abuse and physical abuse at some time in their lives than women in either of the pain-free or chronic headache groups. This was also true for experiencing physical abuse in both childhood and adulthood. When the association between the various categories of abuse (childhood sexual abuse, childhood physical abuse, adulthood sexual abuse, adulthood physical abuse) and the outcome variables of somatization, depression, and anxiety were examined, the correlations between childhood physical abuse and both depression and anxiety were significant, while those for childhood sexual abuse were not. On the basis of these results, it appears that inferences concerning the singularly pathogenic nature of childhood sexual abuse in women with chronic pelvic pain have been premature. More research is clearly needed.

MULTIDISCIPLINARY APPROACH TO CHRONIC PELVIC PAIN

The inadequacy of the traditional medical model for guiding treatment of chronic pelvic pain is seen in the reliance on hysterectomy as a standard treatment modality. The long-term efficacy of hysterectomy performed for chronic pelvic pain is unknown. In spite of its frequent utilization, there are no data to support the effectiveness of hysterectomy as a treatment for chronic pelvic pain. In fact, in a large collaborative review from the United States, histologic diagnoses were discovered in fewer than half (41%) of hysterectomy specimens removed from women with chronic pelvic pain (Lee, Dicker, Rubin, & Ovy, 1984). Between 14% and 25% of women referred to pelvic pain clinics have already undergone hysterectomy and bilateral salpingo-oophorectomy without significant improvement in symptoms or disability. A significant proportion of women who have undergone hysterectomy for chronic pelvic pain will report temporary improvement in symptoms lasting from 2–6 months. This probably represents a transient placebo or denervation response (Slocumb, 1990a). Reevaluation of these patients at 6 months to one year after surgery frequently reveals a recurrence of symptoms (Slocumb, 1990a).

In one of the few follow-up reports to date, Stovall, Ling, and Crawford (1990) studied 99 premenopausal women who had undergone hysterectomy for chronic pelvic pain. All subjects had symptoms and physical examination findings suggestive of uterine disease prior to surgery. Diagnostic laparoscopy had been performed in only 12 of the women. In spite of presurgical assumptions, no histologic pathology was found in 66% of these women. Follow-up pain status was determined by outpatient chart review. Twenty-two (22.2%) of the women reported persistent pelvic pain at follow-up (range 15–64 months). With respect to physical findings, there were no significant differences between women who reported relief of pain and those who did not with respect to preoperative, intraoperative, or histologic findings. The authors note that, due to their reliance on chart review for follow-up data, new symptoms or pain that may have been interpreted as other than gynecologic by the patient could not be ruled out. If this were the case for some of the women whose charts indicated relief of pelvic pain, the actual "success" rate of hysterectomy would be even lower.

On the basis of evidence to date, the need for nonsurgical alternatives for treatment of chronic pelvic pain is clear. Physicians, motivated to alleviate the patient's symptoms, tend to resort to surgical procedures before considering nonmedical diagnoses or seeking alternative therapies. Availability of a multidisciplinary pain clinic facilitates the process of denying or deferring hysterectomy (or other unwarranted medical or surgical intervention) by the primary physician (Reiter, Gambone, & Johnson, 1991; Gambone & Reiter, 1990) and provides the opportunity to tailor therapy to the unique needs of each patient.

There have been relatively few articles within the past decade describing the multidisciplinary evaluation and treatment of women with chronic pelvic pain. Multidisciplinary evaluation and management involves a team composed of the referring physician, gynecologist, psychologist, nurse-specialist and, when indicated, specialists in the areas of urology, gastroenterology, and anesthesiology.

ASSESSMENT

Savitz (1985) has suggested that the physician presented with a chronic pelvic pain patient has a "great advantage" in attempts to establish the presence of a somatic etiology for the pain. This advantage is supposedly provided by the availability of direct access to the structures in question through speculum ex-amination, palpation, culdoscopy, and laparoscopy. The fallacy of this notion should be obvious by now; not only is the correlation between pelvic pathology and chronic pelvic pain notoriously poor (Lee et al., 1984; Rapkin, 1986; Walker et al., 1988), but there are also numerous nongynecologic sources of pain that may be perceived as arising from the pelvis (Reiter & Gambone, 1990b; Slocumb, 1990b). In keeping with a multidisciplinary conceptualization of chronic pelvic pain, evaluation of possible symptom sources includes a thorough medical evalu-ation aimed at both gynecologic and nongynecologic conditions (Gambone & Reiter, 1990; Peters et al., 1991).

The use of laparoscopy in the evaluation of chronic pelvic pain has been an area of controversy, with some researchers recommending universal use of this diagnostic tool (Roseff & Murphy, 1990) and others concluding that laparoscopy plays no significant role in the diagnosis and treatment of pelvic pain (Peters et al., 1991). The truth probably lies somewhere between these two extremes. Although laparoscopy is a relatively safe procedure, it is not without risks. Possible complications include mechanical trauma, electrical or thermal damage, bleeding, and injury to adjacent pelvic structures (Roseff & Murphy, 1990). The frequently poor correlation between laparoscopic findings and the presence or severity of symptoms has already been discussed (see p. 71). Although the risks associated with laparoscopy and questions about the association between laparoscopically visualized pathology and chronic pelvic pain in group studies challenge its use as a routine component of a chronic pelvic pain diagnostic work-up, it may still be helpful in selected cases.

Psychosocial assessment of the chronic pelvic pain patient should routinely include assessment of symptoms of depression and anxiety, the perceived im-pact of the patient's pain on her daily functioning and relationships, her beliefs about her pain (e.g., Is she afraid she might have cancer?; What makes her pain better or worse?; etc.), current life stresses in addition to pain (e.g., marital discord; illness of a family member; financial difficulties; etc.), and history of both sexual and physical abuse. Since many chronic pain patients fear being told (or have already been told) "Your pain is all in your head," it is important to explain that the psychosocial assessment is a standard part of the evaluation. If necessary, it may be pointed out that the health care team recognizes that the patient is much more than a medical diagnosis and that psychological and social factors are also important in determining her overall health. Depending on the constraints of time and available staff, some of the psychosocial assessment (e.g., symptoms of depression and anxiety, stressful life events) can be accomplished with self-report measures. However, interviews are preferable for sensitive issues such as abuse history (see Wyatt & Peters, 1986, for a discussion). Also, diag-nostic interviews are necessary for women in whom psychopathology (e.g., de-pressive disorders, substance abuse, sexual dysfunction) is suspected.

TREATMENT

The importance of a thorough evaluation of the patient with chronic pelvic pain cannot be overstated. It is only after both physical and psychosocial factors have been carefully evaluated that an appropriate treatment plan can be formulated. The management of somatic symptoms is usually straightforward, but long-term improvement from disability requires treatment of psychological and behavioral symptoms as well.

Reiter, Gambone, and Johnson (1991) evaluated the impact of the availability of a multidisciplinary chronic pelvic pain clinic on utilization of hysterectomy for chronic pelvic pain. A 3-year retrospective audit of hysterectomy indications at their institution revealed that a relatively high proportion (16.3%) of hysterectomies were performed for chronic pelvic pain. Following the establishment of a pelvic pain clinic, the rate of hysterectomy for chronic pelvic pain decreased to 5.8%. This reduction was sustained for the entire four-year study interval. It was observed that almost all patients reported subjective improvement of symptoms during and shortly after completion of multidisciplinary therapy. However, a high rate of recurrence of pain (43%) was observed within 6 months. Despite this finding, few of the patients subsequently requested surgery, and most were involved in ongoing psychotherapy.

The Stanford approach uses psychotherapy and biofeedback training in the treatment of chronic pelvic pain. The goal of reducing the pain symptoms is obtained through behavior modification, pain-control training, self-hypnosis, marital therapy, sex therapy, and other psychotherapeutic treatment modalities (Wood et al., 1990). The multidisciplinary approach may also incorporate the concurrent use of antidepressant and neuroleptic medications, operant conditioning programs, and brief or supportive psychotherapy.

Peters et al. (1991) demonstrated the effectiveness of this approach in a randomized prospective trial comparing multidisciplinary to standard medical therapy. In this study, 106 women with chronic pelvic pain were randomly assigned to one of two treatment groups. The first group was treated with a standard medical approach in which organic causes of pain were first excluded and diagnostic laparoscopy was routinely performed. If no somatic cause was found, patients were then referred for pain-control therapy. In the second group, an integrated approach was utilized in which equal attention was devoted to somatic, psychologic, dietary, environmental, and physiologic factors. Laparoscopy was not routinely performed in this group. Evaluation performed one year after the beginning of treatment revealed that patients who were treated with the integrated approach had significantly less pain, disability, and global somatic symptomatology than patients managed by the standard medical approach.

SUMMARY

In spite of the fact that chronic pelvic pain is not well explained by the medical model, many health care professionals continue to adopt this simplistic approach to these patients. If no somatic findings emerge to explain the pain, a psychogenic label is automatically attached to the patient, often with no psychological evidence. Grzesiak and Perrin (1987) have noted four unfortunate consequences of this type of diagnostic labeling. First, failure to obtain affirmative psychological data before diagnosing pain as psychogenic in origin is poor scientific and clinical practice. Second, when applied in this fashion, the psychogenic label is merely descriptive and serves no function in planning treatment for the patient. Third, arbitrarily labeling the patient's pain problem as "psychogenic" frequently alienates the patient and may set off another round of doctor-shopping rather than leading the patient to accept appropriate treatment. Finally, in spite of the existence of the unquestionably "real" nature of other disorders with a psychogenic component (e.g., peptic ulcer; colitis), many professionals continue to believe that "psychogenic" is synonymous with "imaginary" or "unreal" when applied to the experience of chronic pain. The inaccuracy of this belief is addressed by Turner and Romano (1989), who point out that most chronic pain syndromes are highly complex combinations of both somatic and psychological factors and, as such, cannot be divided neatly into mutually exclusive categories of "somatic" and "psychogenic." The more relevant and important tasks are to determine whether psychological processes are playing a role in the development and maintenance of the patient's pain and to plan treatment accordingly.

REFERENCES

Beard R. W., Belsey, E. M., Lieberman, B. A., & Wilkinson, J.C.M. (1977). Pelvic pain in women. *American Journal of Obstetrics and Gynecology, 128*, 566–570.

Benson, R. C., Hanson, K. H., & Matarazzo, J. D. (1959). Atypical pelvic pain in women: Gynecologic–psychiatric considerations. *American Journal of Obstetrics and Gynecology, 77*, 806–825.

Bonica, J. J. (1985). Importance of the problem. In G. M. Aronoff (Ed.), *Evaluation and treatment of chronic pain*. Baltimore: Urban & Schwartzberg.

Crue, B. L., Jr. (1988). Historical perspectives. In J. N. Ghia (Ed.), *The multidisciplinary pain center: Organization and personnel functions for pain management*. Boston: Kluwer Academic.

Dennis, S. G., & Melzack, R. (1977). Pain-signalling systems in the dorsal and ventral spinal cord. *Pain, 4*, 97–132.

Duncan, C. H., & Taylor, H. C., Jr. (1952). A psychosomatic study of pelvic congestion. *American Journal of Obstetrics and Gynecology, 64*, 1–12.

Eysenck, H. J., & Eysenck, S.B.G. (1964). *Manual of the Eysenck Personality Inventory*. London: University of London Press.

Fordyce, W. E. (1976). *Behavioral methods for chronic pain and illness*. St. Louis, MO: Mosby.

Fordyce, W. E. (1989). The cognitive/behavioral perspective on clinical pain. In J. D. Loeser, & K. J. Egan (Eds.), *Managing the chronic pain patient*. New York: Raven Press.

France, R. D., Krishnan, K.R.R., & Houpt, J. L. (1988). Overview. In R. D. France, & K.R.R. Krishnan (Eds.), *Chronic pain*. Washington, DC: American Psychiatric Press.

Gambone, J. C., & Reiter, R. C. (1990). Nonsurgical management of chronic pelvic pain: A multidisciplinary approach. *Clinical Obstetrics and Gynecology, 33*, 205–212.

Gidro-Frank, L., Gordon, T., & Taylor, H. C., Jr. (1960). Pelvic pain and female identity: A survey of emotional factors in 40 patients. *American Journal of Obstetrics and Gynecology, 79*, 1184–1202.

Gross, R. J., Doerr, H., Caldirola, D., Guzinski, G. M., & Ripley, H. S. (1980/1981). Borderline syndrome and incest in chronic pelvic pain patients. *International Journal of Psychiatry in Medicine, 10,* 79–96.

Grzesiak, R. C., & Perrin, K. R. (1987). Psychological aspects of chronic pain. In W. Wu, & L. G. Smith (Eds.), *Pain management: Assessment and treatment of chronic and acute syndromes*. New York: Human Sciences Press.

Lee, N. V., Dicker, R. C., Rubin, G. L., & Ovy, H. W. (1984). Confirmation of the preoperative diagnoses for hysterectomy. *American Journal of Obstetrics and Gynecology, 150*, 283.

Locke, F. R., & Donnelly, J. F. (1947). The incidence of psychosomatic disease from a private referred gynecologic practice. *American Journal of Obstetrics and Gynecology, 54*, 783–790.

Magni, G., Salmi, A., de Leo, D., & Ceola, A. (1984). Chronic pelvic pain and depression. *Psychopathology, 17*, 132–136.

Nathan, P. W. (1976). The gate-control theory of pain: A critical review. *Brain, 99*, 123–158.

Melzack, R., & Wall, P. D. (1965). Pain mechanisms: A new theory. *Science, 150*, 971–979.

Merskey, H. (1978). The patient with chronic pain. *Practitioner, 220*, 237–242.

Peters, A. A., van Dorst, E., Jellis, B., van Zuuren, E., Hermans, & Timbos, J. B. (1991). Randomized clinical trial to compare two different approaches in women with chronic pelvic pain. *Obstetrics and Gynecology, 77*, 740–744.

Rapkin, A. J. (1986). Adhesions and pelvic pain: A retrospective study. *Obstetrics and Gynecology, 68*, 13–15.

Rapkin, A. J., Kames, L. D., Darke, L. L., Stampler, F. M., & Naliboff, B. D. (1990). History of physical and sexual abuse in women with chronic pelvic pain. *Obstetrics and Gynecology, 76*, 92–96.

Reiter, R. C. (1990a). Occult somatic pathology in women with chronic pelvic pain. *Clinical Obstetrics and Gynecology, 33*, 154–160.

Reiter, R. C. (1990b). Chronic pelvic pain. *Clinical Obstetrics and Gynecology, 33*, 117–118.

Reiter, R. C. (1990c). A profile of women with chronic pelvic pain. *Clinical Obstetrics and Gynecology, 33,* 130–136.

Reiter, R. C., & Gambone, J. C. (1990a). Demographic and historical variables in women with chronic pelvic pain. *Obstetrics and Gynecology, 75,* 428–432.

Reiter, R. C., & Gambone, J. C. (1990b). Nongynecologic somatic pathology in women with chronic pelvic pain and negative laparoscopy. *Journal of Reproductive Medicine, 36,* 253–259.

Reiter, R. C., Gambone, J. C., & Johnson, S. R. (1991). Availability of a multidisciplinary pelvic pain clinic and frequency of hysterectomy for pelvic pain. *Journal of Psychosomatic Obstetrics and Gynecology, 12,* 109–116.

Reiter, R. C., Shakerin, L. R., Gambone, J. C., & Milburn, A. K. (1991). Correlation between sexual abuse and somatization in women with somatic and nonsomatic chronic pelvic pain. *American Journal of Obstetrics and Gynecology, 165,* 104–109.

Renaer, M., Vertommen, H., Nijs, P., Wagemans, L., & Van Henelrijck, T. (1979). Psychological aspects of chronic pelvic pain in women. *American Journal of Obstetrics and Gynecology, 134,* 75–80.

Roseff, S., & Murphy, A. (1990). Laparoscopy in the diagnosis and therapy of chronic pelvic pain. *Clinical Obstetrics and Gynecology, 33,* 137–143.

Savitz, D. (1985). Medical evaluation of the chronic pain patient. In G. M. Aronoff (Ed.), *Evaluation and treatment of chronic pain.* Baltimore: Urban & Schwarzenberg.

Slocumb, J. C. (1990a). Operative management of chronic abdominal pelvic pain. *Clinical Obstetrics and Gynecology, 33,* 196–204.

Slocumb, J. C. (1990b). Chronic somatic, myofascial, and neurogenic abdominal pelvic pain. *Clinical Obstetrics and Gynecology, 33,* 145–153.

Steege, J. F., Stout, A. L., & Somkuti, S. G. (1991). Chronic pelvic pain in women: Toward an integrative model. *Journal of Psychosomatic Obstetrics and Gynecology, 12,* Suppl., 3–30.

Stenchever, M. A. (1990). Symptomatic retrodisplacement, pelvic congestion, universal joint, and peritoneal defects...Fact or fiction? *Clinical Obstetrics and Gynecology, 33,* 161–167.

Stovall, T. G., Ling, F. W., & Crawford, D. A. (1990). Hysterectomy for chronic pelvic pain of presumed uterine etiology. *Obstetrics and Gynecology, 75,* 676–679.

Turk, D. C. (1986). *Pain management: A handbook of psychological treatment approaches.* New York: Pergamon Press.

Turk, D. C., Meichenbaum, D., & Genest, M. (1983). *Pain and behavioral medicine: A cognitive–behavioral perspective.* New York: Guilford Press.

Turk, D. C., & Rudy, T. E. (1987). Towards a comprehensive assessment of chronic pelvic pain patients. *Behavioral Research and Therapy, 25,* 237–249.

Turner, J. A., & Romano, J. M. (1989). Behavioral and psychological assessment of chronic pain patients. In J. D. Loeser & K. J. Egan (Eds.), *Managing the chronic pain patient.* New York: Raven Press.

Walker, E.., Katon, W., Harrop-Griffiths, J., Holm, L., Russo, J., & Hickok, L. R. (1988). Relationship of chronic pelvic pain to psychiatric diagnosis and childhood sexual abuse. *American Journal of Psychiatry, 145,* 75–80.

Walker, E., Katon, W., Neraas, K., Jemelka, R. P., & Massoth, D. (1992). Dissociation in women with chronic pelvic pain. *American Journal of Psychiatry, 149*, 534–537.

Walling, M. K. (1992). Sexual abuse and family models of pain/illness in the development of chronic pelvic pain. Unpublished dissertation. Iowa City: University of Iowa.

Wood, D. P., Wiesner, M. G., & Reiter, R. C. (1990). Psychogenic chronic pelvic pain: Diagnosis and management. *Clinical Obstetrics and Gynecology, 33*, 179–195.

Wyatt, G. E., & Peters, S. D. (1986). Methodological considerations in research on the prevalence of child sexual abuse. *Child Abuse and Neglect, 10*, 241–251.

Zung, W.W.K. (1965). A self-rating depression scale. *Archives of General Psychiatry, 12*, 63–70.

5

Gynecologic Surgery

Amy Fuller Stockman

Gynecologic surgery has many of the same psychological concomitants that accompany surgery in general (e.g., stress responses; Wallace, 1984). However, because gynecologic surgery has a direct effect on a woman's reproductive system, and therefore a direct effect on her self-perception, it may create its own distinct psychological difficulties, both preoperatively and postoperatively. Although there are numerous types of gynecologic surgery, most of the literature examines hysterectomy for benign conditions (e.g. menorraghia.) This chapter will address several issues including: a) incidence and prevalence of hysterectomy, b) potential social and psychological explanations for high hysterectomy rates, c) physical and psychological consequences of hysterectomy, and d) clinical implications.

INCIDENCE AND PREVALENCE

Hysterectomy has been intensively studied because of the large numbers of hysterectomies that are performed annually. In a recent two-year review of National Center for Health statistics on hysterectomy, Hufnagel (1988) reported that about 670,000 women receive hysterectomies each year in the United States, and a total of 19.1% of all American women over the age of 15 have had a hysterectomy. Over the course of their lifetime, 50% of women in the United

States are expected to have a hysterectomy (Dennerstein & van Hall, 1986). The annual incidence rate was 6.5 per 1,000 women in 1979 (Dennerstein & van Hall, 1986). Although some Western countries have hysterectomy rates that approach the rate in the U.S., there are still approximately twice as many hysterectomies per capita performed in the United States as elsewhere in the world (Sloan, 1978; Van Keep, Wildemeersch, & Lehert, 1983). Frequently, hysterectomy is performed in conjunction with another gynecologic surgery such as oophorectomy (removal of the ovaries). Very few women have received a bilateral oophorectomy who have not also had a hysterectomy, and 36% of all hysterectomy patients have had a bilateral oophorectomy (Hufnagel, 1988). Therefore, few data are available on the incidence and prevalence of oophorectomy as a distinct entity.

ACCOUNTING FOR GYNECOLOGIC SURGERY

What can account for the large number of hysterectomies performed in the United States? There are several reasons advanced for why women receive hysterectomies at such high rates. In addition to the obvious medical indications, historical biases and psychological indications may play prominent roles.

Medical Indications

The uterus is often removed in order to treat a life-threatening disease, or to improve women's physical quality of life (Gray, 1983). Common indications for hysterectomy include leiomyomata (fibroids) of the uterus, abnormal uterine bleeding, symptoms accompanying pelvic inflammatory disease, ovarian diseases such as endometriosis, carcinoma of the endometrium, and carcinoma of the cervix (Gray, 1983). In addition to these six indications, there is what is called a "combined syndrome" in which women display a multitude of physical and/or psychological symptoms (Gray, 1983). Although each symptom displayed in the "combined syndrome" is not sufficient to indicate the need for a hysterectomy, approximately 30% of hysterectomies are performed as a result of this combination of symptoms (Gray, 1983). However, multiple indications for hysterectomy have been linked to nonconfirmation of diagnosis of actual tissue pathology and this finding suggests that hysterectomy is more appropriately performed when there is a single preoperative indication (Reiter, Gambone, & Lench, 1992).

Medical indications for hysterectomy appear to be fairly uniform across nationalities and studies and have been grouped into five general categories by Reiter et al. (1992). These categories include cancer, acute conditions such as infection or rupture of the uterus, benign disease such as leiomyomata, discomfort problems including chronic pelvic pain, menstrual disorders or urinary incontinence, as well as elective hysterectomies for sterilization or cancer pro-phylaxis.

Negative Views of the Uterus

Historically, the reproductive system has been viewed as the root of practically all physiological and psychological illness in women. In the nineteenth century, the female reproductive organs were perceived as the dominating force in the feminine biological makeup, capable of controlling all of the other organs in the body. The etiologies of the illnesses of most of the internal organs were suggested to be merely a manifestation of uterine dysfunction (Ehrenreich & English, 1979). The uterus was perceived to have a similar negative effect on the emotional functioning of women. Citations in ancient Greek correspondence suggest that emotional lability and mental illness were the result of the 'hysterical' organ—the uterus (Sloan, 1978).

Another view of the uterus and ovaries as serving a purely utilitarian function, that of childbearing, also promotes removal of these organs after the last desired pregnancy. Wright (1969) summed up the prevailing view of his decade when he stated, "The uterus has but one function: reproduction. After the last planned pregnancy, the uterus becomes a useless, bleeding, symptom-producing, potentially cancer-bearing organ, and therefore should be removed" (p. 560). This post-childbearing, "useless uterus syndrome" has been frequently posited as proper indication for hysterectomy by many surgeons in the past (Sloan, 1978).

Psychological Indications

Although there are times when hysterectomy is medically indicated for organic conditions, many women receive a hysterectomy when there is no demonstrable uterine pathology (Dennerstein & van Hall, 1986). In fact, hysterectomy is most often performed because of the patient's belief that her physical condition requires a hysterectomy, rather than an actual objective medical assessment that a hysterectomy is required (Kincey & McFarlane, 1984).

Problems related to menstruation commonly cause women to seek a hysterectomy (Dennerstein & van Hall, 1986). Most of the complaints received from women seeking hysterectomy concerning their menstrual period suggest that they have a decreased tolerance for menstrual symptoms which previously would have been considered acceptable (Dennerstein & van Hall, 1986). Primary among these is a menstrual blood flow which is perceived to be abnormally heavy, often occurring after discontinued use of oral contraceptives. However, when menstrual blood loss was objectively measured, only 50% of women studied showed an increased blood loss during menstruation (Fraser, 1981). In addition, there was no significant correlation between actual and perceived blood loss (Chimbira, Anderson & Turnbull, 1980).

Emotional state has been suggested to be a major factor in influencing women's actual menstrual blood loss and perceptions of menstrual discomfort and perceived blood flow (Dennerstein & van Hall, 1986). In concurrence with this view, Gath, Cooper, and Day (1982) suggest that a combination of emotional distress and a persistent, heavy menstrual flow could increase the likelihood of a gynecologic referral and subsequent selection for gynecologic surgery. However, it is unclear whether the emotional distress women reported in these studies was a product of their heavy menstrual flow, or was a premorbid condition.

Preoperative psychological disorders in hysterectomy patients have a prevalence which is four to five times higher than that in the general population (Gath, 1980). Gath, Cooper, Bond, and Edmonds (1982) found that 58% of hysterectomy patients displayed preoperative psychopathology as measured by the Present State Examination (PSE; Wing, Cooper, & Sartorius, 1974). The high rate of preoperative psychiatric disorders in hysterectomy patients may be due to the fact that many women with psychological disorders somaticize their inner distress, because seeking advice for a physical problem is seen as much more acceptable in our society than seeking advice for a mental health problem (Dennerstein & van Hall, 1986). It is also possible that women who can be diagnosed as having a preoperative psychological disorder repeatedly present with physical complaints of nonorganic origin, prompting the gynecologist to use increasingly more invasive physical treatment methods. Regardless of the reasons for such a high level of preoperative psychological problems, postoperative psychological problems are probably more of a reflection of preoperative morbidity, than of the effects of the hysterectomy itself (Ryan, Dennerstein, & Pepperell, 1989).

CONSEQUENCES OF GYNECOLOGIC SURGERY

Ever since Blundell's observation of continued sexual desire in the patient following his performance of the first documented hysterectomy in 1828 (Blundell, 1892; cited in Kincey & McFarlane, 1984), physicians and researchers alike have been interested in the consequences of hysterectomy. This section presents a selective review of the literature concerning the consequences of hysterectomy, including the postsurgical side effects of this surgery in terms of women's physical, social, and psychological functioning. In order to clarify the inconsistency of earlier reports and more recent studies investigating these associations, methodological inadequacies of some of the older empirical research will be briefly discussed.

Methodological Flaws

In the past, empirical evidence regarding the consequences of gynecologic surgery has been difficult to interpret because of severe methodological inadequacies. These methodological problems include the use of retrospective designs, nonstandardized measures, heterogeneous samples, and delayed postoperative assessments.

Prospective versus retrospective design. Many retrospective studies have suggested that the postsurgical psychological problems seen in many women were the result of the surgery itself. Clearly, knowledge of the baseline, preoperative rate of psychological problems in the study population is crucial to the interpretation of postoperative problems. Several studies (e.g., Gath, Cooper, & Day, 1982; Ryan et al., 1989) have found that a large proportion of hysterectomy patients had psychological problems prior to surgery. Only prospective studies can determine directionality of effect. That is, it is impossible to know whether results reflect the operation itself, the anxiety produced by any surgical procedure, the physical condition (if any) which necessitated the operation, or preexisting psychopathology.

Standardized versus unstandardized measures. In many studies, the only method by which investigators identified postoperative psychological problems was by subjective clinical judgment (e.g., Richards, 1974). It is doubtful that there was adequate interrater reliability, or that this was a valid assessment for many subjects, as judgment was likely to be affected by individual training. Also, since experimenters were not blind to the hypothesis, they were likely to have expectations about the postsurgery outcome leading to prominent observer bias. Recently, there has been a move toward use of established standardized assessments, such as the Present State Examination (PSE; Wing et al., 1974), or the Profile of Mood States (POMS; McNair, Lorr, & Droopleman, 1971) to determine postsurgical morbidity.

Non-homogeneous samples. The use of mixed samples, such as having subjects undergoing surgery for malignant and benign conditions in the same study population (e.g., Barker, 1968), is not appropriate. A patient's response to a malignant condition could bring about greater psychiatric problems than the surgery itself. Also, many studies have grouped together women undergoing hysterectomy and oophorectomy with women undergoing hysterectomy only. Oophorectomy has hormonal consequences that may have effects beyond those of hysterectomy alone.

Immediate versus delayed postoperative assessment. The timing of postoperative assessments can seriously confound the validity of interpretations of postsurgery morbidity. For example, symptoms of emotional distress detected in patients immediately after surgery could be more a reflection of anxiety, pain, or reactions to the anesthesia than of persistent psychological pathology. On the other hand, assessments made several years after surgery might not have any relation to the previous surgery, and certainly many intervening variables would have contaminated any data collected after such a lengthy period.

Recent studies have been much more methodologically sophisticated, and allow for more valid generalizations about the consequences of gynecological surgery.

Postsurgical Side Effects

Surgery is stressful for most patients regardless of their preoperative condition (Bradley, 1982; O'Hara, Ghoneim, Hinrichs, Mehta, & Wright, 1989). Also, the patient's preoperative behaviors such as abuse of alcohol can adversely affect postoperative morbidity (Felding, Jensen, & Tonnesen, 1992). Women undergoing gynecological surgery face additional unique physical and psychological consequences.

Removal of healthy ovaries during hysterectomy has been a common practice, usually performed because it is believed that there is no ovarian function after menopause, or to avoid future ovarian cancer (Hufnagel, 1988). However, this practice is increasingly controversial. The ovaries continue to produce estrogen for 12 or more years after menopause and androgens are produced indefinitely (Asch & Greenblatt, 1977). Ovarian cancer is the most rare of all gynecologic cancers, accounting for only 4% of all female cancers (Hufnagel, 1988). Premature loss of estrogen can have devastating consequences on the health of affected women, increasing risk of heart disease (Centerwall, 1981), and osteoporosis (Schiff & Ryan, 1980).

Two obvious side effects of hysterectomy are the cessation of menstruation and subsequent loss of reproductive function. Discussions of posthysterectomy sequelae are replete with mention of these two concerns, yet there is little methodologically sound empirical evidence from which to draw any conclusions.

Menstruation has been described as the "badge of femininity" (Dennerstein & van Hall, 1986), and as the visible indicator that the uterus is alive and well (Sloan, 1978). An early study found that a majority of women viewed menstruation as a valuable and necessary function, equating its loss to a loss of femininity (Drellich & Bieber, 1958). Conversely, another early study reported that women either were unconcerned or reported positive feelings following cessation of menstruation (Jacobs, Daily, & Wills, 1957).

Loss of reproductive functioning may be viewed as negative or positive depending on the situation of the woman experiencing it. Younger women, especially those still hoping to have children, have particularly poor adaptive responses to hysterectomy (Kaltreider, Wallace, & Horowitz, 1979). A more positive response to hysterectomy may be characteristic of women who wish to eliminate the possibility of an undesired pregnancy and the use of birth control techniques (Drellich & Bieber, 1958). In a study of American army wives who received a hysterectomy primarily for contraceptive purposes, Hampton and Tarnasky (1974) found that the majority were satisfied with the operation and did not miss their reproductive function. Cultural and generational differences may also have an effect on how women perceive loss of reproductive function, and make it difficult to draw any general conclusions about the issue (Kincey & McFarlane, 1984).

Changes in sexual functioning have also been examined as a consequence of hysterectomy. For some women, hysterectomy brings permanent relief to the fears of pregnancy or uterine disease. However, for others, hormonal and anatomical changes associated with removal of the uterus and ovaries create new problems in sexual functioning, such as vaginal dryness or scar tissue, which make intercourse painful (Bachman, 1990; Huffman, 1985). Overall, posthysterectomy sexual dysfunction is most often found in women who perceive the uterus as integral to their femininity, youth, and attractiveness (Milburn & Reiter, 1993).

Some of the earlier studies examining posthysterectomy sexual functioning reported a reduction in sexual libido (i.e., Utian, 1975). Others obtained mixed results, such as a retrospective study completed by Dennerstein and Burrows (1977). They found that 37% of subjects reported a decrease in their overall satisfaction with sexual relations in the areas of sexual desire, sexual enjoyment, ability to climax, vaginal lubrication, and dyspareunia, although 34% reported improvement in their overall satisfaction with sex. Variables which they found to be related to a worse overall sexual outcome postsurgically included infrequent (less than one time per week) sexual intercourse presurgically, and high anxiety levels about being "sexually altered" by the operation.

In a study of 156 women undergoing gynecologic surgery, Gath, Cooper, and Day (1982) did not find a decrease in sexual functioning following hysterectomy. In fact, at the six-month follow-up, 56% of subjects actually reported an increase in frequency of sexual intercourse, and 39% reported an increase in enjoyment of sexual intercourse. Because of the use of prospective data, as well as validated and reliable assessment measures, the results of this study are probably much more representative of posthysterectomy sexual functioning.

The most widely studied result of hysterectomy is its association with psychological disorders. Most early studies noted an increased rate of psychiatric morbidity in women who had undergone hysterectomy and concluded that psychological disorders, depression in particular, were caused by the hysterectomy itself (Ackner, 1960; Barker, 1968; Bragg, 1965; Richards, 1973; Stengel, Zeitlyn, & Rayner, 1958). However, as discussed earlier in this chapter, methodological inadequacies plagued these studies, most notoriously the fundamental error that association implies causation.

Much of the recent work in this field tends to refute a causal link between hysterectomy and subsequent psychological disorders. Martin, Roberts, Clayton, and Wetzel (1977) were the first to suggest that preoperative psychopathology was the best predictor of posthysterectomy psychological disorders, and that hysterectomy did not cause psychiatric illness. Following preoperative interviews with 49 women undergoing hysterectomy for benign conditions, 57% of the subjects were diagnosed as being psychiatrically ill. Of the women diagnosed as having postoperative depression or "post-hysterectomy" syndrome, almost all had demonstrated psychopathology (depression or Briquet's syndrome) prior to surgery. Martin, Roberts, and Clayton (1980) concluded that as a group, the posthysterectomy patients were less symptomatic than before the procedure. Women who were symptomatic postsurgically were mainly those who had displayed psychiatric illness preoperatively, in particular "hysteria" (Briquet's somatization disorder). No significant changes in sexual, marital, or occupational functioning were found.

Gath and his colleagues conducted prehysterectomy interviews of 148 women with menorrhagia (excessive menstrual bleeding) of benign origin with follow-up interviews occurring at six and 18 months (Gath, Cooper, Bond, & Edmonds, 1982; Gath, Cooper, & Day, 1982). They found a strong association between preoperative mental problems and posthysterectomy psychiatric diagnosis. They also concluded that hysterectomy was not the cause of psychiatric disorders for this population. Not only did psychiatric morbidity not increase as a result of hysterectomy, but it actually decreased by 50% postoperatively according to PSE criteria (Gath, Cooper, & Day, 1982). Of the 43 cases of psychiatric disorder determined at 18-month follow-up, only 9 were non-cases preoperatively. Levels of psychosexual functioning, general well-being, and social functioning were seen to improve as well. However, the level of psychiatric morbidity found in this sample of hysterectomy patients was significantly higher than in the general population, although lower than in a psychiatric population (Gath, Cooper, & Day, 1982).

The incidence of depression after hysterectomy was studied by Lalinec-Michaud, Engelsmann, and Marino (1988) by comparing hysterectomy, cholecystectomy, and other pelvic operations groups. Preoperative depression was found to be predictive of postoperative depression. Hysterectomy patients displayed significantly more depressive symptoms preoperatively than did cholecystectomy patients, although they were not found to have a higher rate of preoperative psychiatric morbidity (i.e., contacts with psychiatrists, treatment with antidepressants). Women undergoing other pelvic operations displayed less depression and fewer cases of mental illness pre- and postoperatively than did hysterectomy patients, but reported more symptomatology than cholecystectomy patients. This finding indicates that gynecologic operations in general were more stressful than other types of operations (Lalinec-Michaud et al., 1988). Depression scores generally decreased postsurgically over a one-year period, suggesting that hysterectomy did not cause mental disorders, but actually improved the general health of women in this study (Lalinec-Michaud et al., 1988).

A prospective study by Ryan et al. (1989) analyzed the pre- and postoperative morbidity rates of hysterectomy for benign conditions, and also investigated psychosocial and gynecologic factors associated with psychological outcome. They found a preoperative psychiatric morbidity rate that was comparable to that described by Gath, Cooper, and Day (1982) and Martin et al. (1977), and that was considerably higher than the psychiatric morbidity rate in the general population. They also concluded that hysterectomy did not cause postsurgical psychological problems, and in fact tended to bring about a decrease in symptomatology displayed by patients.

Based on the most recent methodologically sound studies, there is little evidence that hysterectomy causes psychological disorders. In fact, psychological disorders may be improved by hysterectomy. However, the high rate of psychological morbidity among women who receive hysterectomies raises interesting questions. Do the conditions indicative of the need for a hysterectomy (i.e., chronic pain; menorrhagia) create a higher rate of psychological morbidity, or do the patient's psychological problems (i.e., anxiety; depression; hysteria) increase her likelihood of experiencing and presenting symptoms and receiving a hysterectomy? Available data do not provide the answer to these questions and, thus, more research is needed in this area.

IMPLICATIONS FOR PRACTITIONERS

Preoperative Screening

Since many of the studies reviewed indicate a significant relation between preoperative and postoperative condition, what can the practitioner do preoperatively to lessen the likelihood of adverse physical and psychiatric sequelae following hysterectomy? Many of the variables related to poor posthysterectomy outcome have been defined, and would be helpful in creating a screening procedure to identify patients who are most at risk. There is a need for a cooperative effort between psychologists and gynecologists in order to develop an approach to identify patients for whom preoperative psychological intervention is necessary.

Several conditions should raise "red flags," leading the practitioner to examine more closely the individual situation in order to determine proper treatment or the need for referral. These conditions include numerous previous surgeries, chronic pelvic pain, menstruation concerns, a history or current evidence of a mental disorder, and multiple indications for surgery.

The polysurgical patient is particularly vulnerable to negative psychological reactions to hysterectomy (Youngs & Wise, 1980). This patient is one who repeatedly requests, and usually obtains, surgical treatment, usually for vague physical complaints without verified organic pathology. Repeated surgeries for nonorganic pathology can be a symptom of somatization disorder (formerly Briquet's Syndrome) found in the American Psychiatric Association's (1987) *Diagnostic and Statistical Manual of Mental Disorders, Third Edition–Revised* (DSM–III–R). In fact, many studies of hysterectomy note a high preoperative level of somatization disorder followed by denial of relief after a hysterectomy (Martin et al., 1980). Therefore, a thorough medical history, including reasons for previous surgeries as well as postsurgical satisfaction, should be taken and psychiatric referrals made as necessary.

Also at increased vulnerability to posthysterectomy dissatisfaction is the patient suffering from chronic pelvic pain (Youngs & Wise, 1980). This patient may or may not have organic pathology, but like the polysurgical patient, has made repeated visits to the doctor for treatment. Surgery for this type of patient often fails to provide permanent relief from her complaints, and frequently leads to dissatisfaction with the services provided and more rarely to an increase in perceived pain (Stovall, Ling, & Crawford, 1990). A behavioral approach incorporating modifications in diet, exercise, and coping with pain and stress through relaxation and other techniques could provide more appropriate and permanent relief from chronic pelvic pain than hysterectomy (Hanson & Gerber, 1990; Nadelson, Notman, & Ellis, 1983). In fact, in the only randomized prospective trial comparing multidisciplinary nonsurgical management to traditional medical management for women with chronic pelvic pain, women receiving the former experienced significantly lower pain severity, disability, and total somatic symptomatology (Peters et al., 1991). In addition, many women suffering from chronic pelvic pain were victims of childhood sexual abuse (Walker, Katon, Harrop-Griffiths, & Holm, 1988). Health care professionals working with chronic pelvic pain patients should always include questions on this topic in their routine history and consider a mental health referral prior to hysterectomy if abuse is an issue (see Chapter 4).

Patients with a previous history of mental disorders, or who are currently displaying symptoms of psychopathology (in particular, anxiety or depression) are at increased risk for postoperative difficulties (Gitlin & Pasnau, 1989), although in the literature reviewed earlier in this chapter, some significant questions have been raised about possible interpretations of this relationship. Thus it would be wise to include a mental health history as part of the routine physical health history prior to treatment. Important factors to consider in screening include personal and family history of mental illness, including treatment modality and response to treatment. To assess for the existence of current psychopathology, physicians also need to be aware of some of the basic symptoms of depressive, anxiety and somatization disorders (e.g., lethargy and loss of appetite for depression) as delineated by *DSM–III–R (APA, 1987)*.

Finally, the physician should take into consideration whether there is a single medical condition necessitating hysterectomy, or whether the patient is presenting a multitude of symptoms, of which no one is sufficient indication for surgery. Approximately one third of all hysterectomies are performed because of this "combined syndrome" (Gray, 1983). Yet, there is recent support for the hypothesis that surgeons are more likely to list multiple indications for cases in which tissue pathology is not expected and for which appropriate nonsurgical management has not been utilized (Reiter et al., 1992).

Identifying patients who have any of these risk factors could help eliminate not only postsurgical psychological morbidity and dissatisfaction, but also some unnecessary surgeries. However, given that many hysterectomies are medically indicated, and that close to a million of these operations are performed each year, it also appears wise to try to improve the outcome for those women who do choose to undergo this procedure. One such way of trying to improve postoperative outcome that is potentially within the grasp of medical personnel is that of pre-surgical preparation.

Preoperative Preparation

Presurgical preparation of hysterectomy patients can have benefits both before and after the operation (Wallace, 1986). Direct intervention measures, such as the use of a highly informational preoperative preparatory booklet have been found to increase knowledge and decrease anxiety about surgery preoperatively (Wallace, 1986). Recently the Oregon Medical Association (OMA) has been piloting a pamphlet to provide information about hysterectomy surgery, including basic information about the female reproductive system, the conditions and diseases which affect it, and their usual treatments before hysterectomy is recommended. A preliminary evaluation of this pamphlet elicited a positive response from patients and physicians (Rose, 1992).

Using objective measures of positive outcome, presurgical preparation increased the performance of self-care and rehabilitation exercises by hysterectomy patients postoperatively (Williams, Gloria, Saavedra, Ferry, & Zaldivar, 1988). Behavioral preparation, consisting of training in muscle relaxation and information about the sensations patients would experience in association with their surgery, was found to reduce hospital stay, pain, and pain medication use in surgical patients (Wilson, 1981). Less pain and faster return to normal activities postoperatively have also been attributed to informational presurgical preparation (Wallace, 1984).

Preoperative education regarding the role of the uterus in sexual functioning, and physiological changes which might affect sexuality postoperatively is considered crucial for both the patient and her sexual partner (Huffman, 1985; Milburn & Reiter, 1993). Concurrent with this education should be an exploration of both partners' expectations and possible misconceptions of postoperative sexual functioning.

Although preoperative preparation generally has positive implications for the hysterectomy patient, some research suggests that individual coping style can turn a potentially helpful intervention into a negative one. For example, Cohen and Lazarus (1973) found that patients who avoided information presurgically spent fewer days in the hospital and had fewer postsurgical complications than those who sought out information. Another study found that providing too much information to individuals who try to distract themselves from surgery, and not enough information to information seekers can lead to high levels of psychophysiological arousal (Miller & Mangan, 1983). Thus a quick assessment of coping style (e.g., "How have you dealt with stressful situations in the past?") through interviews with the patient and her family can provide information necessary to create an effective preoperative intervention.

Because a variety of informational and behavioral preparation techniques are beneficial to patients, both before and after surgery, a plan which incorporates more than one modality (i.e., informational material, stress-reduction techniques) will provide more opportunities to meet patient needs.

CONCLUSIONS

The high incidence rate (above that which could be expected for the rate of gynecological pathology) of gynecologic surgery suggests clearly that it is not solely a medical problem. There are also numerous psychological and sociological concomitants of the procedure that are suggested in the literature. Proper assessment of both the physical and mental condition of the potential hysterectomy patient is essential in order to avoid some of the negative sequelae commonly associated with gynecologic surgery. Preoperative preparation designed for each patient can also decrease negative responses to surgery. Overall, a multidisciplinary approach which integrates the knowledge and expertise from both physical and mental health domains is most likely to be effective in meeting the needs of patients seeking gynecologic surgery.

REFERENCES

Ackner, B. (1960). Emotional aspects of hysterectomy. *Advanced Psychosomatic Medicine, 1,* 248–252.

American Psychiatric Association (1987). *Diagnostic and statistical manual of mental disorders.* 3rd Edition–Revised (DSM–III–R). Washington, DC: Author.

Asch, R., & Greenblatt, R. (1977). Steroidogenesis in the post-menopausal ovary. *Clinical Obstetrics and Gynaecology, 4*, 85.

Bachmann, G. A. (1990). Psychosexual aspects of hysterectomy. *Women's Health Issues, 1*, 41–49.

Barker, M. G. (1968). Psychiatric illness after hysterectomy. *British Journal of Medicine, 2*, 91–95.

Bradley, C. (1982). Psychological factors affecting recovery from surgery. In J. Watkins & M. Salo (Eds.), *Trauma, stress and immunity in anesthesia and surgery* (pp. 335–361). Woburn, MA: Butterworths.

Bragg, R. L. (1965). Risk of admission to mental hospital following hysterectomy or cholecystectomy. *American Journal of Public Health, 5*, 1403–1410.

Centerwall, B. (1981). Premenopausal hysterectomy and cardiovascular disease. *American Journal of Obstetrics and Gynecology, 139*, 58–61.

Chimbira, T. H., Anderson, A.B.M., & Turnbull, A. C. (1980). Relation between measured menstrual blood loss and patients' subjective assessment of loss, duration of bleeding, number of sanitary towels used, uterine weight and endometrial surface area. *British Journal of Obstetrics and Gynaecology, 87*, 603–609.

Cohen, F., & Lazarus, R. S. (1973). Active coping processes, coping dispositions, and recovery from surgery. *Psychosomatic Medicine, 35*, 375–389.

Dennerstein, M. B., & Burrows, G. D. (1977). Sexual response following hysterectomy and oophorectomy. *Obstetrics and Gynecology, 49*, 92–96.

Dennerstein, L., & van Hall, E. (1986). *Psychosomatic gynecology*. Park Ridge, NJ: Parthenon Publishing.

Drellich, M.G., & Bieber, I. (1958). The psychologic importance of the uterus and its functions. *Journal of Nervous and Mental Disease, 126*, 322–336.

Ehrenreich, B., & English, D. (1979). *For her own good: 150 years of the experts' advice to women*. London: Pluto Press.

Felding, C., Jensen, L. M., & Tonnesen, H. (1992). Influence of alcohol intake on postoperative morbidity after hysterectomy. *American Journal of Obstetrics and Gynecology, 166*, 667–670.

Fraser, I. (1981). Perceptions of menstrual cycle symptomatology. In L. Dennerstein & G.D. Burrows (Eds.), *Obstetrics, gynaecology and psychiatry* (pp. 97–104). Melbourne, AU: York Press.

Gath, D. (1980). Psychiatric aspects of hysterectomy. In L. Robins, P. Clayton, & J. Wing (Eds.), *The social consequences of psychiatric illness* (pp. 33–45). New York: Brunner/ Mazel.

Gath, D., Cooper, P., Bond, A., & Edmonds, G. (1982). Demographic psychiatric and physical factors in relation to psychiatric outcome. *British Journal of Psychiatry, 140*, 343–350.

Gath, D., Cooper, P., & Day, A. (1982). Hysterectomy and psychiatric disorder: Levels of psychiatric morbidity before and after hysterectomy. *British Journal of Psychiatry, 140*, 335–350.

Gitlin, M. J., & Pasnau, R. O. (1989). Psychiatric syndromes linked to reproductive function in women: A review of current knowledge. *American Journal of Psychiatry, 146*, 1413–1422.

Gray, L. A. (1983). *Vaginal hysterectomy: Indications, technique, and complications*. Springfield, IL: Charles C Thomas.

Hampton, P. T., & Tarnasky, W. (1974). Hysterectomy and tubal ligation: A comparison of the psychological aftermath. *American Journal of Obstetrics and Gynecology, 119*, 949–952.

Hanson, R. W., & Gerber, K. E. (1990). *Coping with chronic pain*. New York: Guilford Press.

Huffman, J. W. (1985). Sex after hysterectomy. *Medical Aspects of Human Sexuality, 19*, 171–179.

Hufnagel, V. G. (1988). The conspiracy against the uterus. *Journal of Psychosomatic Obstetrics and Gynaecology, 9*, 51–58.

Jacobs, W. M., Daily, H. I., & Wills, S. H. (1957). The effect of hysterectomy on young women. *Surgical Gynecology and Obstetrics, 104*, 307–309.

Kaltreider, N. B., Wallace, A., & Horowitz, M. (1979). A field study of the stress response syndrome: Young women after hysterectomy. *Journal of the American Medical Association, 242*, 1499–1503.

Kincey, J., & McFarlane, T. (1984). Psychological aspects of hysterectomy. In A. Broome & L. Wallace (Eds.), *Psychology and gynaecological problems* (pp.142–160). London: Tavistock Publications.

Lalinec-Michaud, M., Engelsmann, F., & Marino, J. (1988). Depression after hysterectomy: A comparative study. *Psychosomatics, 29*, 307–314.

Martin, R. L., Roberts, W. V., & Clayton, P. J. (1980). Psychiatric status after hysterectomy. *Journal of the American Medical Association, 244*, 350–353.

Martin, R. L., Roberts, W. V., & Clayton, P. J., & Wetzel, R. (1977). Psychiatric illness and non-cancer hysterectomy. *Diseases of the Nervous System, 38*, 974–980.

McNair, D. M., Lorr, M., & Droopleman, L. F. (1971). *Profile of mood states*. San Diego: Educational and Industrial Testing Service.

Milburn, A., & Reiter, R. (1993). Women's sexual health and sexual dysfunction. In T. R. Moore, R. C. Reiter, R. W. Rebar, & W. Baker (Eds.), *Gynecology and obstetrics: A longitudinal approach* (pp. 845–855). New York: Churchill Livingstone.

Miller, S. M., & Mangan, C. E. (1983). Interacting effects of information and coping style in adapting to gynecologic stress: Should the doctor tell all? *Journal of Personality and Social Psychology, 45*, 223–236.

Nadelson, C. C., Notman, M. T. & Ellis, E. A. (1983). Psychosomatic aspects of obstetrics and gynecology. *Psychosomatics, 24*, 871–884.

O'Hara, M. W., Ghoneim, M. M., Hinrichs, J. V., Mehta, M. P., & Wright, E. J. (1989). Psychological consequences of surgery. *Psychosomatic Medicine, 51*, 356–370.

Peters, A. A., van Dorst, E., Jellis, B., van Zuuren, E., Hermans, J., & Trimbos, J. B. (1991). Randomized clinical trial to compare two different approaches in women with chronic pelvic pain. *Obstetrics and Gynecology, 77*, 740–744.

Reiter, R. C., Gambone, J. D., & Lench, J. B. (1992). Appropriateness of hysterectomies performed for multiple preoperative indications. *Obstetrics & Gynecology, 80*, 902–905.

Richards, D. H. (1973). Depression after hysterectomy. *Lancet, 2*, 430–433.

Richards, D. H. (1974). A post-hysterectomy syndrome. *Lancet, 2*, 983–985.

Rose, B. K. (1992). Informed consent and hysterectomy: Enhancing the right to know. *American Journal of Public Health, 82*, 609–610.

Ryan, M. M., Dennerstein, L., & Pepperell, R. (1989). Psychological aspects of hysterectomy: A prospective study. *British Journal of Psychiatry, 154*, 516–522.

Schiff, I., & Ryan, K. (1980). Benefits of estrogen replacement. *Obstetrical and Gynecological Survey Supplement, 35*, 202.

Sloan, D. (1978). The emotional and psychosexual aspects of hysterectomy. *American Journal of Obstetrics and Gynecology, 131*, 598–605.

Stengel, E., Zeitlyn, B. B., & Rayner, E. H. (1958). Post-operative psychoses. *Journal of Mental Science, 104*, 389–402.

Stovall, T. G., Ling, F. W., & Crawford, D. A. (1990). Hysterectomy for chronic pelvic pain of presumed uterine etiology. *Obstetrics and Gynecology, 75*, 676–679.

Utian, W. H. (1975). Effect of hysterectomy, oophorectomy and estrogen therapy on libido. *Journal of Gynaecology and Obstetrics, 13*, 97–100.

Van Keep, P. A., Wildemeersch, D., & Lehert, P. (1983). Hysterectomy in six European countries. *Maturitas, 5*, 69–75.

Walker, E., Katon, W., Harrop-Griffiths, J., & Holm, L. (1988). Relationship of chronic pelvic pain to psychiatric diagnoses and childhood sexual abuse. *American Journal of Psychiatry, 145*, 75–80.

Wallace, L. M. (1984). Psychological preparation as a method of reducing the stress of surgery. *Journal of Human Stress, 10*, 62–79.

Wallace, L. M. (1986). Communication variables in the design of pre-surgical preparatory information. *British Journal of Clinical Psychology, 25*, 111–118.

Williams, P. D., Gloria, M. D., Saavedra, L. D., Ferry, T. C., & Zaldivar, S. B. (1988). Effects of preparation for mastectomy/hysterectomy on women's post-operative self-care behaviors. *International Journal of Nursing Studies, 25*, 191–206.

Wilson, J. (1981). Behavioral preparation for surgery: Benefit or harm? *Journal of Behavioral Medicine, 4*, 79–102.

Wing, J. K., Cooper, J. E., & Sartorius, N. (1974). *The measurement and classification of psychiatric symptoms*. London: Cambridge University Press.

Wright, R. C. (1969). Hysterectomy: Past, present and future. *Obstetrics and Gynecology, 33*, 560–565.

Youngs, D. D., & Wise, T. N. (1980). Psychological sequelae of elective gynecologic surgery. In D. D. Youngs & A. A. Ehrhardt (Eds.), *Psychosomatic obstetrics and gynecology* (pp. 255–264). New York: Appleton–Century–Crofts.

6

Gynecologic Cancer

Lynette A. Menefee

Cancer is the second leading cause of death in women following heart disease (Boring, Squires, & Tong, 1991). In 1991, the National Cancer Institute estimated that 12% of cancer deaths in women would result from gynecologic cancer (Boring et al., 1991). In the same year, it was estimated that 71,700 women would be diagnosed with gynecologic cancer (Boring et al., 1991). Research has shown the dramatic psychological, social, and familial effects of cancer on women (e.g., Taylor, 1983; Wortman & Dunkel-Schetter, 1979). Although most studies have documented psychological changes that occur after breast cancer, gynecologic cancer can have equally devastating psychological effects. The purpose of this chapter is to review some of the psychological aspects of gynecologic cancer and their implications for treatment. First, a brief review of the major types of gynecologic malignancies and types of treatment will be provided.

Types of Gynecologic Cancer

The most common type of gynecologic cancer occurs in the endometrium or uterine lining and is called endometrial cancer (Silverberg & Lubera, 1989). Occurring mostly in postmenopausal women, the predominant symptom is vaginal bleeding (Morrow, Curtin, & Townsend, 1993). Risk factors include older age, residency in North America or Northern Europe, higher levels of education or income, white race, obesity, hypertension, diabetes, and a family history of endometrial cancer (Brinton & Hoover, 1992; Gusberg, 1986; Yazigi, 1989).

Malignant neoplasms are also associated with factors related to the unopposed stimulation of the endometrium by estrogen, such as low parity, late menopause, chronic anovulation, long-term estrogen use, or a history of endometrial hyperplasia, which is an abnormal increase in tissue cells (Brinton & Hoover, 1992; Yazigi, 1989). The majority of cases are diagnosed when the tumor is confined to the uterus, and survival in these early cases is quite good. Although specific treatment depends on the histology of the cells and their metastatic extension, a common course of treatment for early-stage disease is a combination of surgery and radiation therapy. Hormonal therapy with or without chemotherapy may be added for recurrent disease (Morrow, Curtin, & Townsend, 1993).

The second most common type of gynecologic neoplasm, which accounts for the most fatalities, is ovarian cancer (Boring, Squires, & Tong, 1991). Usually occurring after age 40, the symptoms are vague and only become apparent as the disease progresses. Women may present with gastrointestinal symptoms, early satiety, or a feeling of abdominal fullness. Associated features include older age, residency in North America or Northern Europe, nulliparity, infertility, early menopause, exposure to asbestos and talc, high socioeconomic or educational status, dietary fat, a female relative with ovarian cancer, and a history of breast cancer (Brinton & Hoover, 1992; Yazigi, 1989). Early-stage disease is usually treated with a total abdominal hysterectomy, bilateral salpingo-oophorectomy, and omentectomy. Women with advanced disease may receive cytoreductive surgery or "debulking" where removal of primary tumors and metastases are the goal (Griffiths, Parker, & Fuller, 1979; Morrow, Curtin, & Townsend, 1993). Adjuvant chemotherapy and/or radiation treatments usually follows surgery (Gusberg, 1986).

Cervical cancer is the third most common gynecologic cancer (Silverberg & Lubera, 1989). Since precancerous lesions can often be detected early by a Pap smear, the incidence of cervical cancer has decreased in the last 40 years. Risk factors include older age, residency in Latin America, Asia, or Africa, low socioeconomic or educational status, smoking, a history of multiple partners, intercourse before the age of 16, African-American, Mexican-American, or American Indian lineage, no previous Pap smear screening, and a history of sexually transmitted diseases, especially herpes simplex or human papillomavirus (Brinton & Hoover, 1992; Gusberg, 1986; Yazigi, 1989). Although regular Pap smears aid in early detection, false negative results have occurred in women diagnosed with cervical cancer (Brinton & Hoover, 1992). Thus women should be treated by physicians who understand the appropriate diagnostic and therapeutic response to normal and atypical Pap smears (Nelson, Averette, & Richart, 1984). Dysplastic (precancerous) lesions, which have not invaded below the surface of the cervix are generally treated with local excision or laser surgery. Locally invasive cervical cancer is treated with radical hysterectomy or radiation therapy.

Recurrent or metastatic disease requires chemotherapy and/or pelvic exenteration (removal of the pelvic viscera including the uterus, tubes, vagina, ovaries, bladder, and rectum). Because this surgery is so extensive, vaginal reconstruction may be necessary (Morrow, Curtin, & Townsend, 1993).

Vulvar and vaginal neoplasms are less common than the gynecologic cancers previously described. Vulvar cancer usually affects postmenopausal women. Symptoms include itching and possible visible abnormalities of the vulva (Hacker, 1986). Risk factors include cigarette smoking and a history of genital warts. Diabetes, obesity, and hypertension have been associated with vulvar cancer in several clinical studies, but have not been confirmed by epidemiologic research assessing these variables (Brinton & Hoover, 1992). Noninvasive vulvar cancer can be treated by local excision of the lesion (Hacker, 1986). Most cancers, however, may require a simple, or even radical vulvectomy, which involves removing vulvar skin and lymph nodes in the groin. Skin grafts from the abdomen, buttocks, or thigh may be necessary. This course of treatment is disfiguring and can be debilitating (Cairns & Valentich, 1986).

Vaginal neoplasms are found most often in women in their sixties, although a small number of young women whose mothers took diethylstilbestrol (DES) have been diagnosed with vaginal cancer (Gusberg, 1986). Vaginal cancer is usually found in the upper third of the vagina and is treated by surgery, which may include vaginal reconstruction surgery or radiation (Morrow, Curtin, & Townsend, 1993).

Surgery, radiation therapy, and chemotherapy are all used to treat gynecologic cancer, although the type or combination of types of treatment vary for each individual based on the type of cancer and the stage. The most common intervention is surgery. A hysterectomy, pelvic lymphadenectomy, vulvectomy, lymph node dissection, or pelvic exenteration may be performed. Radiation therapy may include intracavity radiation treatment, in which radiation is administered through a uterine and/or vaginal implant, or standard external beam therapy (Krouse, 1990). Side effects of this treatment are fatigue, weakness, diarrhea, and changes in the skin (Morrow, Curtin, & Townsend, 1993). Chemotherapy treatments may produce side effects such as fatigue, anemia, alopecia, nausea, vomiting, diarrhea, and decreased resistance to infection (Burish & Lyles, 1981). Each drug has its own constellation of side effects, many of which can be controlled or prevented. Psychological reactions to these treatments will be discussed in the next section.

Each type of gynecologic cancer has different risk factors and prognoses, making generalizations about medical treatments or psychological impact difficult to make. The next section reviews the issues which may be important for women with gynecologic cancer, but the discussion must be placed in the context of the type and stage of cancer and the specific woman's life circumstances.

PSYCHOLOGICAL ASPECTS OF GYNECOLOGIC CANCER

Adjustment to Cancer: Normal Reactions and Psychiatric Morbidity

Approximately 50% of people diagnosed with cancer experience a period of adjustment, which includes depressed and anxious reactions in response to disease or treatments, while the remaining 50% experience more severe distress (Massie & Holland, 1989). A four-stage model that includes descriptions of normal reactions, and indicators of maladaptive coping for women with gynecologic cancer, was described by Krouse (1990). Beginning with the recognition of symptoms and diagnosis (Recognition–Exploration stage), the woman may feel guilt, embarrassment, anxiety, isolation, and denial of disease. Since several gynecologic cancers can be detected early with routine gynecologic examinations, some women may blame themselves for not seeking routine care that might have discovered their condition.

The woman enters the Crisis–Climax stage with the initiation of medical care, in which more diagnostic tests may be completed, treatment given, and the results evaluated. Hospitalization is usually required and this period of time is often stressful for the patient and her family. Anxiety about treatment, the physical effects of treatment, depression, altered body image, and concerns about changing relationships may be present (Krouse, 1990).

Different concerns will be present in different clinical courses. For example, the person who has the potential for long-term survival has different psychological issues than the person for whom no primary treatment is possible. Terminally ill patients often live with extreme exhaustion, increased dependency, and coping with impending death (Holland, 1989a). Elderly women face increased morbidity and mortality during treatment, especially when other diseases, such as cardiovascular disease or diabetes mellitus are present (Kennedy, Flagg, & Webster, 1989).

Following treatment, the woman with gynecologic cancer enters the Adaptation–Maladaptation stage, in which she calls on her repertoire of coping strategies and her social support network. Adapting to functional changes, differences in self-perceptions, relationships, and employment situations are psychological issues relevant to this stage. Maladaptation occurs when coping does not enhance daily functioning and the woman withdraws from relationships (Krouse, 1990). Generally, the first year of adjusting to the medical and psychosocial aspects of gynecologic cancer is crucial, although the type and stage of gynecologic cancer may make the length of normal adjustment longer or shorter.

The general direction of adaptation is evident in the Resolution–Disorganization stage. Resolution indicates a maximal involvement in life and a strengthened sense of self-worth. Disorganization occurs when increased withdrawal from relationships, helplessness, depression, and increased personal doubts persist. Recurrence of disease or further treatments may cause a woman to recycle through the stages of adjustment.

A theory of cognitive adaptation to victimizing events has been applied to women with breast cancer (Taylor, 1983) and may have implications for women with gynecologic cancer as well. According to this theory, cognitive adaptation to cancer centers on three basic themes: a search for meaning in the experience, an attempt to regain mastery over the event and over one's life, and an effort to enhance self-esteem. Women with gynecologic cancer may believe their cancer is punishment for previous sexual behavior, such as masturbation, extramarital affairs, sexually transmitted disease, or abortion (Harris, Good, & Pollack, 1982). The second theme of adaptation involves an attempt to control the environment. Women with gynecologic cancer may believe that a cessation of sexual activities may prevent recurrence. Negotiation of decision making between hospital staff and the woman with cancer regarding self-care while in the hospital may increase her sense of control (Krouse, 1990). The third theme of adaptation involves enhancing self-worth. Social comparison to others who are less fortunate is commonly used by women with cancer to enhance self-worth (Wortman & Dunkel-Schetter, 1979). Empirical studies have yet to determine the usefulness of these models for women with gynecologic cancer, but they provide directions to consider.

Psychiatric morbidity. Psychological reactions that are more severe than the normal fluctuations of crisis and transition expected with a diagnosis of cancer are experienced by approximately 50% of individuals with cancer (Derogatis et al., 1983; Massie & Holland, 1989). The majority of these individuals meet diagnostic criteria for adjustment disorders with depressed or anxious symptoms (American Psychiatric Association, 1987). Delirium related to the effects of the disease or treatment is diagnosed most frequently after adjustment disorders, followed by anxiety and personality disorders. A very small percentage of individuals with cancer are diagnosed with major mental illnesses (Massie & Holland, 1989).

Few empirical studies have concentrated on normal adjustment reactions or psychiatric morbidity in women with gynecologic cancer. In a longitudinal investigation of women with early-stage gynecologic cancer, women with benign tumors, and healthy controls, the women with cancer reported more depression and confusion than did women in the other groups (Andersen, Anderson, & deProsse, 1989b). Women in the cancer and benign tumor groups reported more anxiety and fatigue than did healthy controls during the initial testing period. Emotional distress, however, improved for the cancer and benign tumor groups by four months. No significant differences were found between these groups at the 4-, 8- and 12-month assessments. This study lends support for the transitory nature of emotional distress in survivable gynecologic cancer. In addition, anxiety may be related to anticipation of difficult treatment, rather than to the diagnosis of a malignancy (Andersen, Anderson, & deProsse, 1989b; Karlsson & Andersen, 1986).

In general, a small number of cancer patients are referred for psychiatric consultation by oncologists. The institution of a psychiatric liaison program in a gynecologic oncology unit was reported to increase the rates of consultation by 5% and the detection of minor psychiatric disorders increased by 11% (McCartney et al., 1989). Increased use of screening instruments may be helpful in detecting psychological difficulties. Golden et al. (1991) found the Carroll Rating Scale to be an effective screening instrument for clinical depression in individuals with nonovarian gynecologic cancer who were not severely disabled and who were not receiving treatment.

Women with gynecologic cancer appear to have normal reactions to illness and share similar rates of psychiatric morbidity along with other individuals with cancer. The type of gynecologic cancer, the severity of disease, and the type of treatment be important determinants of psychological distress. Empirical studies which address both normal and maladaptive coping are needed with this population.

Psychological Issues and Treatment Implications

A number of studies report the psychological and psychosocial difficulties experienced by women with gynecologic cancer. Some areas, such as sexuality, are more thoroughly researched than other areas, such as changes in close relationships. Descriptions of psychological or psychosocial difficulties are more common in the literature than are empirical studies. Despite the difficulties with descriptive research, some of these studies ask important questions and have implications for psychological intervention. A few of these studies in selected topic areas will be reviewed as areas of potential importance to women with gynecologic cancer.

Psychological responses to medical treatment. The period of time after diagnosis and before surgical treatment can be distressing. One study of women with gynecologic cancer found that marked pretreatment anxiety was present for 68% of women. Younger women were more likely to experience anxiety during this time. Specific worries included the possibility of death, how their families would cope while they were hospitalized, being hospitalized, and fears of operations, treatments and their after effects (Corney, Everett, Howells, & Crowther, 1992).

Moderate anxiety before external radiotherapy was found to facilitate positive adjustment by increasing attentiveness to treatment information, promoting a sense of control, and accepting reassurances from others (Andersen & Tewfik, 1985). Negative mood was reported to increase over the three weeks when radiotherapy was administered, but to decrease by three months following treatment. The severity of side effects was positively correlated with negative mood and disruption of function (Nail, King, & Johnson, 1986).

Palliative chemotherapy for women with advanced cancer may cause physical side effects and psychological difficulties. Psychological difficulties may be conditioned responses to treatment, such as conditioned vomiting before, during, or after chemotherapy treatment, as well as negative mood or affect precipitated by a diagnosis of terminal cancer (Burish & Lyles, 1981; Payne, 1990). Several styles of coping with palliative chemotherapy have been noted, including positive thinking, fighting the disease, acceptance, fearfulness, and hopelessness (Payne, 1990).

A variety of psychological techniques can help women with gynecologic cancer who experience anticipatory nausea and vomiting in reaction to chemotherapy or anxiety in response to treatment. Conditioned immune suppression may also be present, as was found in a study of women receiving cyclic chemotherapy for ovarian cancer (Bovbjerg et al., 1990). Progressive muscle relaxation, biofeedback with imagery, systematic desensitization, and cognitive or attentional distraction are some techniques that were used and shown to be effective for people with cancer (Redd, 1988). Relaxation therapy has been shown to be effective in reducing anxiety, negative affect, and nausea for individuals receiving chemotherapy (Burish & Lyles, 1981). Women who receive internal radiotherapy may be highly anxious posttreatment, even if anxiety was low at pretreatment (Andersen, Karlsson, Anderson, & Tewfik, 1984) and may benefit from behavioral modification techniques or counseling.

Perhaps one of the easiest intervention strategies to deliver during the diagnosis and treatment stages is the providing of information. Although individuals and family members vary in their desire to know about cancer, most women and their families will cope more easily when fully informed about the disease and the treatments (Krouse, 1990). In fact, seeking information was found to promote acceptance of illness and decreased negative affect in four different types of chronic illnesses (including cancer) regardless of the controllability of the disease (Felton & Revenson, 1984).

Fully informing the woman and her family of the possible consequences of treatment, including the physical, psychological, and psychosocial implications will allow her to make the best decisions for herself and prepare her for the future. It may not be appropriate or possible to share all the details during the first stages of illness. Acquainting the woman, however, with a few common psychological reactions (e.g., that she may feel depressed, that sexual relationships may be disrupted for a time) and informing her that there is help for these problems may allow her to feel more comfortable about mentioning these problems if they occur. Information about diagnosis and treatment is most effective if delivered in person and may be better understood with the aid of pelvic models or diagrams (Cain et al., 1983). Providing information to the woman and her family decreases the likelihood that myths will be believed and facilitates relationships with physicians and professionals working in oncology.

Body image. Several investigators have described a change in body image among women with gynecologic cancer (e.g., Holmes, 1987; Krouse, 1990). Concerns about the effects of treatment may be related to the woman's altered body image (Krouse, 1990; Whale, 1991). Although greater disruption of body image may occur in women who receive pelvic exenteration (Andersen & Hacker, 1983b), alterations in body image are present in women with less obvious physical changes (Krouse, 1990). Some women associate the uterus with femininity, sexual drive, and status as a wife and mother (Holmes, 1987). Women with gestational trophoblastic disease may be especially susceptible to distress over the loss of a pregnancy and possible loss of the ability to carry a future pregnancy (Wenzel, Berkowitz, Robinson, Bernstein, & Goldstein, 1992). Belief in myths, early socialization, or the portrayal of women in the media may perpetuate the notion that women must have a "perfect" body to feel good about themselves and their relationships. For instance, women may believe that they will lose their orgasmic ability or their femininity with treatment (Shell, 1990). How fears regarding changes in body image are manifested in everyday relationships has yet to be researched. Women's changed feelings about their bodies as a result of gynecologic cancer, however, may have an impact on their psychological and psychosocial well-being.

The psychologist or mental health professional can help the woman by being sensitive to the fact that an altered body image can lead to lower self-esteem. Listening to the woman's fears and providing a way for her to begin accepting her body may help. Connection with loving interpersonal relationships often helps women who have endured a change in body image because of hair loss during chemotherapy or physical alterations from surgery (Shell, 1990).

Close relationships. Close relationships are affected by the diagnosis of cancer (Lichtman & Taylor, 1986), yet few empirical studies have focused specifically on the close relationships of women with gynecologic cancer. Therefore, general findings of studies of women with cancer that are thought to be relevant to women with gynecologic cancer will be discussed.

Corroborating the findings of the few marital satisfaction assessments given in studies about sexuality in women with gynecologic cancer (e.g., Andersen, Anderson, & deProsse, 1989a; Andersen & Jochimsen, 1985), are studies of the marital relationships of women with breast cancer. These studies show that the majority of marital relationships improve despite fears of death, traumatic medical treatments, role changes, and threats of recurrence (Lichtman & Taylor, 1986; Sewell & Edwards, 1980). The best predictor of dissatisfaction in the marital relationship after cancer treatment may be a history of instability in the relationship before the diagnosis of cancer (Sewell & Edwards, 1980). A lack of communication in the marital relationship concerning gynecologic cancer and its ramifications may contribute to this dissatisfaction (Northouse & Northouse, 1987). Additional stress might be found in couples who have previously operated with strict gender roles and who may be forced, temporarily or permanently, to adjust the rules of responsibility in their relationship.

Differences in coping styles between women with gynecologic cancer and their partners may also contribute to misunderstandings. In a study of 112 individuals with early-stage cervical cancer and advanced breast or gynecologic cancer, and their mates, Gotay (1984) found that partners were more disturbed by the possibility of death than were the women with disease. Both the women and partners reported seeking information as the most frequent coping strategy. However, partners of women with early-stage cancer were more apt to take direct action and talk to others than were the women themselves (Gotay, 1984). Thus communication between the couple, family members, and health professionals is important for optimal coping.

Many variables, including the socioeconomic status of the family, the assistance needed, available social support, the nature of the prior relationship, perceived stress and perceived control over the situation, and the individual's and caregiver's responses to stress, influence the quantity and quality of support given and the strain on the care giver (Sales, Schulz, & Biegel, 1992). A study of 357 women between the ages of 20 and 54 with newly diagnosed breast, endometrial, or ovarian cancer found that the most important member of the support network was a spouse for married women, and relatives for single women (Smith, Redman, Burns, & Sagert, 1986). In this study, few women reported stress in their marriage due to the cancer diagnosis. The majority of women found being able to talk about their disease most helpful. The presence of psychological difficulties in close relationships for women with gynecologic cancer may be related to the type of cancer, the stage of the disease, and the extent of treatment. Following vulvectomy, more than half of the women in one study and approximately half of their partners reported long-term psychological distress (Andreasson, Moth, Buus Jensen, & Bock, 1986). For breast cancer patients, findings of a few studies showed that relationships with family and friends either improved or stayed the same as before the diagnosis of cancer (e.g., Lichtman & Taylor, 1986).

Wortman and Dunkel-Schetter (1979) postulated that troubled interpersonal relationships after cancer are often characterized by the partner's feelings of fear and belief in maintaining an optimistic facade. For instance, individuals in close relationships to women with cancer might avoid talking about cancer by engaging in superficially optimistic conversation. These behaviors inhibited the patient from talking freely.

A psychological intervention that may be helpful in maintaining close relationships is providing information to both the woman with cancer and her partner (Andreasson, Moth, Buus Jensen, & Bock, 1986). Marital or family therapy may assist the couple in understanding their coping styles, adjusting to temporary or permanent effects of treatment, making decisions regarding medical treatment, and learning to express their thoughts and feelings.

Quality of life. Women with metastatic cancer and their families may assess treatment in terms of the quality of the woman's life. The participation of the woman and consideration of her values and preferences should be a critical part of decision making (McCartney & Larson, 1987). Women and their families must decide what types of treatment will be delivered when the treatment would prolong dying (Holland, 1989b; McCartney & Larson, 1987). These decisions are sensitive ones for the family of a terminally ill individual. Professionals working with these families should approach them with care and understanding.

Sexual functioning. One of the most studied aspects specific to gynecologic cancer is that of sexual functioning. Concerns about sexuality are common in most cancer patients, although the type of concern varies with the age of the individual, the type and stage of cancer, cancer treatment, and previous sexual difficulties (Auchincloss, 1989; Burbie & Polinsky, 1992). Similarly, gynecologic cancer patients report concern about sexual functioning, although the ranges vary widely and the relative importance of these concerns has been disputed (Andersen, 1987; Auchincloss, 1989; Bos, 1986: Harris, Good, & Pollack, 1982).

The nature of treatment and physical alterations resulting from treatment can significantly affect sexual behavior (Auchincloss, 1989). Radiation therapy destroys ovarian function and induces menopause for premenopausal women. Vaginal irradiation may cause severe vaginal atrophy and stenosis (Andersen, Karlsson, Anderson, & Tewfik, 1984). In addition, tissue changes resulting from radiation can remain for 36 months following the treatment (Andersen, 1986). Changes in vaginal tissue result in the lack of vaginal lubrication and dyspareunia, or pain on intercourse (Andersen, 1986). Women with cervical cancer treated with irradiation experienced less sexual enjoyment, orgasmic ability, frequency of intercourse, and sexual dreams than women treated with surgery (Seibel, Freeman, & Graves, 1980).

Surgical treatment has also been found to be a factor in the decreased frequency of intercourse for women with gynecologic cancer and benign gynecologic disease (Andersen, Anderson, & deProsse, 1989a). Dramatic effects of surgical treatment can be seen in women with vulvar cancer. Surgical treatment for vulvar cancer can be mutilating and affect sexual arousal even though sexual desire is reported. In fact, 50%–90% of women with vulvar cancer who are treated with radical surgery report cessation of sexual activity (Andersen & Hacker, 1983a). Women who have been treated with pelvic exenteration may be managing two ostomies, surgical wounds from construction of a neovagina, discharge, pain, and bleeding (Cairns & Valentich, 1986). Adjuvant chemotherapy also produces loss of ovarian function and appearance concerns (Auchincloss, 1989).

The significance of gynecological organs, the age of the woman, and fears of pain during sexual activity may be additional considerations for women with gynecologic cancer. Some women may lose the ability to bear children. Older women may face bias about the diminished importance of sexuality, whether or not she has a partner (Shell, 1990). Fears of inadequacy as a sexual partner or feeling less "womanly" after treatment may be present (Shell, 1990). Importantly, physical changes such as fatigue and the expectation of pain during sexual activity have been shown to be factors in sexual functioning. Endometrial cancer patients reported a decrease in the frequency of intercourse and dissatisfaction with their sexual lives, partially related to physical discomfort (Cochran, Hacker, Wellisch, & Berek, 1987). Sexual functioning of the partner or concerns about hurting the woman may also contribute to dissatisfaction with sexual functioning (Andersen, Anderson, & deProsse, 1989a).

Studies of the sexual functioning of gynecologic cancer patients have been criticized for methodological weaknesses. Thomas (1987) detailed three weaknesses of a study by Andersen and Jochimsen (1985). The critique most salient to research in this area is the limited internal and external validity, since noncomparable control groups were used. However, the nature of gynecologic cancer and many topics of study in health psychology necessitates the use of quasiexperimental designs (Andersen & Jochimsen, 1987). These designs are an improvement compared with correlational or descriptive designs used in early studies of gynecologic cancer (Andersen & Hacker, 1983a). Another methodological difficulty is the lack of comparability of the norm groups (white, young, educated) of sexual assessment measures to women with gynecologic cancer (Andersen, 1986). Generalizability is also hindered by little or no racial or ethnic diversity within samples.

One might question the empirical attention sexual functioning has received in the literature. Since gynecologic cancer involves organs that are important for reproductive and sexual functioning and women report concerns about their sexual lives, this attention may be warranted. Some investigators believe, however, that previous research has focused more on the frequency of coitus and orgasms than on the quality of sexual relationships and intimacy between couples (Bos, 1986; Burbie & Polinsky, 1992). Further, the incidence of sexual dysfunction in women in general is not studied in relation to women with gynecologic cancer, perhaps making women with cancer seem more dysfunctional than women in general (Bos, 1986). Cairns and Valentich (1986) question whether vaginal reconstructive surgery is the ideal for some women, since it is based on the assumption that the capacity for vaginal–penile intercourse is the definition of sexual functioning and is recommended with little regard to a woman's age, sexual orientation, or developmental status.

A number of suggestions for talking to a woman and her partner about sexual function morbidity have been proposed (e.g., Andersen, 1985; Auchincloss, 1989: Burbie & Polinsky, 1992; Schover & Fife, 1986). Usually, these models contain an assessment of the couple's previous sexual relationship and current functioning. Difficulties in various stages of the female sexual response cycle are detailed by the type of treatment received in a publication by the American Cancer Society (Schover, 1991). This information may be shared with the woman and her partner. Different psychological interventions may be used for each stage of the sexual response cycle (Berek & Andersen, 1992). For women with gynecologic cancer, sexual difficulties may begin with the onset of cancer symptoms, such as postcoital bleeding and dyspareunia (Harris et al., 1982). Thus normal difficulties with lubrication after radiotherapy may be inaccurately associated with fears of disease recurrence (Andersen, 1985). Finally, recommendations can be made that fit with the difficulties of the couple (e.g., using lubrication, trying different positions, managing ostomies, working on intimacy apart from sexuality) (Shell, 1990). The diagnosis of cancer prompts some couples to reassess their priorities and the importance of an active sexual life. These couples may not report distress over changes in sexual activity and do not prefer intervention (Andersen, 1985).

Coping and Social Support

Although few studies have focused on coping strategies most helpful for women with gynecologic cancer, several generalizations can be made from the psychooncology literature. One consistent finding across studies of individuals with cancer is the increased efficacy of active as opposed to passive coping strategies (Rowland, 1989a). Psychologists can help individuals discover how they can increase active coping strategies, such as using more problem-solving behaviors. Professionals can help a patient negotiate her plan of care by first assisting in eliciting attributions about disease and treatments and then engaging in negotiation of available options and care. The process of negotiation is thought to increase the patient's perceptions of control over her care and encourage active participation (Krouse, 1990).

Increasing perceptions of control may be an important component of adopting an active stance toward disease. A sense of control was found to be adaptive in cancer patients, even when physical outcome was poor (Thompson, Sobolew-Shubin, Galbraith, Schwankovsky, & Cruzen, 1993). Although many individuals in this study felt they could not control the course of their disease, they found different domains in which they could exert control (e.g., symptoms, relationships with others, etc.). One caution is necessary when discussing the role of control and cancer patients. Individuals may be concerned that their treatment could be affected by normal depressed emotions due to an emphasis placed on positive emotions and healing in the popular press (Massie & Holland, 1989). An excellent moderate approach to cancer wellness can be found in Cella (1990).

Predictors of poor coping are: perceived or actual social isolation, low socioeconomic status, alcohol or drug abuse, previous psychiatric history, a history of recent losses, inflexibility and rigidity of coping, a pessimistic philosophy of life, and multiple obligations (Rowland, 1989a). Thus psychologists and mental health professionals should be aware of these characteristics and the possibility of early intervention for individuals with these characteristics.

Several authors have discussed social support and the importance of including family members in interventions (Gates, 1988; Holmes, 1987; Northouse & Northouse, 1987). Most authors advocate some formal or informal assessment process. According to Gates (1988), an important part of this process is the identification of the "most-significant other." Although this person is most often a husband, he/she could also be a parent, child, sibling, lover, friend, neighbor, or employer (Gates, 1988). In addition, social support from friends, coworkers, religious groups, community agencies, self-help groups, and health and mental health professionals has been shown to promote positive adjustment to cancer (e.g., Rowland, 1989b).

Psychologists and mental health workers can help the woman evaluate the quantity and quality of social support she receives from her social support network. Sometimes referrals to community self-help programs or health and welfare professionals are needed. Helping family members define their needs and communicate with each other can help increase the support felt by the woman with cancer (Northouse & Northouse, 1987).

The family and friends of the woman may want to be helpful, but may not know how. Informational brochures about how to talk with a woman with cancer is provided by some hospitals (e.g., Rowland, 1989b) and contain advice such as how to greet and talk to a person in the hospital, and how to know when to leave. Psychologists and mental health professionals can facilitate the assessment of the social support system, suggesting supplemental sources, and defining how to meet the woman's needs. Helping families communicate, acquire and process information, express their feelings, and cope with helplessness are important interventions (Northouse & Northouse, 1987).

Upon completion of treatment, counseling concerning the expectations of others and reentry into life may be helpful (Tross & Holland, 1989). Families may need instruction about how not to be overprotective of the woman. Not knowing what to tell employers or coworkers upon a return to work may also be a dilemma when women with cancer return to their job (Feldman, 1986). Practical advice from individuals who have undergone treatment for the same type of cancer can be very valuable to a woman at this point (Tross & Holland, 1989).

Psychologists working with women with gynecologic cancer and their families can make these interventions directly or help health professionals share information with all parties, communicate hope, and share control over uncertainty of the disease with the woman and her family (Northouse & Northouse, 1987). At some time it may also be necessary for the woman and her family to discuss the treatments and the quality of life which is most desired. Measuring the physical, psychological, social, and economic status of the woman and discussing these issues with family members is imperative (McCartney & Larson, 1987). Family members, as well as individuals with cancer, have found self-help groups beneficial (Lieberman, 1988) and may want a referral to such a group.

Psychologists can also intervene by assessing the woman's concrete service needs and by providing referrals to help them obtain services. Three areas of service needs have been found for individuals with advanced cancer: physical, instrumental, and administrative (Mor, Guadagnoli & Wool, 1987). Physical needs include aiding the individual in accomplishing physical tasks. Instrumental needs include meal preparation, housekeeping, and shopping. Administrative tasks involve completing financial and legal paperwork and obtaining information on illness and services (Mor et al., 1987). Although it is not practical for psychologists to provide each of these services, it is possible for psychologists to help the woman and her family strategize how best to meet these needs. Many questions still need to be answered about what types of social support are most helpful for whom and when these supports are most helpful. Close relationships and social support is an important area for possible intervention.

Issues in psychological intervention. There is no question that the diagnosis of cancer changes the lives of women and their families (Andersen, 1986). Designing psychological interventions for women with gynecologic cancer poses special challenges for the psychologist. In what areas is it most appropriate to intervene? When should these treatments be delivered? Should the woman with cancer, the couple, or the family be the focus of intervention?

Although no literature tests the outcomes of delivering these treatments at different times, most authors suggest that information and interventions performed "sooner" are "better," especially for women at high risk (e.g., Cairns & Valentich, 1986; Northouse & Northouse, 1987). Andersen (1987) suggested implementing preventive interventions for couples at high risk for sexual morbidity and rehabilitative services for women at lesser risk. Gates (1988) recommended a system of automatic referral for individuals who lack emotional support, have emotional difficulties, or have significant others with emotional problems. Evidence suggests that both women who are cured of gynecologic cancer and those who are not cured can benefit from psychotherapeutic interventions (e.g., Andersen & Tewfik, 1985; Bos-Branolte, Zielstra, Rijshouwer, & Duivenvoorden, 1988).

The individuality of each woman with gynecologic cancer must be considered when discussing psychological aspects of cancer. Not all women will have difficulties with body image or sexuality or any other aspect of adjusting to disease, treatment, and surviving with a history of gynecologic cancer. Nor can one psychological intervention or all psychological interventions be recommended for all women.

The inclusion of social environmental factors during and following medical treatment should be included in psychological interventions. Mental health professionals can educate physicians and medical support staff about the psychological and psychosocial needs of the woman and her family. Social support systems can also be analyzed and recommendations can be made.

Women with gynecologic cancer and their families are affected psychologically, socially, and economically by the diagnosis of cancer. Many decisions regarding treatment, quality of life, and future functioning must be made. Psychological and psychosocial difficulties can be a part of these women's experience. More research concerning the specific problems and effectiveness of interventions is needed in order for psychologists to provide the most effective services for these women.

REFERENCES

American Psychiatric Association (1987). *Diagnostic and statistical manual of mental disorders*. 3rd Edition–Revised. (DSM–III–R). Washington, DC: Author.

Andersen, B. L. (1985). Sexual functioning morbidity among cancer survivors: Present status and future research directions. *Cancer, 55*, 1835–1842.

Andersen, B. L. (1986). Sexual difficulties for women following cancer treatment. In B. L. Anderson (Ed.), *Women with cancer: Psychological perspectives* (pp. 257–288). New York: Springer-Verlag.

Andersen, B. L. (1987). Sexual functioning complications in women with gynecologic cancer: Outcome and directions for prevention. *Cancer, 60*, 2123–2128.

Andersen, B. L., Anderson, B., & deProsse, C. (1989a). Controlled prospective longitudinal study of women with cancer: I. Sexual functioning outcomes. *Journal of Consulting and Clinical Psychology, 57*, 683–691.

Andersen, B. L., Anderson, B., & deProsse, C. (1989b). Controlled prospective longitudinal study of women with cancer: II. Psychological outcomes. *Journal of Consulting and Clinical Psychology, 57*, 692–697.

Andersen, B. L., & Hacker, N. F. (1983a). Psychosexual adjustment after vulvar surgery. *Obstetrics & Gynecology, 62*, 457–462.

Andersen, B. L., & Hacker, N. F. (1983b). Psychosexual adjustment following pelvic exenteration. *Obstetrics and Gynecology, 61*, 331–338.

Andersen, B. L., & Jochimsen, P. R. (1985). Sexual functioning among breast cancer, gynecologic cancer, and healthy women. *Journal of Consulting and Clinical Psychology, 53*, 25–32.

Andersen, B. L., & Jochimsen, P. R. (1987). Research design and strategy for studying psychological adjustment to cancer: Reply to Thomas. *Journal of Consulting and Clinical Psychology, 55*, 122–124.

Andersen, B. L., Karlsson, J. A., Anderson, B. A. , & Tewfik, H. (1984). Anxiety and cancer treatment: Response to stressful radiotherapy. *Health Psychology, 3*, 535–551.

Andersen, B. L., & Tewfik, H. H. (1985). Psychological reactions to radiation therapy: Reconsideration of the adaptive aspects of anxiety. *Journal of Personality and Social Psychology, 48*, 1024–1032.

Andreasson, B., Moth, I., Buus Jensen, S., & Bock, J. E. (1986). Sexual function and somatopsychic reactions in vulvectomy-operated women and their partners. *Acta Obstetrica Gynecologica Scandinavica, 65*, 7–10.

Auchincloss, S. S. (1989). Sexual dysfunction in cancer patients: Issues in evaluation and treatment. In J. C. Holland & J. H. Rowland (Eds.), *Handbook of psychooncology: Psychological care of the patient with cancer* (pp. 383–413). New York: Oxford University Press.

Berek, J. S., & Andersen, B. L. (1992). Sexual rehabilitation: Surgical and psychological approaches. In W. J. Hoskins, C. A. Perez, & R. C. Young (Eds.), *Principles and practice of gynecologic oncology* (pp. 401–416). Philadelphia: J.B. Lippincott.

Boring, C. C., Squires, T. S., & Tong, T. (1991). Cancer statistics, 1991. *CA—A Cancer Journal for Clinicians, 41*, 19–36.

Bos, G. (1986). Sexuality of gynecologic cancer patients: Quantity and quality. *Journal of Psychosomatic Obstetrics and Gynaecology, 5*, 217–224.

Bos-Branolte, G., Zielstra, E. M., Rijshouwer, Y. M., & Duivenvoorden, H. J. (1988). Psychotherapy in patients cured of gynecological cancers. *Recent Results in Cancer Research, 108*, 277–288.

Bovbjerg, D. H., Redd, W. H., Maier, L. A., Holland, J. C., Lesko, L. M., Niedzwiecki, C., Rubin, S. C., & Hakes, T. B. (1990). Anticipatory immune suppression and nausea in women receiving cyclic chemotherapy for ovarian cancer. *Journal of Consulting and Clinical Psychology, 58*, 153–157.

Brinton, L. A., & Hoover, R. N. (1992). Epidemiology of gynecologic cancers. In W. J. Hoskins, C. A. Perez, & R. C. Young (Eds.), *Principles and practice of gynecologic oncology* (pp. 3–26). Philadelphia: J.B. Lippincott.

Burbie, G. E., & Polinsky, M. L. (1992). Intimacy and sexuality after cancer treatment: Restoring a sense of wholeness. *Journal of Psychosocial Oncology, 10*, 19–33.

Burish, T. G., & Lyles, J. N. (1981). Effectiveness of relaxation training in reducing adverse reactions to cancer chemotherapy. *Journal of Behavioral Medicine, 4*, 65–78.

Cain, E. N., Kohorn, E. I., Quinlan, D. M., Schwartz, P. E., Latimer, K., & Rogers, L. (1983). Psychosocial reactions to the diagnosis of gynecologic cancer. *Obstetrics and Gynecology, 62*, 635–641.

Cairns, K. V., & Valentich, M. (1986). Vaginal reconstruction in gynecologic cancer: A feminist perspective. *Journal of Sex Research, 22*, 333–346.

Cella, D. F. (1990). Health promotion in oncology: A cancer wellness doctrine. *Journal of Psychosocial Oncology, 8*(1), 17–30.

Cochran, S. D., Hacker, N. F., Wellisch, D. K., & Berek, J. S. (1987). Sexual functioning after treatment for endometrial cancer. *Journal of Psychosocial Oncology, 5*(3), 47–61.

Corney, R. H., Everett, H., Howells, A., & Crowther, M. E. (1992). Psychosocial adjustment following major gynaecological surgery for carcinoma of the cervix and vulva. *Journal of Psychosomatic Research, 36*, 561–568.

Derogatis, L. R., Morrow, G. R., Fetting, J., Penman, D., Piasetsky, S., Schmale, A. M., Henricho, M., & Carnicke, C.L.M. (1983). The prevalence of psychiatric disorders among cancer patients. *Journal of the American Medical Association, 249*, 751–757.

Feldman, F. L. (1987). Female cancer patients and caregivers: Experiences in the workplace. *Women & Health, 11*, 137–153.

Felton, B. J., & Revenson, T. A. (1984). Coping with chronic illness: A study of illness controllability and the influence of coping strategies on psychological adjustment. *Journal of Consulting and Clinical Psychology, 52*, 343–353.

Gates, C. C. (1988). The "most-significant-other" in the care of the breast cancer patient. *CA—A Cancer Journal for Clinicians, 38*, 146–153.

Golden, R. N., McCartney, C. F., Haggerty, J. J., Raft, D., Nemeroff, C. B., Ekstrom, D., Holmes, V., Simon, J. S., Droba, M., Quade, D., Fowler, W. C., & Evans, D. L. (1991). The detection of depression by patient self-report in women with gynecologic cancer. *International Journal of Psychiatry in Medicine, 21*, 17–27.

Gotay, C. C. (1984). The experience of cancer during early and advanced stages: The views of patients and their mates. *Social Science and Medicine, 18*, 605–613.

Griffiths, C. T., Parker, L. M., & Fuller, A. F. (1979). Role of cytoreductive surgical treatment in the management of advanced ovarian cancer. *Cancer Treatment Reports, 63*, 235–243.

Gusberg, S. B. (1986). Cancer of the female reproductive tract. In A. I. Holeb, G. J. Subak-Sharpe, W. H. White, & P. Kasofsky (Eds.), *The American Cancer Society cancer book: Prevention, diagnosis, treatment, rehabilitation, cure* (pp. 479–508). New York: Doubleday & Company.

Hacker, N. F. (1986). Vulvar and vaginal cancer. In N. F. Hacker & J. G. Moore (Eds.), *Essentials of obstetrics and gynecology*, (pp. 498–508). Philadelphia: W. B. Saunders.

Harris, R., Good, R. S., & Pollack, L. (1982). Sexual behavior of gynecologic cancer patient. *Archives of Sexual Behavior, 11*, 503–510.

Holland, J. C. (1989a). Clinical course of cancer. In J. C. Holland & J. H. Rowland (Eds.), *Handbook of psychooncology: Psychological care of the patient with cancer* (pp. 75–100; 134–135). New York: Oxford University Press.

Holland, J. C. (1989b). Radiotherapy. In J. C. Holland & J. H. Rowland (Eds.), *Handbook of psychooncology: Psychological care of the patient with cancer* (pp. 134–145). New York: Oxford University Press.

Holmes, B. C. (1987). Psychological evaluation and preparation of the patient and family. *Cancer, 60*, 2021–2024.

Karlsson, J. A., & Andersen, B. L. (1986). Radiation therapy and psychological distress in gynecologic oncology patients: Outcomes and recommendations for enhancing adjustment. *Journal of Psychosomatic Obstetrics and Gynecology, 5*, 283–294.

Kennedy, A. W., Flagg, J. S., & Webster, K. D. (1989). Gynecologic cancer in the very elderly. *Gynecologic Oncology, 32*, 49–54.

Krouse, H. J. (1990). Psychological adjustment of women to gynecologic cancers. *NAACOGS Clinical Issues in Perinatal and Women's Health Nursing, 1*, 495–512.

Lichtman, R. R., & Taylor, S. E. (1986). Close relationships and the female cancer patient. In B. L. Andersen (Ed.), *Women with cancer: Psychological perspectives* (pp. 233–256). New York: Springer-Verlag.

Lieberman, M. A. (1988). The role of self-help groups in helping patients and families cope with cancer. *CA—A Cancer Journal for Clinicians, 38,* 163–168.

Massie, M. J., & Holland, J. C. (1989). Overview of normal reactions and prevalence of psychiatric disorders. In J. C. Holland & J. H. Rowland (Eds.), *Handbook of psychooncology: Psychological care of the patient with cancer* (pp. 273–282). New York: Oxford University Press.

McCartney, C. F., Cahill, P., Larson, D. B., Lyons, J. S., Wada, C. Y., & Pincus, H. A. (1989). Effect of a psychiatric liaison program on consultation rates and on detection of minor psychiatric disorders in cancer patients. *American Journal of Psychiatry, 146,* 898–901.

McCartney, C. F., & Larson, D. B. (1987). Quality of life in patients with gynecologic cancer. *Cancer, 60,* 2129–2136.

Mor, V., Guadagnoli, E., & Wool, M. (1987). An examination of the service needs of advanced cancer patients. *Journal of Psychosocial Oncology, 5*(3), 1–17.

Morrow, C. P., Curtin, J. P., & Townsend, D. E. (Eds.) (1993). *Synopsis of gynecologic oncology* (4th ed.). New York: Churchill Livingstone.

Nail, L. M., King, K. B., & Johnson, J. E. (1986). Coping with radiation treatment for gynecologic cancer: Mood disruption in usual function. *Journal of Psychosomatic Obstetrics and Gynaecology, 5,* 271–281.

Nelson, J. H., Averette, H. E., & Richart, R. M. (1984). Dysplasia, carcinoma in situ, and early invasive cervical carcinoma. *CA—A Cancer Journal for Clinicians, 34,* 306–327.

Northouse, P. G., & Northouse, L. L. (1987). Communication and cancer: Issues confronting patients, health professionals, and family members. *Journal of Psychosocial Oncology, 5*(3), 17–46.

Payne, S. A. (1990). Coping with palliative chemotherapy. *Journal of Advanced Nursing, 15,* 652–658.

Redd, W. H. (1988). Behavioral approaches to treatment-related distress. *CA—A Cancer Journal for Clinicians, 38,* 138–145.

Rowland, J. H. (1989a). Intrapersonal resources: Coping. In J. C. Holland & J. H. Rowland (Eds.), *Handbook of psychooncology: Psychological care of the patient with cancer* (pp. 44–57). New York: Oxford University Press.

Rowland, J. H. (1989b). Interpersonal resources: Social support. In J. C. Holland & J. H. Rowland (Eds.), *Handbook of psychooncology: Psychological care of the patient with cancer* (pp. 58–71). New York: Oxford University Press.

Sales E., Schultz, R., & Biegel, D. (1992). Predictors of strain in families of cancer patients: A review of the literature. *Journal of Psychosocial Oncology, 10*(2), 1–26.

Schover, L. R. (1991). *Sexuality and cancer for the woman who has cancer, and her partner.* New York: American Cancer Society.

Schover, L. R., & Fife, M. (1986). Sexual counseling of patients undergoing radical surgery for pelvic or genital cancer. *Journal of Psychosocial Oncology, 3*(3), 21–41.

Seibel, M. M., Freeman, M. G., & Graves, W. L. (1980). Carcinoma of the cervix and sexual function. *Obstetrics and Gynecology, 55,* 484–487.

Sewell, H. H., & Edwards, D. W. (1980). Pelvic genital cancer: Body image and sexuality. *Frontiers in Radiation Therapy and Oncology, 14*, 35–41.

Shell, J. A. (1990). Sexuality for patients with gynecologic cancer. *NAACOGS Clinical Issues in Perinatal and Women's Health Nursing, 1*, 479–494.

Silverberg, E., & Lubera, J. (1989). Cancer statistics. *CA—A Cancer Journal for Clinicians, 39*, 3–20.

Smith, E. M., Redman, R., Burns, T. L., & Sagert, K. M. (1986). Perceptions of social support among patients with recently diagnosed breast, endometrial, and ovarian cancer: An exploratory study. *Journal of Psychosocial Oncology, 3*(3), 65–81.

Taylor, S. E. (1983). Adjustment to threatening events: A theory of cognitive adaptation. *American Psychologist, 38*, 1161–1173.

Thomas, J. (1987). Problems in a study of the sexual response of women with cancer: Comment on Andersen and Jochimsen. *Journal of Consulting and Clinical Psychology, 55*, 120–121.

Thompson, S. C., Sobolew-Shubin, A., Galbraith, M. E., Schwankovsky, L., & Cruzen, D. (1993). Maintaining perceptions of control: Finding perceived control in low-control circumstances. *Journal of Personality and Social Psychology, 64*, 293–304.

Tross, S., & Holland, J. C. (1989). Psychological sequelae in cancer survivors. In J. C. Holland & J. H. Rowland (Eds.), *Handbook of psychooncology: Psychological care of the patient with cancer* (pp. 101–116). New York: Oxford University Press.

Wenzel, L., Berkowitz, R., Robinson, S. Bernstein, M., & Goldstein, D. (1992). The psychological, social, and sexual consequences of gestational trophoblastic disease. *Gynecologic Oncology, 46*, 74–81.

Whale, Z. (1991, March). A threat to femininity?: Minimizing side-effects in pelvic irradiation. *Professional Nurse*, 309–312.

Wortman, C. B., & Dunkel-Schetter, C. (1979). Interpersonal relationships and cancer: A theoretical analysis. *Journal of Social Issues, 35*, 120–155.

Yazigi, R. (1989). Early diagnosis of gynecologic cancer. *Texas Medicine, 85*, 42–45.

7

Contraception

Kristen K. Brewer

Contraception is important to virtually all heterosexually active women, and has been throughout history (Zatuchni, 1989). A woman may want to prevent pregnancy for any number of reasons. She may not be financially or emotionally prepared to have a child. She may have a career, and choose to delay having children until later in life, or she may not want any children at all. Motherhood is no longer necessary to womanhood. Therefore, birth control can assist a woman in the timing of pregnancy so that when it does occur, she will be ready for it.

Contraception is also important in the context of two significant social problems. One is sexually transmitted diseases (STDs), and AIDS in particular. While abstinence is the only sure way of preventing the sexual transmission of these diseases, some forms of contraception, especially the condom, can greatly reduce the risk (Greydanus & Lonchamp, 1990).

Teenage pregnancy is another important health and social problem. American adolescents are engaging in more premarital sex at an earlier age than ever before (Fisher, Byrne, Edwards, Miller, Kelly, & White, 1979). Frequently this sexual activity results in undesired pregnancy, which can pose a serious health risk in addition to the emotional and social implications (see Chapter 15).

In addition to these specific problem areas, it is widely accepted that about 50% of all pregnancies are unintended. This chapter will address some of the psychological and practical contraceptive issues facing women and their health care providers, including research findings in this area.

CONTRACEPTIVE METHODS

Following are brief descriptions of birth control methods, along with some relevant characteristics of each.

Sterilization

Female sterilization involves a surgical procedure during which the fallopian tubes are blocked or severed so that sperm cannot pass and fertilize an ovum. This is considered permanent, although reversal of sterilization is possible in many cases (Papera, 1990). Most reversal procedures are less than 50% successful, although when clips have been used to clamp off the fallopian tubes, without actually cutting them, reversibility can increase to 90% (Rioux, 1989). Complications of the sterilization procedure are rare, occurring in less than 4% of cases, and can include bleeding, uterine perforation, or bowel trauma (Porter, Waife, & Holtrop, 1983). The main advantage of sterilization is that it is a very effective method of birth control that does not require any activity on the part of either partner once the procedure is performed.

Oral Contraceptives

"The pill" is the most widely prescribed medication today (Steinberg, 1989). It contains a combination of estrogen and progestin, now at much lower doses than when first introduced in the 1950s. The combination pill works primarily by suppressing ovulation; it also changes the cervical mucus, making it resistant to penetration by sperm, and alters the uterine lining, making the implantation of a fertilized egg more difficult (Clarke, 1990). The risks associated with taking the pill are actually quite small, especially with the newer low-dose pills. When evaluating the risks and benefits of taking the pill, it is important to remember that most studies were carried out using the higher-dose pills (Ellsworth & Leversee, 1990). Women taking the low-dose pill may have slightly increased risk of thromboembolic disease, hypertension, stroke, myocardial infarction, and hepatic and breast neoplasia (Steinberg, 1989). Far more common, but less severe side effects include headache, acne, breast tenderness, weight gain, nausea, and breakthrough bleeding (Shearin & Boehlke, 1989). There is strong evidence that the pill also has many noncontraceptive benefits, including the regulation of menstrual flow, and the reduction of the risk of ovarian cancer, endometrial cancer, benign breast disease, ovarian cysts, pelvic inflammatory disease, dysmenorrhea, and anemia (Hankinson et al., 1992; Kaunitz, 1992; Steinberg, 1989). Some of these benefits can last for up to ten years after discontinuation of the pill (Steinberg, 1989). There are certain instances when oral contraceptives are contraindicated. Absolute contraindications include thromboembolic disease, stroke, coronary artery disease, liver disease, pregnancy, and cancer of the breasts or reproductive system (Porter et al., 1983). Relative contraindications, those for which the prescribing physician must evaluate each case individually, include significant hypertension, severe migraine, age over 45, cervical dysplasia, diabetes, and gall bladder disease (Ellsworth & Leversee, 1990; Porter et al., 1983). In general, the pill should not be prescribed for women over the age of 35 who smoke.

There is also a progestin-only pill known as the "mini-pill." Although the mini-pill is not widely used, it may be an option for women who are unable to take the estrogen found in the combined pill (Shearin & Boehlke, 1989). These women may include those who are breast-feeding (Chi, Robbins, & Balogh, 1992), diabetics, and women with hypertension (Greydanus & Lonchamp, 1990).

Oral contraceptives have the advantage of being a very effective and reversible form of contraception. Because the pill is not coitus-dependent, it does not interfere with sexual spontaneity, though the woman does have to remember to take it at roughly the same time every day in order for it to be effective.

Vaginal Spermicides

Spermicides can come in many forms including jellies, creams, suppositories, foaming tablets, and aerosol foams. They can be used alone or in combination with the barrier contraception methods. Vaginal spermicides generally contain nonoxynol–9, which inactivates sperm, and an inert substance, which disperses the nonoxynol–9 in the vagina and provides a partial barrier to sperm (Porter et al., 1983). Vaginal spermicides can be purchased without a prescription, act as a lubricant during intercourse, and the nonoxynol–9 may provide some protection against STDs, including HIV (Bounds, 1989). This method is generally less effective than other contraceptives and is seen by many women as inconvenient because the spermicide must be applied before each intercourse and because the spermicide remains effective for a relatively short period of time.

Diaphragm

The diaphragm is a small dome-shaped rubber device that fits across the upper vagina, covering the cervix and creating a partial barrier to sperm as well as serving as a carrier for spermicide (Delvin & Barwin, 1989). The diaphragm should be filled with spermicide and inserted before intercourse and must be left in place for at least six hours following intercourse. Additional spermicide must be applied before each additional act of intercourse (Delvin & Barwin, 1989). A woman must be professionally fitted for a diaphragm, which is available in a wide range of sizes. Refitting may be required after significant weight loss or gain or after pregnancy (Greydanus & Lonchamp, 1990).

Cervical Cap

The cervical cap is a thimble-shaped latex device about half the size of a diaphragm (Greydanus & Lonchamp, 1990). Usually used with a spermicide, it fits tightly around the cervix by suction and prevents sperm from entering the cervix (Delvin & Barwin, 1989). The cervical cap has much in common with the diaphragm, with a few important differences. The cap can be left in place longer, requires less spermicide, and need not be refit after a weight change (Corsaro & Lichtman, 1990). However, not all women will be able to be fitted with a cervical cap, because only four sizes are currently available (Delvin & Barwin, 1989).

Vaginal Contraceptive Sponge

The sponge is dome-shaped, fits over the cervix much like the cap or diaphragm, and contains nonoxynol–9. Adding two tablespoons of water before insertion activates the spermicide. The sponge works in three ways: a) it is a physical barrier to sperm; b) the spermicide inactivates sperm; and c) the sponge absorbs semen (Eichhorst, 1988). This method has the advantage of being available without a prescription and does not require fitting. The sponge may be inserted up to 24 hours before intercourse, so it does not interfere with sexual spontaneity, and it is effective for an unlimited number of coital acts without adding spermicide (Bounds, 1989). Studies generally indicate that the sponge offers some protection against the transmission of HIV and other STDs (Rosenberg, Davidson, Chen, Judson, & Douglas, 1992), although there have been reports to the contrary (Kreiss et al., 1992). Reports of toxic shock syndrome have been associated with sponge use, but it seems that the risk is very small and can be reduced if the sponge is not left in for more than 24 hours and is not used during menstruation (Greydanus & Lonchamp, 1990).

Condom

The condom is a latex sheath that is rolled onto the erect penis and works by preventing the ejaculate from entering the vagina. Condoms are widely available and perhaps one of the most well-known methods of birth control. An important advantage of the condom is that it provides the best protection against STDs, especially condoms with nonoxynol–9 (Greydanus & Lonchamp, 1990). However, some couples complain that condoms interfere with sexual spontaneity or reduce sensation (Eichhorst, 1988). An important consideration for women is that the cooperation of the male partner is essential.

The female condom has recently become available. This is a loose-fitting polyurethane sheath with two flexible rings, one at either end. The smaller ring (found at the closed end) is inserted over the cervix much like a diaphragm and the larger ring remains outside the vagina (Kulig, 1989). It can be inserted any time prior to intercourse, is available without a prescription, and is estimated to be as effective as the male condom (Franklin, 1990). In recent trials, women generally reported favorable attitudes toward the female condom, especially because it enables women to have more control over their own protection than they have with the male condom (Gregersen & Gregersen, 1990; Shilling, El-Bassel, Leeper, & Freeman, 1991). On the other hand, common complaints about the female condom have been that it is too big, messy, inconvenient, and difficult to insert (Sakondhavat, 1990).

Intrauterine Device (IUD)

The IUD is a small plastic device with nylon threads attached which is inserted into the uterus by a medical professional, and is effective for up to eight years. There are two types of IUDs available in the United States: the Progestasert, which releases progesterone, and the Paraguard (copper T), which contains copper. The mechanism by which they prevent pregnancy is unclear, but it is generally believed that two processes are at work. First, having a foreign body in the uterus causes an inflammatory response, making the lining of the uterus inhospitable to the implantation of an ovum. Second, both the progesterone and the copper ions released by IUDs increase the viscosity of the cervical mucus, making it more difficult for sperm to penetrate (Tatum & Connell, 1989). The IUD is very effective and it does not affect sexual spontaneity. Several side effects have been associated with the IUD, including pain during insertion, perforation of the uterine wall, cramping, bleeding, and an increased risk of pelvic inflammatory disease (Clarke, 1990). Most of these problems occur only in rare cases, although cramping and breakthrough bleeding are more common, especially in the first few months after insertion (Tatum & Connell, 1989).

Norplant

This device consists of six capsules filled with the progestin levonorgestrel (Shoupe & Mishell, 1989). The capsules are implanted subdermally in the woman's arm during a short surgical procedure under local anesthesia (Eichhorst, 1988). Levonorgestrel is released gradually, providing contraception for five years by suppressing ovulation and changing the cervical mucus so that penetration by sperm is less likely (Shoupe & Mishell, 1989). Norplant's possible side effects include changes in bleeding patterns, headaches, acne, and breast discharge (Shoupe & Mishell, 1989). This method offers the advantage of being an extremely effective and reversible contraceptive without the problem of compliance.

Injectables

Depot medroxyprogesterone acetate (DMPA or Depo Provera), the most common long-acting injectable, has only recently been approved for widespread contraceptive use in the United States, although it has been used worldwide for over ten years (Shearin & Boehlke, 1989). DMPA contains a progestin and is given every three months (Franklin, 1990). This method is very effective, long-lasting, and reversible. However, some side effects are common: menstrual changes are universal and often unpredictable, except that amenorrhea becomes increasingly common with duration of use; some women experience headache, dizziness, bloating of the abdomen or breasts, mood changes, and weight gain (Kaunitz, 1989).

Periodic Abstinence

This method is also known as the *rhythm method* or natural family planning and prevents pregnancy by allowing the woman to identify the time in her cycle during which she is most fertile, so that intercourse can be avoided. Natural family planning involves three activities, used separately or in combination. With the calendar method, the woman avoids sex during the time she is likely to be ovulating, days 10–19 of her cycle for a woman with 28–30 day cycles (Eichhorst, 1988). The basal body temperature will rise $1/2$–1 degree F as an indicator of ovulation (Greydanus & Lonchamp, 1990). In the Billing ovulation method, the woman watches for changes in her cervical mucus; during her fertile period there will be an increase in mucus and it will be clear and stretchy (Eichhorst, 1988). Periodic abstinence may be the method of choice for those women who object to artificial methods for religious or other reasons. However, this method involves careful planning and self-control on the part of both partners in order to be effective. Also, some women, especially after pregnancy and menarche and before menopause, do not have regular cycles, so watching the calendar will not help them to know when they are ovulating.

Withdrawal

Also known as *coitus interruptus*, the male withdraws his penis from the vagina before ejaculation so that semen is not deposited in the vagina. Withdrawal is not usually considered an effective method of contraception, because of the presence of sperm in the preejaculatory fluid (Kulig, 1989).

PSYCHOLOGICAL ISSUES

Research on the psychological aspects of contraception has focused largely on adolescents and young adults; therefore that is where this section will be focused. When looking at this body of research it is important to note that samples are generally nonrandom and unrepresentative, consisting of mostly white, middle-class subjects. Most studies utilize relatively accessible clinic and university populations. An additional problem that contributes to unrepresentative samples in studies of adolescents is that parents are often reluctant to give consent for their children to participate in studies having to do with sex, the concern being that this will lead the teens to engage in more sexual behaviors.

Information Sources

One topic that has been investigated is where adolescents get information about contraception. The media is not an unimportant source. While American teens view thousands of sexual references and behaviors on television each year (Strasburger, 1989), they see little to do with contraception or sexually transmitted diseases. Television may be the first time that children get a glimpse of sex, and they get a very unrealistic view. On television contraception is rarely mentioned, and characters almost never become pregnant or contract STDs (Lowry & Towles, 1989). Basically, television gives the impression that sex should be spontaneous and unplanned. Many adolescents may believe that what they see on television is real, and they may use it as a model for their own behavior. However, since AIDS has become a problem, some television shows have begun addressing the issue of contraception. It is interesting to note that even though teenage pregnancy has been recognized as a problem for years, it has taken a problem with life-or-death consequences for the networks to stop censoring references to contraception.

People are also an important source of contraception information for adolescents, although one consistent finding of descriptive studies is that parents are usually the least important source (Morrison, 1985). Peers, physicians, and educators are consistently cited as more important (Milan & Kilman, 1987). One factor may be that parents, even when they do talk to their children about contraception, are vague and do not discuss specific methods. The information that is reaching adolescents from various sources is apparently inadequate, because at least half of all adolescents have inaccurate beliefs about the onset of fertility, the timing of fertile periods within a woman's cycle, or the magnitude of risk involved in unprotected intercourse (Morrison, 1985).

One suggestion for educating adolescents has been to use computer games with realistic situations requiring decision making. Paperney and Starn (1989) have designed two computer games to educate teens about the realities of having a baby and about contraception. Both games provide factual information and correct common misconceptions using an interactive/responsive format. Initial research on the utility of these games has yielded positive results. From pre- to posttest, subjects using the games showed significant improvements in knowledge and attitudes about pregnancy and contraception. Educational programs like this may be effective for many reasons: adolescents do not have to actually talk to anyone about sensitive topics which may be embarrassing for them; they have exposure to real-life situations and the possible consequences of their decisions, without having to live with those consequences; and because it is in the form of a game it may be seen as fun. Educational games may be better at holding adolescents' attention than reading pamphlets or listening to someone talk.

Predictors of Contraceptive Nonuse

In addition to the lack of accurate information, there are a number of other reasons that sexually active teens do not use contraception. Teens give many reasons for nonuse including: they just do not like it, they find it embarrassing, it is messy, it interferes with enjoyment, they have religious objections to using it, they believe that contraception is dangerous, or they just feel that the other partner is responsible (Morrison, 1985).

Correlational studies have attempted to identify predictors of contraceptive behavior. Personality variables hypothesized to be associated with contraceptive behavior include locus of control and self-esteem. The hypothesis with respect to locus of control is that an internal locus of control should predict more responsible contraceptive behavior, and someone with an external locus of control would be more likely to leave herself in the hands of fate. In fact, this variable has been shown to discriminate between users and nonusers of contraception, with an internal locus of control being associated with users. However, locus of control is not related to the effectiveness of the method chosen or consistency of use (Morrison, 1985).

There is not much evidence that self-esteem is a useful predictor. The hypothesized relation is that women with higher self-esteem will be more likely to assume responsibility for contraception as a consequence of being better able to acknowledge their sexuality and needing less social approval. However, studies addressing this variable have had inconclusive results (Morrison, 1985).

Sex guilt has consistently been associated with less frequent contraceptive use, nonuse at last intercourse, and less effective use (Strassberg & Mahoney, 1988). If adolescents feel guilty about having sex, they are less likely to plan for it, and contraception requires planning ahead. This perspective suggests that just telling teens that premarital sex is wrong may contribute to irresponsible sex. If they go ahead and engage in sexual activity anyway, they may be more likely to feel guilty about it if they have been convinced that it is wrong, and therefore be less likely to use birth control.

Sex guilt is very similar to the construct of erotophobia (Fisher, Byrne, & White, 1983), which refers to negative emotional response to sexual cues. Byrne (1983) has identified five steps in acquiring and using contraception, each of which may be seen as a sexual cue: a) acquire, process, and retain accurate contraceptive information; b) acknowledge the likelihood of engaging in sexual intercourse; c) obtain the relevant contraceptive; d) communicate with the sexual partner about contraception; and e) utilize the chosen method of contraception. Byrne argues that because each of these steps is, in itself, a sexual cue, erotophobes will be less likely to perform each step. Byrne and his colleagues found that subjects scoring high on their erotophobia–erotophilia scale were less likely to possess accurate information about conception and contraception, acknowledge the possibility that they may have intercourse in the near future, communicate with their sexual partners, or use contraception consistently (Fisher et al., 1983). Erotophobes also have more negative attitudes toward contraception in general, when compared with erotophilic subjects (those having a more positive emotional response to sexual cues).

Another concept related to contraceptive nonuse is what has been termed the illusion of unique invulnerability (Perloff & Fetzer, 1986). To some extent, everyone seems to have this misconception that bad things only happen to other people, but it is even more common among adolescents. Burger and Burns (1988) found that a teen who estimates the probability that she will become pregnant as less than that of others is less likely to use effective birth control. One possible explanation is that the thought that she might become pregnant causes anxiety, so she convinces herself that she will not, thereby reducing the anxiety. Another possible explanation is that she may have a stereotypical image of an unwed mother which does not resemble the image she has of herself (Burger & Burns, 1988). A more recent study (Whitley & Hern, 1991) replicated the finding that young women tend to estimate their own likelihood of becoming pregnant as lower than that of others. However, unlike Burger and Burns (1988), these researchers found that the less likely a woman perceived herself to become pregnant, the *more* likely she was to use effective contraception (Whitley & Hern, 1991).

Communication is also related to contraceptive use. First, there is a consistent positive relation between communication within the sexual dyad and effective use of contraception (Morrison, 1985). In addition, it has been shown that communication between mothers and daughters is related to consistent birth control use (Kotva & Schneider, 1990).

Decision Making and Contraceptive Use

Other researchers have attempted to apply decision making models to contraceptive decisions. Fishbein's attitude model (Ajzen & Fishbein, 1980) states that behavior is best predicted by intention, which is a function of both the attitude toward performing the act and normative beliefs about the act. Research generally supports this model (e.g., Adler, Kegeles, Irwin, & Wibblesman, 1990). In a study extending this model to contraceptive attitude change, McCarty (1981) found that using a persuasive message about the advantages of a particular birth control method not only changed subjects' attitudes toward a method, but also their intentions to use that method.

Luker (1975) applied a model of subjective expected utility to contraceptive decision making. According to this model, what the individual perceives as the costs and benefits of each option will determine the decision made. It is important that the perceived costs and benefits are considered—researchers often mistakenly assume that using contraception has many benefits and few costs, whereas nonuse has many costs and few benefits (Luker, 1975). Teenagers especially may focus on the immediate instead of long-term costs and benefits. They may see the inconvenience of using contraception much more clearly than the relatively distant possibility of getting pregnant. The probabilities associated with each outcome are also subjective. The actual probability that one will become pregnant in a particular instance of intercourse is relatively low and may be perceived as even lower by an adolescent who is uninformed or who has been "getting away with it" for a while already.

While males generally have more decision-making power in dyadic relationships, this is not the case when it comes to contraception. Gerrard, Breda, and Gibbons (1990) asked both partners of the sexual dyad individually about their preferred methods of contraception and then asked about actual use. Actual contraceptive practice was much closer to what the females had said was preferred. This may not be surprising, given that women tend to know more factual information about contraception, most methods are used by the woman, and men cannot get pregnant. It is in the best interest of the woman to make sure that birth control is used, since she has more at stake.

Sexually Transmitted Diseases (STDs)

An issue that has only recently been addressed in the research literature is contraception and the prevention of HIV and other STDs. It appears that most adolescents are aware of AIDS, but some do not know that sexual intercourse is a mode of transmitting HIV, and even more do not know that using a condom can decrease the risk of transmission (Rickert, Jay, Gottlieb, & Bridges, 1989). Even those who are knowledgeable about the risk of HIV are not likely to alter their behavior. This may be another instance of the illusion of unique invulnerability.

One focus of the attempt to prevent the spread of HIV is to change attitudes toward condoms, in order to increase their use. Tanner and Pollack (1988) demonstrated that receiving erotic condom instructions improved attitudes toward condoms for subjects of both sexes. The authors hypothesize that contraception is usually associated with punishment (pregnancy and disease), and we should try to change this so that it is instead associated with sexual pleasure. This idea is congruent with the concept of erotophobia (Fisher et al., 1983).

Recently, Bandura (1990) has proposed a self-efficacy model of safer sex practices, in which sexual risk reduction is related to an individual's belief that he or she has the ability to effectively carry out the safer behavior. Wulfert and Wan (1993) applied this model to condom use and found that self-efficacy did indeed predict condom use, while sexual attitudes, AIDS knowledge, and perceived vulnerability did not.

CLINICAL CONSIDERATIONS

Many women, even after deciding to seek contraceptive advice, may be hesitant. Establishing rapport with the woman is an important first step. Confidentiality is a concern for many women; this is why women's clinics are so popular, especially for adolescents, who are often afraid that a family member will find out if they seek contraceptives from the family doctor. From the beginning it is important to ensure confidentiality in order to make the woman feel more at ease.

Education is the next step. Young women are usually misinformed about reproduction and fertility. Many young women believe that they cannot become pregnant the first time they have intercourse. They are also misinformed about the timing of fertility in the menstrual cycle. Correcting these misconceptions needs to be done as soon as possible, preferably before the young woman is sexually active, because half of all premarital pregnancies occur in the first six months of sexual activity (Zabin, Kantner, & Zelnik, 1979).

Jay, DuRant, and Litt (1989) report an increase in teen pregnancies even among those considered to be contraceptive users. They suggest the following reasons for this: use of unreliable methods of birth control, contraceptive method switching, and noncompliance. These are areas in which service providers might focus their efforts in educating adolescents.

Women approaching menopause may also have special contraceptive concerns. While these women are not as fertile as younger women, the occurrence of anovulatory cycles is unpredictable (Jarrett & Lethbridge, 1990) and the risks associated with pregnancy are greater (Fortney, 1987). About 40% of women over forty are protected by contraceptive sterilization, but there remains a large number who need other forms of birth control (Fortney, 1987). For these women using other methods, it is generally recommended that they continue to use contraception for two years after cessation of menses if it occurs before age 49 and for one year if it occurs after age 50 (Jarrett & Lethbridge, 1990).

For a woman of any age, written information (e.g., pamphlets), in language she can understand, may be useful. A woman should be aware of all of the contraceptive options available to her, as well as important facts about each. Once she has this information, she may need assistance sorting through it all. When trying to match a woman with the best form of birth control for her, important considerations include effectiveness, contraindications, whether she is at risk for STDs, frequency of intercourse, and motivation to comply.

A common concern is how effective a method will be at preventing pregnancy (Harvey, Beckman, & Murray, 1991). Table 7.1 lists failure rates for the various methods. Contraception efficacy studies can be difficult to interpret, because results vary widely from study to study. Results can be influenced by the sample used, which is usually self-selected, and by how long the women have been using the method being tested. Most failure rates decline with duration of use, probably because more experience with a method leads to more correct use (Trussel et al., 1990). This brings up another important effectiveness issue. Contraception is much more effective if it is used correctly and consistently. Unfortunately, this is not always the case. Therefore a distinction is often made between theoretical effectiveness and use effectiveness. "Theoretical effectiveness" refers to how effective a method would be if it were used perfectly every time, while "use effectiveness" is how effective a method is in actual use, given that not everyone uses it perfectly.

What constitutes "acceptable" effectiveness varies according to the individual. It is more important to some women that they not become pregnant than it is to other women, and therefore effectiveness will be of different levels of importance for different women. For example, for a married woman planning on having children in the near future, effectiveness probably is not as important an issue as it is for an unwed adolescent who is not in a serious relationship, or for the woman who may suffer a serious health consequence as a result of pregnancy.

Contraindications and safety of methods are also important in choosing a contraceptive method (Harvey et al., 1991). Contraindications to using the pill are listed earlier in this chapter. In addition, there are physical reasons that a woman may not be able to use some of the other methods. For example, she or her partner may have an allergy to nonoxynol–9 or to the rubber of which diaphragms are made. And because the cervical cap is available in only a few sizes, not all women will be able to be fitted.

The risk of HIV infection and other STDs increases as the number of partners increases, and becomes even greater if the partners are at risk. All women, but especially those at risk, should be educated about the transmission of STDs and

TABLE 7.1 Lowest Expected and Typical Percentages of Accidental Pregnancy in the United States during the First Year of Use of a Method (adapted from Trussel et al., 1990)

	% Accidental Pregnancy	
Method	Lowest	Typical
Chance	85	85
Sterilization	0.2	0.4
Pill	0.1	3
Periodic abstinence	*	20
calendar	9	*
ovulation method	3	*
sympto-thermal	2	*
Withdrawal	4	18
Spermicides	3	21
Diaphragm	6	18
Cervical cap	6	18
Sponge		
parous women	9	28
nulliparous women	6	18
Condom	2	12
IUD		
Progestasert	2	3
copper T	0.8	*
Norplant	0.04	0.04
Depo Provera	0.3	0.3

Note. Figures for the cervical cap and diaphragm are when used with spermicide; figures for the condom are without spermicide; sympto-thermal refers to the ovulation method supplemented by the calendar and basal body temperature methods.

* Data not available.

ways to reduce the risk. Contraceptives utilizing the spermicide nonoxynol–9 offer some protection against STDs, but condoms are the best protection because they prevent the exchange of bodily fluids. Female condoms protect in the same way.

A woman having intercourse only infrequently does not need contraception continuously and therefore may opt for a coitus-dependent method. On the other hand, a woman engaging in frequent intercourse may find it inconvenient to have to deal with contraceptives for every coital act, in which case she might prefer a method that offers continuous protection and is not directly connected to coitus (e.g., the pill, IUD, Norplant).

Some methods require more motivation and/or planning than others. In order to be a successful contraceptor, a woman must remember to take a pill every day, use a condom/diaphragm/sponge whenever she has intercourse, or be strict about abstaining during her fertile period. When a health care professional suspects that a woman may not be able or likely to comply with these contraceptive regimens, methods requiring less motivation should be considered. The IUD and Norplant are very effective options which require virtually nothing of the woman once in place.

Jay and colleagues (1989) have made several suggestions for improving compliance, including establishing a good relationship with the patient, providing her with a thorough explanation of the contraceptive, and reducing barriers to compliance such as long waiting times or inconvenient hours. Cost can be another barrier, especially for adolescents. Norplant, in particular, is quite expensive initially, so may not be an option for many women.

A group of women with special needs are the chronically mentally ill and mentally retarded. McCullough, Coverdale, Bayer, and Chervenak (1992) have recently proposed family planning guidelines for female patients with chronic mental illness, based on the patients' ability to make decisions autonomously. They recommend that patients with impaired autonomy first be counseled in an attempt to help them become able to make an informed contraceptive decision. If this is not possible, the patient can be presented with options the clinician believes are consistent with the patient's values. The authors emphasize that forced surgical sterilization is not justifiable; they recommend Norplant as a safe, effective, and reversible method which may be appropriate for this population (McCullough et al., 1992). Other authors have made similar recommendations (David & Morgall, 1990).

More work needs to be done to identify and establish the usefulness of specific steps that might be taken to improve contraceptive compliance. Other practical issues might also be addressed in the research. For example, studies have investigated adolescents' decisions regarding whether or not to use contraception, but little attention has been given to how a particular method is chosen. Also most studies focus solely on adolescents and college-age women, with women beyond their mid-twenties receiving virtually no attention at all. There may be important differences in the psychological aspects of the contraceptive behavior of different age groups. The more we know about all the aspects of contraceptive behavior, especially what influences decision making, the better we will be able to assess and fulfill the contraceptive needs of women.

REFERENCES

Adler, N. E., Kegeles, S. M., Irwin, C. E., & Wibbleman, C. (1990). Adolescent contraceptive behavior: An assessment of the decision processes. *Journal of Pediatrics, 116*, 463–471.

Ajzen, I., & Fishbein, M. (1980). *Understanding attitudes and predicting social behavior*. Englewood Cliffs, NJ: Prentice-Hall.

Bandura, A. (1990). Perceived self-efficacy in the exercise of control over AIDS infection. *Evaluation and Program Planning, 13*, 9–17.

Bounds, W. (1989). Male and female barrier contraceptive methods. In M. Filshie & J. Guillebaud (Eds.), *Contraception: Science and practice* (pp. 172–202). London: Butterworths.

Burger, J. M. & Burns, L. (1988). The illusion of unique invulnerability and the use of effective contraception. *Personality and Social Psychology Bulletin, 14*, 264–270.

Byrne, D. (1983). Sex without contraception. In D. Byrne & W. A. Fisher (Eds.), *Adolescents, sex and contraception* (pp. 3–31). Hillsdale, NJ: Lawrence Erlbaum.

Chi, I.-C., Robbins, M., & Balogh, S. (1992). The progestin-only oral contraceptive—its place in postpartum contraception. *Advances in Contraception, 8*, 93–103.

Clarke, H. (1990). Intrauterine devices. In R. Lichtman & S. Papera (Eds.), *Gynecology: Well-woman care* (pp. 109–126). Norwalk, CT: Appleton & Lange.

Corsaro, M., & Lichtman, R. (1990). Barrier methods. In R. Lichtman & S. Papera (Eds.), *Gynecology: Well-woman care* (pp. 71–90). Norwalk, CT: Appleton & Lange.

David, H. P., & Morgall, J. M. (1990). Family planning for the mentally disordered and retarded. *Journal of Nervous and Mental Disease, 178*, 385–391.

Delvin, M. C., & Barwin, B. N. (1989). Barrier contraception. *Advances in Contraception, 5*, 197–204.

Eichhorst, B. C. (1988). Contraception. *Primary Care, 15*, 437–459.

Ellsworth, A. J., & Leversee, J. H. (1990). Oral contraceptives. *Primary Care, 17*, 603–622.

Fisher, W. A., Byrne, D., Edwards, M., Miller, C. T., Kelley, K., & White, L. A. (1979). Psychological and situation-specific correlates of contraceptive behavior among university women. *Journal of Sex Research, 15*, 38–55.

Fisher, W. A., Byrne, D., & White, L. A. (1983). Emotional barriers to contraception. In D. Byrne & W. A. Fisher (Eds.), *Adolescents, sex and contraception* (pp. 207–242). Hillsdale, NJ: Lawrence Erlbaum.

Fortney, J. A. (1987). Contraception for American women 40 and over. *Family Planning Perspectives, 19*, 32–34.

Franklin, M. (1990). Recently approved and experimental methods of contraception. *Journal of Nurse-Midwifery, 35*, 365–376.

Gerrard, M., Breda, C., & Gibbons, F. X. (1990). Gender effects in couples' sexual decision making and contraceptive use. *Journal of Applied Social Psychology, 20*, 449–464.

Gregersen, E., & Gregersen, B. (1990). The female condom: A pilot study of the acceptability of a new female barrier method. *Acta Obstetrica Gynecologica Scandinavica, 69*, 73–77.

Greydanus, D. F., & Lonchamp, D. (1990). Contraception in the adolescent: Preparation for the 1990s. *Medical Clinics of North America, 74*, 1205–1224.

Hankinson, S. E., Colditz, G. A., Hunter, D. J., Spencer, T. L., Rosner, B., & Stampfer, M. J. (1992). A quantitative assessment of oral contraceptive use and risk of ovarian cancer. *Obstetrics & Gynecology, 80*, 708–714.

Harvey, S. M., Beckman, L. J., & Murray, J. (1991). Perceived contraceptive attributes and method choice. *Journal of Applied and Social Psychology, 21*, 774–790.

Jarrett, M. E., & Lethbridge, D. J. (1990). The contraceptive needs of midlife women. *Nurse Practitioner, 15,* 34–39.

Jay, M. S., DuRant, R. H., & Litt, I. F. (1989). Female adolescents' compliance with contraceptive regimens. *Pediatric Clinics of North America, 36,* 731–746.

Kaunitz, A. M. (1989). Injectable contraception. *Clinical Obstetrics and Gynecology, 32,* 356–368.

Kaunitz, A. M. (1992). Oral contraceptives and gynecological cancer: An update for the 1990s. *American Journal of Obstetrics and Gynecology, 167,* 1171–1176.

Kotva, H. J., & Schneider, H. G. (1990). Those "talks"—general and sexual communication between mothers and daughters. *Journal of Social Behavior and Personality, 5,* 603–613.

Kreiss, J., Ngugi, E., Holmes, K., Ndinya-Achola, J., Waiyaki, P., Roberts, P. L., Ruminjo, I., Sajabi, R., Kimata, J., Fleming, T. R., Anzala, A., Holton, D., & Plummer, F. (1992). Efficacy of nonoxynol 9 contraceptive sponge use in preventing heterosexual acquisition of HIV in Nairobi prostitutes. *Journal of the American Medical Association, 268,* 477–482.

Kulig, J. W. (1989). Adolescent contraception: Nonhormonal methods. *Pediatric Clinics of North America, 36,* 717–730.

Lowry, D. T., & Towles, D. E. (1989). Soap opera portrayals of sex, contraception, and sexually transmitted diseases. *Journal of Communication, 39,* 76–83.

Luker, K. (1975). *Taking chances: Abortion and the decision not to contracept.* Berkeley: University of California Press.

McCarty, D. (1981). Changing contraceptive usage intentions: A test of the Fishbein model of intention. *Journal of Applied Social Psychology, 11,* 192–211.

McCullough, L. B., Coverdale, J., Bayer, T., & Chervenak, F. A. (1992). Ethically justified guidelines for family planning interventions to prevent pregnancy in female patients with chronic mental illness. *American Journal of Obstetrics and Gynecology, 167,* 19–25.

Milan, R. J., & Kilman, P. R. (1987). Interpersonal factors in premarital contraception. *Journal of Sex Research, 23,* 289–321.

Morrison, D. M. (1985). Adolescent contraceptive behavior: A review. *Psychological Bulletin, 98,* 538–568.

Papera, S. (1990). Sterilization. In R. Lichtman & S. Papera (Eds.), *Gynecology: Well-woman care* (pp. 465–472). Norwalk, CT: Appleton & Lange.

Paperney, D. M., & Starn, J. R. (1989). Adolescent pregnancy prevention by computer games: Computer-assisted instruction of knowledge and attitudes. *Pediatrics, 83,* 742–752.

Perloff, L. S., & Fetzer, B. K. (1986). Self-other judgments and perceived vulnerability to victimization. *Journal of Personality and Social Psychology, 50,* 502–520.

Porter, C. W., Waife, R. S., & Holtrop, H. R. (1983). *Contraception: The health provider's guide.* New York: Grune & Stratton.

Rickert, V. I., Jay, M. S., Gottlieb, A., & Bridges, C. (1989). Adolescents and AIDS: Females' attitudes and behaviors toward condom purchase and use. *Journal of Adolescent Health Care, 10,* 313–316.

Rioux, J.-E. (1989). Female sterilization and its reversal. In M. Filshie & J. Guillebaud (Eds.), *Contraception: Science and practice* (pp. 275–291). London: Butterworths.

Rosenberg, M. J., Davidson, A. J., Chen, J.-H., Judson, F. N., & Douglas, J. M. (1992). Barrier contraceptives and sexually transmitted diseases in women: A comparison of female-dependent methods and condoms. *American Journal of Public Health, 82*, 669–674.

Sakondhavat, C. (1990). The female condom. *American Journal of Public Health, 80*, 498.

Shearin, R. B., & Boehlke, J. R. (1989). Hormonal contraception. *Pediatric Clinics of North America, 36*, 697–715.

Shilling, R. F., El-Bassel, N., Leeper, M. A., & Freeman, L. (1991). Acceptance of the female condom by Latin- and African-American women. *American Journal of Public Health, 81*, 1345–1346.

Shoupe, D., & Mishell, D. R. (1989). Norplant: Subdermal implant system for long-term contraception. *American Journal of Obstetrics and Gynecology, 160*, 1286–1292.

Steinberg, W. M. (1989). Oral contraception: Risks and benefits. *Advances in Contraception, 5*, 219–228.

Strasberger, V. C. (1989). Adolescent sexuality and the media. *Pediatric Clinics of North America, 36*, 747–773.

Strassberg, D. L., & Mahoney, J. M. (1988). Correlates of the contraceptive behavior of adolescents/young adults. *Journal of Sex Research, 25*, 531–536.

Tatum, H. J., & Connell, E. B. (1989). Intrauterine contraceptive devices. In M. Filshie & J. Guillebaud (Eds.), *Contraception: Science and practice* (pp. 144–171). London: Butterworths.

Tanner, W. M., & Pollack, R. H. (1988). The effect of condom use and erotic condom instructions on attitudes toward condoms. *Journal of Sex Research, 25*, 537–541.

Trussel, J., Hatcher, R. A., Cates, W., Stewart, F. H., & Kost, K. (1990). A guide to interpreting contraceptive efficacy studies. *Obstetrics & Gynecology, 76*, 558–567.

Whitley, B. E., Jr., & Hern, A. L. (1991). Perceptions of vulnerability to pregnancy and the use of effective contraception. *Personality and Social Psychology Bulletin, 17*, 104–110.

Wulfert, E., & Wan, C. K. (1993). Condom use: A self-efficacy model. *Health Psychology, 12*, 346–353.

Zabin, L. S., Kantner, J. F., & Zelnik, M. (1979). Risk of adolescent pregnancy in the first months of intercourse. *Family Planning Perspectives, 11*, 215–226.

Zatuchni, G. I. (1989). Advances in contraception. *Advances in Contraception, 5*, 193–196.

8

Sexually Transmitted Diseases

Alison Milburn and Kristen K. Brewer

Sexually transmitted diseases (STDs) are a major public health problem in this country. Each year in the United States there are approximately 12 million new cases of STDs, and about one in six adults have an STD (American Social Health Association, 1991). Increasingly, these diseases are incurable. Whereas gonorrhea and syphilis used to be of greatest concern, now rates of viral infections, including genital herpes, human papillomavirus (HPV) and human immunodeficiency virus (HIV), are increasing (Cates & Toomey, 1990). In addition to the obvious medical and public health consequences of STDs, a number of psychological variables are important, such as adjustment to having an STD, treatment-seeking behavior, and prevention of the spread of STDs. In this chapter we will discuss the psychological reactions to having an STD in general, and describe some of the more common STDs, along with the psychological implications unique to those diseases. Finally, we will present strategies for the prevention of STDs.

There has always been a stigma attached to having a sexually transmitted disease. People with STDs traditionally have been seen as immoral and promiscuous; indeed, sometimes even as deserving of disease. Because of the stigma associated with STDs, many individuals may delay seeking treatment out of fear, embarrassment, or guilt (Romanowski & Piper, 1988). Health professionals may also be uncomfortable discussing STDs with patients (Romanowski & Piper, 1988; Wertheimer, Balduzzi, & Minghetti, 1991).

Psychological reactions to the diagnosis of an STD can vary greatly, and are not well understood (Ross, 1990). Some of the most common psychological responses include anxiety, guilt, anger, and relationship difficulties (Ross, 1990; Wardropper & Woolley, 1991). In addition, sexual dysfunction is relatively common, and includes coital orgasmic dysfunction, loss of libido, dyspareunia, and vaginismus (Wardropper & Woolley, 1990).

HERPES SIMPLEX VIRUS

Herpes Simplex Virus (HSV) has been the most widely studied sexually transmitted disease with regard to its psychological contributors and effects. HSV is characterized by painful vesicular eruptions of the skin and mucosa of the genital region. It occurs in two types: type 1 accounts for 10–15% of cases and type 2 for the remaining 85–90%. Approximately 16.4% of persons ages 15–74 are infected with HSV type 2, with 25 million Americans affected (Swanson & Chenitz, 1990). HSV rates are highest in those between ages 20–44, women, African-Americans, those of low education level and socioeconomic status, those residing in cities, those residing in the southern part of the U.S., and men in the military. Most cases of HSV are asymptomatic, identified only by the presence of antibodies indicating prior infection (Swanson & Chenitz, 1990).

During the primary HSV infection vesicles rupture, exposing shallow tender ulcers that crust and heal. This process is often associated with genital discomfort. If the lesions occur on the cervix or in the vagina, the woman may experience watery discharge and dysuria. Other symptoms can include neuralgic pain, fever, malaise, and headaches. The primary infection usually resolves within one to three weeks, but the infection can still be transmitted for another six to eight weeks (Nettina & Kauffman, 1990).

When not active, HSV migrates via nerve pathways to the sacral ganglia, where it remains latent. Reactivations occur by unknown mechanisms (Hoon et al., 1991). HSV type 2 accounts for 98% of recurrences. HSV will recur in 60–90% of patients and recurs at an average rate of five to eight attacks per year, with a gradual reduction in the recurrence rate. There is wide variability in the rate of recurrences both across individuals and within individuals over time (Kemeny, Cohen, Zegans, & Conant, 1989).

The symptoms associated with recurrent episodes are typically less severe than symptoms that occur with the primary infection. Prodromal symptoms such as pain, itching, or burning can occur prior to the vesicular skin eruption. There has been a great deal of speculation about possible causes for the recurrence of the infection. Suggested triggers include emotional distress, sunburn, fever, menses, systemic infection, or immunosuppression. There has been little systematic study of these possible triggers, so this speculation has been based primarily on anecdotal evidence (Kemeny et al., 1989).

HSV infections have been associated with a variety of negative medical outcomes. Recurrent cervical herpes is associated with an increased risk of cervical dysplasia. Women with herpes show an increased rate of spontaneous abortion and premature delivery. Neonatal infection is also a risk. Cesarean section may be required if the infection is active at the time of delivery (Chenitz & Swanson, 1989).

The diagnosis of HSV requires obtaining a tissue culture at the time of an active infection. The presence of antibodies indicating prior infection can be detected in asymptomatic individuals (Swanson & Chenitz, 1990), but this test is of little practical use. There is currently no cure for herpes infection. The treatment of herpes at this time primarily involves the use of acyclovir, an antiviral medication which can be administered orally, topically, or intravenously. Given orally, acyclovir increases the rate of shedding of the infection and decreases the healing time of lesions and the duration of pain. Given continuously it has been shown to decrease the rate of recurrences. Condoms have been shown to be protective against the transmission of the HSV infection, depending on their proper use and the location of the herpes lesions. Nonoxynol–9, a spermicide, may also decrease transmission of the infection (Chenitz & Swanson, 1989).

The association between psychological stress and HSV recurrences has been a source of significant controversy. The presumed relationship is thought to be mediated by immune functioning. There is increasing evidence that psychological stress in various forms is associated with changes in immune status. Acute stressors have been shown to activate the two major stress systems in the body, the sympathetic adrenal-medullary system (SAM) and the hypothalamic-pituitary-adrenocortical system (HPAC) (O'Leary, 1990). Most of the hormones released by these systems have been shown to be stress responsive and to have immunologic effects. Evidence from studies of normal subjects undergoing psychological stress shows consistent change in immune status from stress, independent of the dietary and sleep changes that sometimes accompany stress. Acute stressors activate both SAM and HPAC systems, causing variable effects on lymphocytes. There is further evidence that prolonged stress may result in prolonged immunosuppression. In some studies, depression, loneliness, and isolation have also been found to be related to immunosuppression (O'Leary, 1990).

O'Leary (1990) argues for a specific connection between psychological stress and herpes recurrences. She states that " . . . cellular control over latent herpes viruses is impaired under conditions of stress, leading to increased levels of herpes antibody in stressed individuals. Presumably this effect, if large enough, could result in an actual outbreak of lesions" (p 373).

A large majority of people with herpes (83–86%) believe that their recurrences are stress related, but empirical studies of this relationship have been mixed (Hoon et al., 1991). Rand, Hoon, Massey, and Johnson (1990) had 64 herpes patients complete prospective charting of psychological stressors and herpes symptoms daily for one month. Results showed that recurrences were not related to increased levels of normal daily stress. Kemeny and colleagues (1989) prospectively studied 36 individuals with herpes. Stress measures used in the study included those of acute life events, ongoing stressors, and anticipated stressors. In this study, both stress and negative mood were significantly negatively correlated with immune function assays. Stress, infections, menstrual cycle, and fatigue were not related, however, to herpes recurrences. The most depressed subjects did have twice as many recurrences as did the least depressed. Alcohol use was related to recurrences, but not to immune functioning. These and other studies have produced mixed results as to the relationship between psychological factors and herpes recurrence.

Psychological responses to HSV infection have been well identified. Clinicians describe a "herpes syndrome" in infected individuals, which is characterized by depression, decreased self-esteem, shame, and guilt, although there is clearly a great deal of variability in response to the disease (Keller, Jadack, & Mims, 1991). The diagnosis of herpes has been associated with feelings of helplessness, inadequacy, denial, anger, guilt, anxiety, shame, depression, a feeling of victimization, decreased self-esteem, and distress associated with sexual activity (Chenitz & Swanson, 1989).

Adjustment to the diagnosis and chronic nature of herpes is predicted by a variety of social and psychological factors. High levels of social support, the use of a partner for positive support, and the use of cognitive coping strategies, such as planful problem-solving, have been associated with improved adjustment. A focus on attributions of blame for the disease, either to the individual herself or to the person who infected the individual, is associated with poor psychological outcomes (Keller et al., 1991; Swanson & Chenitz, 1990). Denial of the disease and wishful thinking are also predictors of poor outcome.

Relationship problems are a prominent complication of HSV infection. Suspicions of infidelity in the partner are common in herpes patients, who search to find the cause of their misfortune. Blaming the current partner for the infection can result in relationship strain or loss. The fear of telling a new sexual partner is the most frequently identified disease-related stressor in those with herpes (Keller et al., 1991). This fear often results in avoidance of situations likely to result in sexual intimacy (Swanson & Chenitz, 1990).

The research on the psychological issues involved in HSV infections has implications for the care of infected individuals. Attention to emotional concerns should be a part of treatment for HSV. The sense of isolation newly diagnosed individuals often feel can be reduced by providing complete information about rates of infection, transmission of the disease, and available treatments. Emotional social support is infrequently used by those with herpes, but its importance in adjustment to the disease has been well established (Keller, Jadack, & Mims, 1991). In addition, keeping herpes a secret can reinforce a negative self-image in the patient, which can have a negative effect on mood and coping (Swanson & Chenitz, 1990). Discussion about how to disclose to others and seek social support can help to improve adjustment.

The utility of psychotherapy in reducing herpes recurrences is unclear. Some studies have suggested this effect. In one investigation of 4,000 individuals with HSV, "conscious stress management" was reported to be the respondents' "most lasting therapy" (Bierman, 1985). Psychotherapy has been shown to reduce the anxiety, depression, and sense of isolation often associated with herpes. Intervention may include reframing (that is, changing the perception of the event without changing the event itself), dealing with grief, guilt, and shame; and self-care and management. This might include a healthy life-style, the use of acyclovir, acquisition of knowledge about the disease, and work on disclosure of the disease to potential sexual partners (Swanson & Chenitz, 1990). Support groups may not be the best form of intervention because of the herpes patient's tendency to identify himself or herself as part of a "deviant" subculture, thereby promoting a negative self-image (Keller, Jadack, & Mims, 1991).

HUMAN PAPILLOMAVIRUS/CONDYLOMA ACUMINATUM

The symptoms associated with the human papillomavirus (HPV) have been recognized since ancient Greek and Roman times. Despite this, few studies have examined the extent and effects of this disease (Becker, Stone, & Alexander, 1987). More than 60 serotypes of the virus have now been detected. Carcinoma has been associated primarily with HPV types 16 and 18; additional types also associated with cervical intraepithelial neoplasia (CIN) or carcinoma include 31, 33, 35, 39, 45, 51, 52 (Bauer et al., 1991).

Condyloma acuminatum are genital warts caused by HPV types 6 and 11. The symptoms associated with condyloma acuminatum include small, soft, fleshy vegetating growths (resembling cauliflower) in the genital, perianal, inguinal, and urethral areas. Condyloma can be diagnosed clinically with the use of a dilute white vinegar solution which highlights lesions. A Pap smear is used to detect cervical lesions. At times condyloma are clinically asymptomatic, but approximately 85% of those exposed will develop warts (Story, 1987). The incubation period for condyloma is long, most often ranging from three weeks to nine months, but sometimes lasting up to three years.

In the past 15 years there has been a large increase in office visits for HPV. Of sexually transmitted diseases, only chlamydia is more common in the United States (Story, 1987). One study of HPV in college-age women found 46% of the study population to be affected (Bauer et al., 1991). Risk factors for HPV infection include cigarette smoking, use of oral contraceptives, multiple sexual partners, and sexual activity at an early age (Daling, Sherman, & Weiss, 1984). Treatment for HPV and condyloma can include trichloroacetic acid (TCA) solution applied to the surface of the condyloma, CO_2-laser ablation, cryotherapy, topical chemotherapy, and interferon-x injections. Condyloma can recur without reinfection due to a weakening of the immune system (for example, from stress, immune system defects, or disease), can be refractory to treatment, and can have a prolonged course (Enterline & Leonardo, 1989).

The diagnosis of HPV has been associated with feelings of embarrassment, shame, and betrayal (Enterline & Leonardo, 1989). One might also expect anxiety (particularly regarding the increased risk of carcinoma) and/or depression in response to the diagnosis. One study by Filiberti et al. (1993) failed to identify depression in a small sample of individuals with HPV, but did find cancer fears in a significant minority (27.5%) of the sample.

Relationship difficulties are another potential negative effect of HPV diagnosis, with increased suspicion and blaming of the partner, fighting, and avoidance of sexual intercourse. Filiberti et al. (1993) found such relationship problems in 16% of their participants. A study of women who attended a colposcopy clinic and were treated for HPV found a significant increase in negative feelings toward sexual intercourse or toward a regular sexual partner after diagnosis (Campion et al., 1988). Abstinence or condom use during HPV treatment may be required, which requires partner acceptance and cooperation. A majority of patients in the Filiberti et al. study described their sexual lives as worsened following diagnosis and treatment (57%), with one-third of those completely interrupting their sex life. Fears cited by participants in the study included that of possible reinfection or possible transmission of the disease. The required use of condoms also played a role in decreased sexual desire in these women. Pain was infrequently cited as a cause of sexual changes (Filiberti et al., 1993).

Women with condyloma or HPV have a significant need for information about their disease. Although its incidence is widespread and growing, general knowledge about HPV is limited, especially as compared with HSV. Counseling of patients should include information about symptoms, transmission, potential risks, and treatment, as well as attention to fears of cancer and changes in sexuality.

CHLAMYDIA, GONORRHEA, AND SYPHILIS

Chlamydia is currently the most common curable STD in the United States (Felts, White, & Marshburn, 1991) and is more common in women than in men (Cates & Toomey, 1990), affecting about two million women each year (Millar, 1987). Symptoms include nonspecific symptoms of infection, such as headaches and fever, and a papule, which develops into a painless vulvovaginal ulcer (Gunning, 1986). However, 50–70 percent of women infected with chlamydia are asymptomatic, including 7–9 percent of women presenting for routine pelvic exams (Felts, White, & Marshburn, 1991). Diagnosis is relatively difficult because *Chlamydia trachomatis* lives only intracellularly (Millar, 1987), so cultures do not always detect it. Treatment is usually tetracycline, except in pregnant women, where erythromycin is usually used (Moy & Clasen, 1990).

Early detection and treatment of chlamydia are of vital importance because of the possible complications of untreated infection. Chlamydia accounts for 20–40 percent of recognized cases of pelvic inflammatory disease (PID), which can result in infertility and includes acute or chronic endometritis, and acute salpingitis (infection of the fallopian tubes). PID may result in chronic pelvic pain (Millar, 1987). Among pregnant women, chlamydia increases the risk of ectopic pregnancy, premature labor, and rupture of membranes, and can be passed on to the neonate in the form of conjunctivitis and chlamydial pneumonia (Millar, 1987).

There are approximately one million new cases of gonorrhea in the United States each year, affecting more men than women at a ratio of about 1.5 to one (Fogel & Nettles-Carlson, 1987). Over the past decade there has been a decrease in cases caused by penicillin-sensitive organisms, but an increase in the number and variety of penicillin-resistant strains of *Neissera gonorrhoeae*, making treatment more difficult (Cates & Toomey, 1990). Symptoms of gonorrhea include vaginal discharge, dysuria, and intermenstrual bleeding, but as is the case in chlamydia, many women may be asymptomatic (Elgart, 1992). Symptoms are generally worse after menses (Moy & Clasen, 1990). Diagnosis is made on the basis of cultures and treatment usually consists of penicillin. Because approximately 45 percent of patients with gonorrhea also have chlamydia, it is recommended that gonorrhea-infected patients also routinely be treated for chlamydia (Fogel & Nettles-Carlson, 1987; Moy & Clasen, 1990). Possible complications of gonorrhea include PID, ectopic pregnancy, and infertility (Moy & Clasen, 1990).

The prevalence of syphilis declined markedly in the 1940s after the introduction of penicillin; however, during the second half of the 1980s there was a rapid increase in the incidence of syphilis (Cates & Toomey, 1990). Symptoms of syphilis appear 10–90 days after exposure, in the form of a chancre; the secondary stage follows in six weeks to six months (if it has not been treated) and includes a widespread rash and lesions, most commonly on the palms and soles (Elgart, 1992). A blood test is used to make a diagnosis and penicillin is usually used for treatment (Elgart, 1992; Gunning, 1986). Because the chancres increase the odds of transmission of HIV, it has been recommended that all patients with syphilis also be tested for HIV (Vilarino & Schulte, 1992).

There are a number of important factors to consider in the treatment of chlamydia, gonorrhea, and syphilis. Compliance with treatment is very important in order to eradicate the infection. It is widely recommended that patients schedule a follow-up visit for a test of cure about 5–14 days after treatment is complete (Moy & Clasen, 1990). Patients also need to be educated about risk of reinfection. One of the most sensitive issues may be the identification and treatment of partners, which is important for prevention of reinfection in patients, spread of infection to other partners, as well as for the health of the partners. Fogel and Nettles-Carlson (1987) recommend that clinicians take extra time to counsel patients and make specific suggestions to them regarding how to tell sexual contacts about the disease. In many areas the local health department will assist in the confidential notification of sexual partners. It is important to inform patients when STDs must be reported to the health department.

HUMAN IMMUNODEFICIENCY VIRUS (HIV) AND ACQUIRED IMMUNODEFICIENCY SYNDROME (AIDS)

Acquired Immunodeficiency Syndrome (AIDS) is a multifactoral disease consisting of a number of severe illnesses that can result in diminished cognitive function, weakness, fevers, weight loss, blindness, opportunistic infections, and cancer (Fawzy, Fawzy, & Pasnau, 1991). It is the result of the presence of the Human Immunodeficiency Virus (HIV) and is as yet incurable. Currently about one million Americans are infected with this fatal disease (Centers for Disease Control, 1993). AIDS occurs most frequently in younger adults, with the greatest number of AIDS cases occurring in the 20 to 39 age group (66% of men and 69% of women) (Cefali, 1990).

The proportion of people with AIDS who are women went up from 3.2% in 1981 to 11.5% in 1991. The annual rate of transmission for cases reported October 1992 through September 1993 was 14.0 per 100,000 population (CDC, 1993). The most common avenue of transmission among women is intravenous (IV) drug use (51%), followed by heterosexual contact (33%) and blood transfusions (9%) (Ickovics & Rodin, 1992). Transmission of HIV through sexual contact occurs more readily from males to females than from females to males (Pizzi, 1992). Women with AIDS are rarely diagnosed with Kaposi's Sarcoma, which is common in men. However, AIDS in women is associated with a wide variety of infections and malignancies, including cervical cancer.

Cefali (1990) identifies three stages of the HIV infection, beginning with the asymptomatic phase. Testing for the virus at this stage is not provoked by physical symptoms, and so a diagnosis may be particularly stressful. Of those in this group, 10–20% will develop AIDS. The second stage, AIDS-related complex (ARC), occurs when physical symptoms develop. Finally, full-blown AIDS precedes the terminal phase of the disease. There is evidence that patients with asymptomatic HIV or ARC are more psychologically distressed than those with AIDS (Bialer, Wallack, & Snyder, 1991). Because there is no cure available for AIDS, medical professionals can only offer treatments to manage symptoms and prolong life. Thus attention to the psychosocial issues accompanying the disease is crucial (Cefali, 1990).

The psychological impact of AIDS begins even prior to diagnosis with the decision to be tested for the virus. The decision to test is often accompanied by considerable anxiety and the possibility of receiving a positive result seems higher to the individual once she decides her risk level is high enough to make testing advisable. While a negative test result is associated with feelings of relief, a positive result promotes numerous fears, including fears of death, contagion, loss of physical attractiveness, increased dependency, isolation, and stigmatization (Cefali, 1990).

Nichols (1985) described four stages of psychosocial adaptation to AIDS in men. These include the *Initial Crisis*, in which patients experience extreme anxiety, guilt, anger, and sadness. During the *Transitional* phase, these emotions persist and attention is focused on past behavior, resulting in distress, confusion, and self-devaluation. In the *Deficiency State—Acceptance* phase, there is a reassessment of values and focus on spirituality, relationships, and quality of life. Finally, during the *Preparation for Death* phase, the individual focuses on resolving unfinished business, including preparation of wills, other financial arrangements, resolving emotional issues with loved ones, and feelings about dependency and death.

Women infected with HIV face a shortened life-span and diagnosis-related emotional chaos, as do men. HIV-infected women express feelings of futility, hopelessness, helplessness, and loss of control. Women with HIV may also face issues that are unique to them. For example, women are more likely than men to be responsible for dependent minor children and so must make decisions about care of their children in their planning. Women also face decisions regarding their childbearing potential. The risk of transmission of HIV infection to an unborn child is believed to be between 20 and 30 percent in any given pregnancy. An infected woman faces complex issues in deciding to initiate, terminate, or complete a pregnancy (Arras, 1990). It has recently been shown in a placebo-controlled study, that AZT taken by the mother during pregnancy and delivery, and by the infant for the first six weeks of life, reduced the rate of transmission to 8.3%, as compared to 25.5% in the control group (Thomas, 1994).

There is no consistent pattern of psychiatric diagnoses in HIV-positive individuals (Bialer, Wallack, and Snyder, 1991). Depression is common and it is often hard to differentiate between major depression and organic mood disorder, depressed type, in these patients. Both disorders are seen. Also common are various types of adjustment disorders. Anxiety occurs frequently, but anxiety disorders are infrequent. Neuropsychological impairment occurs in a large percentage of AIDS patients. Referred to as "AIDS Dementia Complex" (ADC), changes in behavior, cognition, and motor skills are frequent. The pathophysiology of this syndrome is not yet known (Bialer, Wallack, & Snyder, 1991).

Management of HIV-infected patients requires the providing of information and opportunities for emotional support, perhaps in the form of support groups (Cefali, 1990). Fawzy, Fawzy, and Pasnau (1991) present a model for psychosocial intervention for HIV-positive individuals. Their model includes four components: health education, stress management, enhancement of coping skills, and psychological support in the form of individual or group counseling. Interventions such as these have been shown to have a positive effect on coping and affective state in AIDS patients and in other medical populations (e.g., cancer patients).

PREVENTION

Given the high incidence of STDs, the potential negative health consequences for women and their children, and the recent increase in incurable STDs, prevention strategies are very important. This section will address strategies for primary prevention in the uninfected population and in STD patients.

Primary prevention involves altering behaviors in order to minimize the risk of exposure to STDs. Behaviors involved in primary prevention include abstinence, careful selection of sexual partners, and the use of condoms, spermicides, and diaphragms (Stone, 1990).

As is often reported in the popular media, abstinence is the only 100% effective means of preventing STDs. This strategy is not appealing to many people, however, as the power of sexual gratification can be quite strong (McGregor, French, and Spencer, 1989). Stone (1990) points out that it is often mistakenly assumed that abstinence means refraining from all sexual activity. She asserts that abstinence refers to "specific avoidance of penetrative genital–anogenital or oral–anogenital contact" (p. 791). In other words, there are a variety of sexual behaviors that do not significantly increase the risk of STDs; Stone advocates promotion of these behaviors as alternatives to higher-risk activities.

Women can reduce their risk of STDs by limiting their number of sexual partners and by careful selection of partners. Women can ask potential partners about their sexual history and about symptoms of STDs. Also, examination of the partner's genitals may reveal symptoms of STDs (Stone, 1990). However, individuals may not be honest about their sexual history and may be asymptomatically infected. When a woman decides to engage in sexual intercourse, she can reduce her risk of contracting an STD from an infected partner by using barrier methods of contraception and spermicide. Condoms have been shown to be impervious to most sexually transmitted pathogens and have been shown in clinical trials to reduce significantly the risk of STDs (Cates & Stone, 1992a). Spermicides, used alone or in conjunction with a diaphragm or vaginal sponge, have been shown, in both laboratory and clinical studies, to be protective against STDs (Cates & Stone, 1992a). A recent correlational study found lower rates of STDs in women using the diaphragm or sponge than in women relying on the condom (Rosenberg, Davidson, Chen, Judson, & Douglas, 1992). The authors propose that women who use female-dependent methods may use them more consistently and correctly than women who rely on condoms, which require the cooperation of the male partner. It is important to note that the methods of contraception that are most effective at preventing STD transmission are not the same methods best at preventing pregnancy (Cates & Stone, 1992a, 1992b). Women may want to use two contraceptive methods in order to prevent effectively both STDs and unwanted pregnancy.

Adolescents are at highest risk for nearly all STDs (Biro & Rosenthal, 1992). Individuals in this age group may be engaging in risky sexual activities because adolescents are not future-oriented and therefore may not see the possible long-term consequences of their behavior (i.e., STD or pregnancy). Also, they may not be skilled in negotiating and communicating about sexual issues (Biro & Rosenthal, 1992).

Many authors have suggested increasing STD education for high school and college students as an important component of prevention (e.g., Calamidas, 1990; Cates & Toomey, 1990). Instilling fear of contracting an STD is not considered an effective technique and may actually undermine prevention programs (Cates & Toomey, 1990). Herold, Fisher, Smith, and Yarber (1990) have outlined a program for school-based STD education, emphasizing health behavior and the positive aspects of sexuality. In addition to increasing students' knowledge about ways to avoid STDs, it is important to make sure that they have the skills necessary to put this knowledge into practice. There is some indication that, although college students possess adequate knowledge about STDs, this knowledge does not always translate into behavior (Baldwin & Baldwin, 1988). A possible explanation for the discrepancy between knowledge and behavior is that individuals may not possess the skills they need to carry out the desired behaviors. For example, research on contraceptive behavior has found that the level of communication with the sexual partner is predictive of contraceptive use (Morrison, 1985). Herold, Fisher, Smith, and Yarber (1990) call for STD education programs to include activities that will improve the skills necessary to engage in the preventive behaviors outlined above. These activities include modeling and role-playing communication with potential partners about STDs, sexual decision making, and training in sexual assertiveness (Herold et al., 1990).

Women currently infected with STDs are a group for whom prevention strategies are particularly important. In addition to being counseled about the ways to prevent future infections, it is important that these patients comply with treatment, including returning for "test of cure" appointments, and identify sexual contacts who may need to be treated to prevent reinfection. Strategies for counseling patients about these issues are discussed earlier in this chapter.

CONCLUSION

Rates of both bacterial and viral STDs are rising and the health consequences of these diseases can be profound. All carry with them the potential for negative psychological effects. Psychologists, as well as medical professionals such as physicians and nurses, must be able to intervene to manage these effects. Psychologists can also play an important role in promoting the behavioral changes necessary to prevent the spread of these diseases. In the treatment and prevention of STDs, emotional and behavioral factors can be as important as medical ones.

REFERENCES

American Social Health Association (1991). *STD: Questions and answers*. Research Triangle Park, NC: Author.

Arras, J. D. (1990). AIDS and reproductive decisions: Having children in fear and trembling. *Millbank Quarterly, 68*(3), 353–382.

Baldwin, J. D., & Baldwin, J. I. (1988). Factors affecting AIDS-related sexual risk-taking behavior among college students. *Journal of Sex Research, 25*, 181–196.

Bauer, H. M., Ting, Y., Greer, C. E., Chambers, J. C., Tashiro, C. J., Chimera, J., Reingold, A., & Manos, M. M. (1991). Genital human papillomavirus infection in female university students as determined by a PCR-based method. *Journal of the American Medical Association, 265*(4), 472–477.

Becker, T. M., Stone, K. M., & Alexander, E. R. (1987). Genital human papillomavirus infection: A growing concern. *Obstetrics and Gynecology Clinics of North America, 14*(2), 389–396.

Bialer, P. A., Wallack, J. D., & Snyder, S. L. (1991). Psychiatric diagnosis in HIV-spectrum disorders. *Psychiatric Medicine, 9*(3), 361–375.

Bierman, S. (1985). Recurrent genital herpes simples infection: A trivial disorder. *Archives of Dermatology, 121*, 513–517.

Biro, F. M., & Rosenthal, S. L. (1992). Psychological sequelae of sexually transmitted diseases in adolescents. *Obstetrics and Gynecology Clinics of North America, 19*, 209–218.

Calamidas, E. G. (1990). AIDS and STD education: What's really happening in our schools? *Journal of Sex Education and Therapy, 16*, 54–63.

Campion, M. J., Brown, J. R., Atia, W., Edwards, R., Cuzick, J., & Singer, A. (1988). Psychosexual trauma of an abnormal cervical smear. *British Journal of Obstetrics and Gynecology, 95*, 175–181.

Cates, W., Jr., & Stone, K. M. (1992a). Family planning, sexually transmitted diseases and contraceptive choice: A literature update—Part I. *Family Planning Perspectives, 24*, 75–84.

Cates, W., Jr., & Stone, K. M. (1992b). Family planning, sexually transmitted diseases and contraceptive choice: A literature update—Part II. *Family Planning Perspectives, 24*, 122–128.

Cates, W., Jr., & Toomey, K. E. (1990). Sexually transmitted diseases: Overview of the situation. *Primary Care, 17*, 1–27.

Cefali, F. E. (1990). Psychosocial aspects of Human Immunodeficiency Virus Infection. *Natural Immunity and Cell Growth Regulation, 9*, 137–142.

Centers for Disease Control. (October, 1993). *HIV/AIDS Surveillance Report*. Atlanta: Author.

Centers for Disease Control. (1993). *Surgeon General's report to the American public on HIV infection and AIDS*. Atlanta: Author.

Chenitz, W. C., & Swanson, J. M. (1989). Counseling clients with genital herpes. *Journal of Psychosocial Nursing, 27*(9), 11–17.

Daling, J. R., Sherman, K. J., & Weiss, N. S. (1984, Jan.–Mar.). Risk factors for condyloma acuminatum in women. *Sexually Transmitted Diseases, 11*, 16–18.

Elgart, M. L. (1992). Sexually transmitted diseases of the vulva. *Dermatologic Clinics, 10*, 387–403.

Enterline, J. A., Leonardo, J. P. (1989). Condyloma acuminata (genital warts). *Nurse Practitioner, 14*(4), 8–16.

Fawzy, F. I., Fawzy, N. W., & Pasnau, R. O. (1991). A model of a psychiatric intervention for AIDS patients. *Psychiatric Medicine, 9*(3), 409–419.

Felts, W. M., White, D. M., & Marshburn, D. (1991). Genital *Chlamydia trachomatis* infection among university students: Review and recommendations. *Journal of College Student Development, 32*, 541–545.

Filiberti, A., Tamburini, M., Stefanon, B., Merola, M., Bandieramonte, G., Ventafridda, G., & DePalo, G. (1993). Psychological aspects of genital human papillomavirus infection: A preliminary report. *Journal of Psychosomatic Obstetrics and Gynecology, 14*, 145–152.

Fogel, C. I., & Nettles-Carlson, B. (1987). Gonorrhea in women: A serious health problem. *Health Care for Women International, 8*, 75–86.

Gunning, J. (1986). Vaginal and vulvar infections. In N.F. Hacker & J.G. Moore (Eds.), *Essentials of obstetrics and gynecology*, Philadelphia: W.B. Saunders.

Herold, E. S., Fisher, W. A., Smith, E. A., & Yarber, W. A. (1990). Sex education and the prevention of STD/AIDS and pregnancy among youths. *Canadian Journal of Public Health, 81*, 141–145.

Hoon, E. F., Hoon, P. W., Rand, K. H., Johnson, J., Hall, N. R., & Edwards, N. B. (1991). A psychobehavioral model of genital herpes recurrence. *Journal of Psychosomatic Research, 35*(1), 25–36.

Ickovics, J. R., & Rodin, J. (1992). Women and AIDS in the United States: Epidemiology, natural history, and mediating mechanisms. *Health Psychology, 11*, 1–16.

Keller, M. L., Jadack, R. A., & Mims, L. F. (1991). Perceived stressors and coping responses in persons with recurrent genital herpes. *Research in Nursing and Health, 14*, 421–430.

Kemeny, M. E., Cohen, F., Zegans, L. S., & Conant, M. A. (1989). Psychological and immunological predictors of genital herpes recurrence. *Psychosomatic Medicine, 51*, 195–208.

McGregor, J. A., French, J. I., & Spencer, N. E. (1989). Prevention of sexually transmitted diseases in women. *Obstetrics and Gynecology Clinics of North America, 16*, 679–702.

Millar, M. I. (1987). Genital chlamydial infection: A role for social scientists. *Social Science and Medicine, 25*, 1289–1299.

Morrison, D. M. (1985). Adolescent contraceptive behavior: A review. *Psychological Bulletin, 98*, 538–568.

Moy, J. G., & Clasen, M. E. (1990). The patient with gonococcal infection. *Primary Care, 17*, 59–83.

Nettina, S. L., & Kauffman, F. H. (1990). Diagnosis and management of sexually transmitted genital lesions. *Nurse Practitioner, 15*(1), 20–39.

Nichols, S. E. (1985). Psychosocial reactions of persons with the acquired immunodeficiency syndrome. *Annals of Internal Medicine, 103*, 765–767.

O'Leary, A. (1990). Stress, emotion, and human immune function. *Psychological Bulletin, 108*(3), 363–382.

Pizzi, M. (1992). Women, HIV Infection and AIDS: Tapestries of life, death and empowerment. *American Journal of Occupational Therapy, 46*(11), 1021–1027.

Rand, K. H., Hoon, E. F., Massey, J. K., & Johnson J.H. (1990). Daily stress and recurrence of genital herpes simplex. *Archives of Internal Medicine, 150*, 1889–1893.

Romanowski, B., & Piper, G. (1988). Sexually transmitted diseases: An overview. *Journal of Social Work and Human Sexuality, 6*, 7–20.

Rosenberg, M. J., Davidson, A. J., Chen, J. H., Judson, F. N., & Douglas, J. M. (1992). Barrier contraceptives and sexually transmitted diseases in women: A comparison of female-dependent methods and condoms. *American Journal of Public Health, 82*, 669–674.

Ross, M. W. (1990). Psychological perspectives on sexuality and sexually transmitted diseases. In K. K. Holmes, P.-A. Mardh, P. F. Sparling, P. L. Wiesner, W. Cates, Jr., S. M. Lemon, & W. E. Stamm (Eds.), *Sexually transmitted diseases* (pp. 55–60). New York: McGraw-Hill.

Stone, K. M. (1990). Avoiding sexually transmitted diseases. *Obstetrics and Gynecology Clinics of North America, 17*, 789–799.

Story, B. (1987, Dec.). Condyloma acuminata: An epidemic with malignant potential. *Physician Assistant, 11*, 13–23.

Swanson, J. M., & Chenitz, W. C. (1990). Psychosocial aspects of genital herpes: A review of the literature. *Public Health Nursing, 7*(2), 96–104.

Thomas, E., Jr. (1994, February 22). AZT reduces likelihood mother with AIDS will transmit virus to child. *Wall Street Journal*, p. B2.

Villarino, M. E., & Schulte, J. M. (1992). Diagnosis and therapy for common sexually transmitted diseases. *Dermatologic Clinics, 10*, 459–468.

Wardropper, A. G., & Woolley, P. D. (1991). Psychosexual problems in a genitourinary clinic. *Stress Medicine, 7*, 143–144.

Wertheimer, A. I., Balduzzi, M., & Minghetti, P. (1991). Reactions of community pharmacists to questions by patients with a stigmatized disease. *Journal of Clinical Pharmacy and Therapeutics, 16*, 435–442.

PART III
Obstetrics

9

Infertility

Robin L. Davisson

THE PROBLEM OF INFERTILITY

Approximately ten to fifteen percent of the American population of childbearing age is infertile (Houghton, 1984). Without contraceptive practices, it is estimated that pregnancy can be achieved within 12 months by 80% of couples. For this reason the American Fertility Society considers a couple to be infertile when a successful pregnancy, resulting in a live birth, has not occurred within one year of "normal" sexual relations without contraception (Mazor & Simons, 1984). About 50 percent of all infertility problems are related to factors in the female (mostly disorders of ovulation and tubal pathology), while 30 percent of possible etiologies can be traced to the male partner. The diagnostic workup for the remaining 20 percent indicates either combined problems for the couple, or discovery of no anatomical, physiological, or pathological cause, leaving the infertility "unexplained" (Mazor & Simons, 1984; Menning, 1977). In the past the investigation and treatment processes included only one partner, usually the female (Shapiro, 1988). Infertility is, however, a problem of two people, indicating that evaluation and management (both medical and psychological) should be of the couple as a unit.

More consideration is given to the problem of infertility now than a decade ago, partly because discussion of sexual matters has become more acceptable. An apparent increase in the rate of infertility over the last three decades has been the major impetus for research and clinical interest in problems of reproduction (Mazor & Simons, 1984). This increase is due to several factors. The trend of delaying marriage and childbearing for the development of careers or other socioeconomic reasons results in many couples attempting to conceive beyond their maximally fertile mid-twenties. As the prevalence of sexually transmitted diseases rises, so does the incidence of reproductive tract scarring resulting from pelvic or genital infections (Shapiro, 1988). In addition, factors such as substance abuse (including smoking), environmental toxins, and extremely vigorous exercise may play a role in the increasing rates of infertility (Shapiro, 1988).

These factors contribute to infertility as a result of their interaction with ovulation, fallopian tubal function, or semen quality. Therefore, evaluation of the infertile couple involves assessment of each of these basic reproductive functions in order to determine which factors require further diagnosis or treatment. Ovulation can be assessed by determining if the patient has symptoms of ovulation, examining a basal body temperature record for the characteristic postovulation rise, and demonstrating an elevation in serum progesterone level during the mid-luteal phase of the cycle, or showing characteristic microscopic changes in the endometrium obtained by uterine bioposy (Pepperell, Hudson, & Wood, 1987). Recognition of an ovulatory disorder is crucial since this is a curable problem which is often reversed with relatively simple treatments. Induction of ovulation with "simple" drug therapies such as clomiphene citrate (Clomid) or bromocriptine, or more complex treatment with gonadotrophins or gonadotrophin-releasing hormone (GnRH), has been shown to be relatively successful (Simpson, 1988).

Another essential feature of the reproductive process is the transport of the egg from the ovary to the outer portion of the fallopian tube where union with the sperm occurs. Any factor which compromises ovum pick-up and transport by the tubes may contribute to infertility (Paterson & Petrucco, 1987). Fiberoptic technology has made direct investigation of tubal anatomy via laparoscopy safe and effective. In the past the investigation and treatment processes included only one partner, usually the female (Shapiro, 1988). Tubal microsurgery allows surgeons to repair adhesions, create openings in the tube if total occlusion is present, and perform uterotubal implantations to bypass severely damaged segments (Patton, 1988). However, tubal pathology often cannot be effectively repaired by tubal surgery. Until the early 1980s, a couple diagnosed with irremediable tubal disease was almost certainly destined to remain childless unless adoption was possible. However, the ability of reproductive scientists successfully to transfer an ovum fertilized *in vitro* into the uterus of the mother has given new hope for these patients (D'Amico & Gambone, 1989). The proliferation of *in vitro* fertilization (IVF) clinics is evidence of the current and projected success of this method of treating infertility. It is now estimated that 15 to 20% of women conceive during the *in vitro* fertilization cycle, and 50% of these conceptions result in live births (Pepperell et al., 1987).

Unfortunately, determination of the causes of infertility and development of treatments for infertility in men have not been as successful as in women. While semen analysis has improved over the past decade and is recognized as being indispensable in the evaluation of male fertility, it still leaves numerous unsolved problems. The lack of standard criteria for judging semen quality, the use of crude manual assessment of sperm numbers and motility, and the unpredictable variation of semen quality from week to week all contribute to difficulties in assessing the male partner (Makler, 1988). Despite these problems, examination of absolute number, character of motility, and number of motile sperm is critical in the evaluation of the infertile couple. Decreased number and/or quality of sperm in the ejaculate (oligospermia) constitutes the majority of cases of male subfertility (D'Amico & Gambone, 1989). While sexually transmitted diseases leading to genital infection, varicose veins in the scrotum, and immunological disorders may be involved in reducing the quality of the semen, the precise etiology of oligospermia is not well understood. Hence, treatment of any of these factors has not been very successful. What can be offered to couples in whom the male partner has untreatable sperm pathology is artificial insemination by donor sperm (AID) (D'Amico & Gambone, 1989). For those couples prepared to accept it, AID is the treatment of choice for overcoming childlessness in this situation.

Although advances in medical knowledge about problems of reproduction have far surpassed those in the behavioral sciences, it has become clear that consideration of the psychological features of the infertile couple must be an integral part of the management process (Mahlstedt, 1985). The relationship between psychological functioning and infertility may be causal, consequential, or both. Although it is very difficult to establish a causal link between psychological factors and infertility, there is some evidence indicating that extremes of behavior influence reproductive capacity (e.g., Bell, 1983; Edelmann & Connolly, 1986). What is easier to establish is that infertility itself provokes alterations in psychological functioning to varying degrees (e.g., Siebel & Taymor, 1982; Wright et al., 1991). The impact of the extensive diagnostic process and subsequent treatment regimens appears to have a substantial effect on psychological adjustment. The rest of this chapter will focus on the psychological aspects of infertility, and the associated implications for clinical intervention in the management of the infertile couple.

PSYCHOLOGICAL FACTORS AS CAUSES OF INFERTILITY

Over the past two decades, less and less emphasis has been placed on psychological factors as causes of infertility. In the past, a diagnosis of "psychogenic" infertility was made in patients whose infertility remained unexplained after the completion of diagnostic tests (Templeton & Penney, 1982). However, as advances in medical research have led to a better understanding of reproductive physiology and improved diagnostic techniques, a diagnosis can now be established for 90 percent of infertile couples (Mazor & Simons, 1984). For this reason, investigation of psychogenic factors as causes of infertility has diminished.

As appreciation for the complexity of interactions between human central nervous system functioning and neuroendocrinology has increased, however, a rationale for the contribution of psychological factors to infertility is apparent. There are central sites at which emotional states or personality factors can potentially alter the precise neuroendocrine regulation of reproductive processes (Mai, Munday, & Rump, 1972; Pepperell, Hudson, & Wood, 1980). Mozley (1976) proposed that eventually most cases of infertility will be traced to structural, physiological, or chemical malfunctioning in some aspect of the emotional center of the brain, the limbic system. One structure of the limbic system, the hypothalamus, is known to be involved in physiological responses to environmental stressors (Shapiro, 1988). Through the production of GnRH, the hypothalamus also interacts with the pituitary gland and ovaries to achieve fertile ovulations, as well as to influence spermatogenesis (Pepperell et al., 1987). Environmental stress may influence ovulatory and sperm functioning through its interaction at the hypothalamus (Shapiro, 1988).

The difficulty in establishing a causal link between psychological factors such as stress and infertility lies in the inability to distinguish between stress as a result of infertility and stress as a causal factor. For example, Berger (1980) reported impotence in some males after prolonged stress associated with infertility diagnostic evaluations. The psychopathology of the male's inability to maintain an erection, failure to ejaculate, and premature ejaculation has been investigated extensively (e.g., Rothman & Kaplan, 1972). However, the interaction between psychological factors and spermatogenesis is less known. It has been reported that, after repeated exposures to the emotional stress of infertility clinic investigations, male partners show reductions in sperm motility and numbers as compared with initial values (Christie & Pawson, 1987; Rothman & Kaplan, 1972). Also of interest is the finding that approximately 10 percent of infertile males show an improvement in their semen quality after cessation of all diagnostic and treatment processes (Siebel & Taymor, 1982). Although the direction of the effect of stress cannot be determined in these studies, it is apparent that stress can be involved at some level in the production of infertility.

Pennington and Atlay (1972) reported a study suggesting that the reassurance associated with a caring, systematic evaluation procedure may be enough to cause some women to conceive. Of 117 women with primary infertility referred to an endocrine investigation clinic, 72 elected to have stimulant drug therapy with Clomid, while the remaining 45 chose not to take drug therapy but underwent the same diagnostic work-up. At a 2-year follow-up evaluation, 56 percent of the 72 drug-therapy patients had conceived, a success rate similar to that found in other studies. Surprisingly, 42 percent of the 45 control patients also had conceived within two years. The investigators suggested that the enthusiasm and hope associated with the early stages of the infertility work-up may have contributed to the increased fertility in the control group.

There is much anecdotal information concerning psychological stress as a cause of infertility. Christie and Pawson (1987) describe a 30-year-old career woman with primary infertility and no apparent organic pathology. During a psychological assessment, it was suggested that perhaps her competitive life-style might be in conflict with her desires for motherhood. Soon after the discussion she quit her job, took a job helping at a local kindergarten, and conceived within the same month. Such anecdotes are plentiful in gynecological practice (Christie & Pawson, 1987; Edelmann & Connolly, 1986).

A number of investigators have attempted to demonstrate differences between infertility patients and comparison groups on various psychological and psychiatric characteristics (Downey et al., 1989; Edelmann & Connolly, 1986; Freeman, Garcia, & Rickels, 1983; Garcia, et al., 1985; Mai, Munday, & Rump, 1972; Paulson, Haarmann, Salerno, & Asmar, 1988). These studies have not consistently demonstrated that psychological impairment is associated with infertility. Although patients undergoing infertility treatment do report high levels of psychological distress (McEwan, Costello, & Taylor, 1987; Wright et al., 1991) and psychiatric symptoms such as anxiety and depression (Lalos, Lalos, Jacobsson, & Von Schoultz, 1986), few studies have established pretreatment psychological functioning which is necessary to establish causation. Daniluk's (1988) study is an exception. Previously undiagnosed couples were interviewed immediately after their first visit to an infertility clinic, four weeks later, within one week of diagnosis, and 6 weeks after diagnosis. Patients reported higher levels of anxiety and depression at the time of the first visit and at diagnosis (in the partner in which the disorder was found) than at other times. However, the interaction of these symptoms with the infertility itself is unclear, owing to the lack of a control group. In a prospective study, Downey et al. (1989) compared pretreatment psychological functioning in women presenting for infertility treatment versus routine gynecologic care. They found that infertility patients and controls were not significantly different on psychiatric symptomatology, depressive episodes, sexual functioning, or self-esteem. However, 75 percent of infertility patients reported mood changes which they attributed to their infertility. While the longitudinal follow-up data collection is not yet complete, they anticipate that, over time, the infertility patients will experience more anxiety, depression, and other psychiatric symptoms if treatment is unsuccessful.

In summary, there is little evidence at this time that psychological impairment causes infertility. Patients presenting for infertility evaluation and treatment are not significantly different from comparison groups on psychological functioning. Emotional stress can be involved in infertility, however, the direction and mechanisms of its effect are not known.

IMPACT OF INFERTILITY ON PSYCHOLOGICAL FUNCTIONING

The process of diagnosing and treating infertility has a profound impact on the lives of the people involved. Couples must cope not only with the intrusive medical evaluations and procedures, but also with the private pain of being childless in a predominantly family-oriented society. Added to the personal struggle are pressures from relatives, friends, and coworkers who recognize parenthood as an integral part of of the development of most adults. And, by its very definition, infertility is a symptom of a medical problem that has been present for at least one year. Facing the problem of infertility is a prolonged ordeal involving repeated attempts and failures, often over many years. The impact of diagnosis, treatment, and long-term consequences of infertility on psychological functioning is a complex matter which has important implications for the clinical care of the infertile couple.

Impact of Diagnosis

A diagnostic work-up can continue for months or years, and the length of time the couple must endure this process is directly related to the amount of psychological distress experienced (Lalos et al., 1986). Women in their thirties or forties report feeling anxious about reaching a diagnosis soon, so as to not waste any more precious months in achieving pregnancy (Shapiro, 1988). Each month acts as a reminder of the infertile couple's problem as the woman begins her period again. The couple must face constant decisions about the risks, costs, and privations of each new procedure.

Because women are more accustomed than men to receiving routine reproductive health care (annual Pap smears, breast and pelvic exams), they appear to withstand the initial diagnostic protocol without much affect on psychological functioning (Shapiro, 1988). However, as there is an increase in number of tests, expenses, and time spent in obtaining a diagnosis, anxiety and distress also rise (Mahlstedt, 1985; Mazor & Simons, 1984). Later tests such as hormone assays, laparoscopy, and endometrial biopsy may leave the woman feeling probed and manipulated (Christie & Pawson, 1987). In addition, charting daily basal body temperature causes some women to experience stress as a result of being constantly reminded of her inability to conceive (Shapiro, 1988).

Men, on the other hand, are much less accustomed to seeking medical care for their reproductive health. General apprehensions about seeing a physician are often intensified by the prospect of having to produce a semen sample by masturbation. This process has been reported to provoke feelings of guilt, inadequacy, and anxiety in the male partner (Mahlstedt, 1985). A poor semen analysis result often comes as a profound shock for both partners. Berger (1980) found that 63 percent of males experienced some form of impotency which lasted for 1 to 3 months after being diagnosed with oligospermia. Most of the wives reported feeling some anger toward their husbands. The process of having his sperm counted and evaluated can be threatening to even the most secure male ego (Menning, 1977).

Two diagnostic tests are particularly intrusive upon the couple's personal and sexual relationship. The postcoital test, where just prior to ovulation the woman must visit her physician within a few hours after having intercourse for evaluation of the cervical mucus–sperm interaction, can be highly stressful for both partners. Potency problems often arise for the male partner as he is aware of the expectations to "perform" upon demand (Christie & Pawson, 1987; Rosenfeld & Mitchell, 1979). Although loss of sexual drive is more obvious in the male partner at such times, the female partner can also experience it. Similar problems can arise when the couple is charting the woman's basal body temperature in order to determine the day of ovulation. Again, the male is required to have sexual intercourse on a schedule, and may experience what Drake and Grunert (1979) refer to as a "mid-cycle pattern of sexual dysfunction."

Impact of Treatment

Beginning a treatment program signifies a simultaneous hope for cure and confirmation of loss of important bodily functions (Mahlstedt, 1985; Shapiro, 1988). A person who has been physically and emotionally healthy enters infertility treatment and suddenly becomes a "patient". Various medications and surgeries cause both men and women suddenly to view their bodies as being damaged or defective, visions which are incompatible with usual images of health and youth (Mahlstedt, 1985). And, there may be actual loss of physical health as a cumulative result of the entire diagnostic and treatment process. Side effects from medications and recovery from surgery can cause physical illness.

The psychological impact of treatment is largely determined by the level of success expected to be associated with a particular treatment (Christie & Pawson, 1987; Shapiro, 1988). Thus it is the physician's responsibility not only to inform the couple of aspects of the procedure, but also to provide accurate information about predicted outcome. As Christie and Pawson (1987) point out, perhaps more than in any other field, the experience of helping the infertile couple can arouse strong feelings of elation, frustration, and anger in the physician. The physician's desire for success must always be balanced by communication of factual information to the patient.

The couple is usually eager for quick and successful treatment, and the physician may be tempted to respond accordingly. This is especially the case with a simple ovulatory disorder diagnosis where treatment can be effective relatively quickly (Brown, Pepperell, & Evans, 1987). It can be difficult for the physician and the couple to explore all other potential etiologies and treatments (Karp, 1972).

Long-Term Adjustment to Infertility

Long-standing infertility is a significant source of stress that produces a host of psychosocial consequences (Kraft et al., 1980). The experience of infertility without diagnosis or treatment is viewed as encompassing a series of losses including loss of important bodily functions, status, self-esteem, sense of control, security, dreams of experiencing pregnancy and childbirth and, of course, a child (Mahlstedt, 1985; Shapiro, 1988). The response of a couple being told that their infertility is caused by a problem for which there is no medical cure almost universally resembles that of mourning a death; that is, there are feelings of anxiety, anger, alienation, guilt, and depression (Mahlstedt, 1985; Menning, 1977; Shapiro, 1982). However, the loss of fertility or of an unborn child usually goes unrecognized by society (Shapiro, 1988). There are no rituals for formalizing the grief of the infertile couple. Friedman and Gradstein (1982) point out that infertility can be a silent, unrecognized loss that many couples struggle with alone.

It appears that there are certain risk factors associated with particularly poor coping responses to failed infertility treatments (Sabourin, Wright, Duchesne, & Belisle, 1991; Strauss, Appelt, Bohnet, & Ulrich, 1992). Newton, Hearn, and Yuzpe (1990) assessed psychological functioning in men and women pre- and post-*in vitro* fertilization. They found a significant subgroup of patients who appeared to be particularly vulnerable to anxiety and depressive episodes. Childless women with high levels of pre-IVF anxiety and depression were found to be at a greater emotional risk for poor coping responses post-IVF. The authors suggest that intervention in the form of grief counseling and assistance in gathering emotional support and coping resources may be especially necessary for these individuals.

Implications for Clinical Care

The emotional consequences of diagnosing, treating, and adjusting to infertility represent a significant struggle for many couples. Importantly, the couples' feelings and attitudes regarding this process can influence the outcome (Mahlstedt, 1985; Menning, 1977; Rosenfeld & Mitchell, 1979). Understanding and attending to the psychological component of infertility is as necessary as providing quality medical care.

During the diagnostic period, open discussion and full explanation of all investigative procedures by the physician appears to minimize the psychological trauma which can occur during this process (Christie & Pawson, 1987; Mahlstedt, 1985). In general, gathering information is an important step in coping with crisis and preparing to make decisions in order to confront a problem (Moos & Schaefer, 1986). The physician should inquire about couples' emotional reactions during each stage of the diagnostic process, and acknowledge the experience of such emotions as common, and probably normal, during the infertility testing process (Edelmann & Connolly, 1986; Mahlstedt, 1985). In situations where a patient or partner requires more emotional support than the physician is able to offer, professional psychological counselling should be arranged in order to facilitate integration of diagnostic information with future life plans (Shapiro, 1988). Such counseling usually consists of two- to three-month group sessions in which a physician, counselor or clinical psychologist, and couples discuss information concerning the procedures, and emotional and sexual problems encountered (Edelmann & Connolly, 1986).

The actions of the treating physician can have a substantial impact on psychological functioning during the infertility treatment program. It is the physician's responsibility not only to discuss and explain all procedures fully, but also to communicate realistic expectations with regard to outcomes and explore all treatment possibilities, regardless of his/her own eagerness for quick success for the couple (Christie & Pawson, 1987). In addition, encouragement of both partners to become involved during the treatment process is an important task of the physician. Sharing the responsibility of understanding the procedures, deciding the course of action, and providing emotional support appears to lessen the burden of the experience of infertility for the patient (Mahlstedt, 1985; Shapiro, 1988).

In the case of failed infertility treatment, it is extremely important that the infertile couple work through and resolve the emotional reactions they are experiencing before considering alternative approaches to parenthood (Christie & Pawson, 1987; Newton, Hearn, & Yuzpe, 1990; Shapiro, 1988). It is during this period of grief that the couple will require access to the appropriate professional counseling facilities and self-help organizations. When resolution of the grief and adjustment to the situation has occurred to some degree, the physician can then help the couple decide whether to explore other options for parenthood, and what those possibilities entail. Introduction of the various alternative methods for achieving parenthood (artificial insemination by husband or donor, in vitro fertilization, gamete intrafallopian transfer, and adoption) raise a wide array of emotional and moral problems for the infertile couple. Typical concerns include dealing with the feeling of achieving pregnancy in a noncoital way, the relatively low success rates of most of these procedures, the clinical atmosphere surrounding the procedures, religious and moral objections to technological reproduction, the capacity for emotional attachment to a child conceived in a nontraditional way, and long evaluation and waiting periods associated with adoption (Shapiro, 1988).

Helping a couple to adjust to the long-term consequences of infertility may be the most difficult aspect of the entire diagnostic–treatment process, and the one for which gynecologists are least prepared (Christie & Pawson, 1987). Professional counseling should be made available for such couples. Infertile couples considering alternative pathways to parenthood also need continuing preparation and support. Community self-help groups for IVF and artificial insemination patients exist in many places throughout the world (Christie & Pawson, 1987).

CONCLUSION

Proper management of infertility requires the evaluation of the couple as a unit in terms of possible etiologic factors and also awareness of the psychological and emotional factors precipitated by the investigation, treatment, and long-term adjustment. Unlike some diagnoses, infertility has definite medical and psychological components which appear to be inseparable. The professional who recognizes the intricate interaction of the intrusiveness of medical procedures, the personal pain associated with the inability to conceive, and the impact of external social relationships, will be most successful in managing the infertile couple.

REFERENCES

Bell, J. S. (1983). Psychological aspects. In T.B. Hargreave (Ed.), *Male infertility* (pp. 46–55). Berlin: Springer-Verlag.

Berger, D. M. (1980). Impotence following the discovery of azoospermia. *Fertility and Sterility, 34* , 154–156.

Brown, J. B., Pepperell, R. J., & Evans, J. H. (1987). Disorders of ovulation. In R. J. Pepperell, B. Hudson, & C. Wood (Eds.), *The infertile couple*. Edinburgh: Churchill Livingstone.

Christie, G. L., & Pawson, M. E. (1987). The psychological and social management of the infertile couple. In R. J. Pepperell, B. Hudson, & C. Wood (Eds.), *The infertile couple*. Edinburgh: Churchill Livingstone.

D'Amico, J. F., & Gambone, D. O. (1989). Advances in the management of the infertile couple. *American Family Physician, 39*, 257–264.

Daniluk, J. C. (1988). Infertility: Intrapersonal and interpersonal impact. *Fertility and Sterility, 49,* 982–994.

Downey, J., Yingling, S., McKinney, M., Husami, N., Jewelewica, R., & Maidman, J. (1989). Mood disorders, psychiatric symptoms, and distress in women presenting for infertility evaluation. *Fertility and Sterility, 52,* 425–432.

Drake, T. S., & Grunert, G. M. (1979). A cyclic pattern of sexual dysfunction in the infertility investigation. *Fertility and Sterility, 32,* 542–545.

Edelmann, R. J., & Connolly, K. J. (1986). Psychological aspects of infertility. *British Journal of Medical Psychology, 59,* 209–219.

Freeman, E. W., Garcia, C. R., & Rickels, K. (1983). Behavioral and emotional factors: Comparison of anovulatory infertile women with fertile and other infertile women. *Fertility and Sterility, 40,* 195–201.

Friedman, R., & Gradstein, B. (1982). *Surviving pregnancy loss.* Boston: Little, Brown.

Garcia, C. R., Freeman, E. W., Rickels, K., Wu, C., Scholl, G., Galle, P. C., & Boxer, A. S. (1985). Behavioral and emotional factors and treatment responses in a study of anovulatory infertile women. *Fertility and Sterility, 44,* 478–484.

Houghton, P. (1984). Infertility: The consumer's outlook. *British Journal of Sexual Medicine, 11,* 185–187.

Karp, L. (1972). Anovulation: What price fertility? *Obstetrics and Gynecology, 40,* 618.

Kraft, A. D., Palumbo, J., Mitchell, D., Dean, C., Meyers, S., & Wright-Schmidt, A. (1980). The psychological dimensions of infertility. *American Journal of Orthopsychiatry, 50,* 618–624.

Lalos, A., Lalos, O., Jacobsson, L., & Von Schultz, B. (1986). Depression, guilt, and isolation among infertile women and their partners. *Journal of Psychosomatic Obstetrics and Gynaecology, 5,* 197.

Mahlstedt, P. P. (1985). The psychological component of infertility. *Fertility and Sterility, 43,* 335–346.

Mai, F.M.M., Munday, R. M., & Rump, E. E. (1972). Psychosomatic and behavioural mechanisms in psychogenic infertility. *British Journal of Psychiatry, 120,* 199–204.

Makler, A. (1988). Modern methods in semen analysis and evaluation. In S. J. Behrman, R. W. Kistner, & G. W. Patton (Eds.), *Progress in infertility* (pp. 633–661). Boston: Little, Brown.

Mazor, M. D., & Simons, H. F. (1984). *Infertility: Medical, emotional, and social considerations.* New York: Human Sciences Press.

McEwan, K. L., Costello, C. G., & Taylor, P. G. (1987). Adjustments to infertility. *Journal of Abnormal Psychology, 96,* 108–116.

Menning, B. E. (1977). *Infertility: A guide for the childless couple.* Englewood Cliffs, NJ: Prentice-Hall.

Moos, R. H., & Schaefer, J. A. (1986). Life transitions and crisis: A conceptual overview. In R. H. Moos (Ed.), *Coping with life crises: An integrated approach* (pp. 3–28). New York: Plenum.

Newton, C. R., Hearn, M. T., & Yuzpe, A. A. (1990). Psychological assessment and follow-up after in vitro fertilization: Assessing the impact of failure. *Fertility and Sterility, 54,* 879–886.

Paterson, P., & Petrucco, O. (1987). Tubal factors and infertility. In R. J. Pepperell, B. Hudson, & C. Wood (Eds.), *The infertile couple*. Edinburgh: Churchill Livingstone.

Patton, G. W. (1988). Microsurgical Reconstruction of the Oviduct. In S. J. Behrman, R. W. Kistner, & G. W. Patton (Eds.), *Progress in infertility* (pp. 125–154). Boston: Little, Brown.

Paulson, J. D., Haarmann, B. S., Salerno, R. L., & Asmar, P. (1988). An investigation of the relationship between emotional maladjustment and infertility. *Fertility and Sterility, 49*, 258.

Pennington, G. W., & Atlay, R. D. (1972). Some surprising results in the investigation and treatment of infertile women. *Journal of Obstetrics and Gynaecology of the British Commonwealth, 79*, 651.

Pepperell, R. J., Hudson, B., & Wood, C. (1980). *The infertile couple*. Edinburgh: Churchill Livingstone.

Pepperell, R. J., Hudson, B., & Wood, C. (1987). *The infertile couple* (2nd ed.). Edinburgh: Churchill Livingstone.

Rosenfeld, D. L. & Mitchell, D. (1979). Treating the emotional aspects of infertility: Counselling services in an infertility clinic. *Americal Journal of Obstetrics and Gynecology, 135*, 177.

Rothman, D., & Kaplan, A. H. (1972). Psychosomatic infertility in the male and female. In J. G. Howells (Ed.), *Modern perspectives in psycho obstetrics* (pp. 31–50). Edinburgh: Oliver and Boyd.

Sabourin, S., Wright, J., Duchesne, C., & Belisle, S. (1991). Are consumers of modern fertility treatments satisfied? *Fertility and Sterility, 56(6)*, 1084–1090.

Shapiro, C. H. (1982). The impact of infertility on the marital relationship. *Social Casework, 63*, 387–393.

Shapiro, C. H. (1988). *Infertility and pregnancy loss*. San Francisco: Jossey-Bass.

Siebel, M. M. & Taymor, M. L. (1982). Emotional aspects of infertility. *Fertility and Sterility, 37*, 137–145.

Simpson, J. L. (1988). Ovarian failure (gonadal dysgenesis). In S. J. Behrman, R. W. Kistner, & G. W. Patton (Eds.), *Progress in infertility* (pp. 239–272). Boston: Little, Brown.

Strauss, B., Appelt, H., Bohnet, H. G., and Ulrich, D. (1992). Relationship between psychological characteristics and treatment outcome in female patients from an infertility clinic. *Journal of Psychosomatic Obstetrics and Gynaecology, 13*, 121–133.

Templeton, A. A., & Penney, G. L. (1982). The incidence, characteristics, and prognosis of patients whose infertility is unexplained. *Fertility and Sterility, 37*, 175–182.

Wright, J., Duchesne, C., Sabourin, S., Bissonnette, F., Benoit, J., & Girard, Y. (1991). Psychosocial distress and infertility: Men and women respond differently. *Fertility and Sterility, 55*, 100–108.

10

Prenatal Diagnosis

Gail L. Rose

INTRODUCTION

Prenatal diagnosis is studied in many different contexts. Physicians and medical researchers recognize its technological advances (e.g., Olds, London, & Ladewig, 1988), while ethicists discuss its link with the eugenics movement and efforts to improve the race by discouraging the birth of handicapped children (de Francisco & Dreyfuss, 1981; Rothman, 1986). The purpose of this chapter is to describe the psychological aspects of the assessment of fetal status during pregnancy. First, some basic information about the medical aspects of prenatal diagnosis will be provided. Next the psychological issues involved in the decision to have prenatal diagnosis, the experience of prenatal diagnosis, and the outcome of prenatal diagnosis will be considered.

MEDICAL ASPECTS

Prenatal Diagnosis and Genetic Counseling

Prenatal diagnosis can be contrasted with genetic counseling, although ideally they are part of the same process. Both of these services involve the assessment of pregnancy risk, but prenatal diagnosis must be performed while the pregnancy is under way. The primary goal of genetic counseling is the assessment of reproductive risk (Abramson, 1981). By assessing maternal age, obtaining the couple's reproductive and medical history, and evaluating each partner's family history of congenital malformation and genetic diseases, a genetic counselor can usually provide the couple with some indication of the degree and type of risks involved in a future pregnancy. Prenatal diagnosis is then offered to parents at high reproductive risk for diagnosable conditions (Donnai, 1987). The goal of prenatal diagnosis is to enable the woman either to continue her pregnancy with confidence that it is unaffected by abnormality, or to allow her to make management decisions in the event of a positive diagnosis (Marteau et al., 1989).

The ideal time for risk assessment is before conception. Discussion of risks and options with the client is facilitated before the stresses and time limitations of pregnancy are imposed (Donnai, 1987).

TECHNIQUES AND PROCEDURES

The four most common methods of prenatal diagnosis are maternal serum alpha-fetoprotein screening, ultrasound, amniocentesis, and chorionic villus sampling. This section will focus on the medical aspects of these four diagnostic techniques.

Maternal Serum Alpha-Fetoprotein (MSAFP) Screening

Alpha-fetoprotein is a protein manufactured by the fetus which can be detected in the mother's blood. Weekly increases in the level of this protein are perceptible (Milunsky, 1986). Deviations from normal levels of maternal serum alpha-fetoprotein can signal fetal abnormality. Elevated levels may indicate the presence of neural tube defects such as anencephaly and spina bifida, while decreased levels can indicate fetal chromosome trisomies, such as Down's Syndrome (DS, trisomy 21) and trisomy 18 (Milunsky, 1986; Nightingale & Goodman, 1990). Maternal serum alpha-fetoprotein screening requires a single tube of blood from the mother, and is optimally performed between 16 and 18 weeks gestation (Milunsky, 1986).

The test for MSAFP is a screen; not a diagnostic test. The screen is designed to signal the need for further diagnostic testing. It cannot correctly diagnose specific birth defects, nor can it guarantee a normal fetus in the event of a negative screen. Elevations and depressions in alpha-fetoprotein levels can be detected for reasons other than fetal abnormality, such as inaccurate gestational age, multiple gestation, maternal weight, and maternal smoking (Milunsky, 1986).

Due to the many influences on MSAFP levels, false positive rates can be quite high. To minimize false positives while maximizing detection of affected fetuses, centers conducting MSAFP screens determine cutoff scores. If the level of MSAFP detected in a screen exceeds the cutoff score, the serum is considered elevated and a second test, obtained at least seven days after the first sample, is usually recommended (Williamson, 1994). Ultrasound is commonly performed in conjunction with the second sample in order to determine gestational age and to detect signs of neural tube defect. If fetal abnormality is suggested by the second phase of testing, amniocentesis is usually recommended (Nightingale & Goodman, 1990).

The accuracy of maternal serum screening for the detection of DS is enhanced by the "triple marker screening" procedure in use at some centers (Wald et al., 1988). Using this procedure, a single sample of maternal blood is analyzed for unconjugated estriol and human chorionic gonadotrophin, in addition to alpha-fetoprotein. In Down's Syndrome pregnancies, levels of unconjugated estriol are lower than normal, while levels of human chorionic gonadotrophin are about twice as high as normal. By examining the combined relative deviations from average of the three products, the practioner can estimate a probability that the fetus is affected. Information derived from this triple screen allows for greater detection of DS with fewer false positives. As with MSAFP screening, abnormal results are typically followed by further diagnostic testing, particularly ultrasound and amniocentesis.

Ultrasound

Ultrasound, or sonography, is performed by passing high-frequency, low-intensity sound waves through the abdomen and/or vagina or labia of the pregnant woman. Echoes are reflected from tissues of varying densities, and can be displayed on a monitor. This procedure enables the practitioner and the pregnant woman to view an image of the fetus *in utero* (Nicolaides & Campbell, 1986; Nightingale & Goodman, 1990).

The tissue, organ, and skeletal imagery obtained with ultrasound provides information that can be used in a number of different ways. Among other things, an ultrasound exam allows for early pregnancy detection, measurement of the fetus and, hence, the determination of fetal age, presence of multiple gestation (e.g., twins, triplets), and detection of congenital anomalies, especially neural tube defects (Nicolaides & Campbell, 1986). Importantly, ultrasound may be used as an adjunct to more invasive procedures, such as amniocentesis and chorionic villus sampling (CVS). For example, using ultrasound, the fetus and placenta can be located and avoided when inserting a needle during amniocentesis.

There are several advantages of ultrasound. It can be performed at any time during pregnancy, it is painless and harmless to both mother and fetus, multiple conditions can be diagnosed with one assessment, and results are obtained immediately (Langer, Ringler, & Reinold, 1988). There are apparently no inherent disadvantages of the procedure.

Amniocentesis

Amniocentesis is an outpatient procedure typically performed between 14 and 16 weeks gestation. Guided by sonography, a long needle is inserted through the woman's abdomen and into her uterus. Amniotic fluid is then removed for chromosomal or enzymatic analysis (Elias & Simpson, 1986). Chromosomal analyses demonstrate any aneuploidy (deviation from a normal set of 46 chromosomes), while enzyme analyses of fetal cells can indicate about 75 diseases of body chemistry (Ampola, 1981), such as Tay-Sachs, a fat-storage disease which causes progressive neurological deterioration and death of the child within four years of birth. Results from amniocentesis are usually available 2 to 4 weeks after the procedure.

The most common reason for performing amniocentesis is to test for DS in women over 35 (Ampola, 1981). The risk of bearing a child with DS increases gradually from a rate of 1/2,400 at age 20, to a rate of 1/40 at age 45 (Ampola, 1981). Amniocentesis for women aged 35 or older became standard practice when the procedure could be performed with a complication rate approximately equal to the risk of bearing a child with DS (i.e., approximately 1/250, or 0.4%). Amniocentesis is also indicated if the parents have had a previous child with aneuploidy, if one of the parents carries a balanced chromosomal translocation, if the mother is a sex-chromosomal mosaic (i.e., she is apparently normal, but may have two or more populations of cells that vary in their sex-chromosomal constitution), if the mother carries a severe sex-linked recessively inherited disease, or if both parents are carriers for a single gene mutation that would produce an inborn error of metabolism in the offspring. All of these conditions place a future child at risk for genetic anomaly (Robinson & Henry, 1985).

Amniocentesis carries with it a degree of risk due to its invasive nature. Maternal and/or fetal infection, trauma to the placenta, and fetal puncture are a few of the rarer complications (Elias & Simpson, 1986). A more common risk is that of inducing an abortion as a result of the procedure. A decade ago, this was occurring in approximately 0.4% to 1.2% of cases (Seeds & Azizkhan, 1990). That is, out of 1,000 pregnancies, there were anywhere between 4 and 12 additional miscarriages after the sixteenth week of pregnancy in women undergoing amniocentesis, compared with those women not undergoing amniocentesis. Now that sonography is being used in conjunction with amniocentesis to guide needle insertion, the complication rate has fallen to approximately 0.25% (R. A. Williamson, personal communication, January 10, 1994).

The main advantage of amniocentesis is its accuracy. Actual fetal chromosomes can be obtained and karyotyped, and alpha-fetoprotein can be analyzed more accurately than with maternal serum screening. In addition, amniocentesis is the only procedure that can diagnose certain metabolic diseases. As a result of the invasiveness of the procedure, however, the woman is put at greater risk of pregnancy loss. An additional disadvantage is the long wait for results. Kolker (1989) reports a typical wait of four weeks for the return of laboratory results, which can be an extremely stressful time for the at-risk mother. In some centers, though, complete cytogenic results are, in most cases, available within two weeks (S. Grant, personal communication, October, 1992). In addition to sometimes having a long wait for results, a woman who decides, upon receiving the results, to terminate her pregnancy must have a second-trimester abortion, which is more emotionally and medically difficult than a first-trimester abortion.

Chorionic Villus Sampling (CVS)

CVS is the newest technique discussed here. This procedure involves the removal of a piece of tissue from the placenta, using a catheter inserted through the cervix (rarely, the abdomen). The basis for this procedure is that the membrane (chorion) surrounding the fetus, and the tissues (villi) responsible for its implantation, are derived from the fetus, and are thus genetically identical to the fetus. For this reason, chorionic villi can be sampled to obtain cells which contain chromosomes identical to those of the fetus (Olds et al., 1988).

The biggest advantage of CVS over amniocentesis is that the procedure can be performed much earlier, at 8–12 weeks instead of 14–18 weeks. In addition, the results are generally available within one week of the procedure, so that the waiting time is reduced. Results are typically obtained in time for a first-trimester abortion, if the woman so chooses (Nightingale & Goodman, 1990). However, the rate of spontaneous abortion in women undergoing CVS is approximately twice that of women having amniocentesis (Kolker, 1989). Also, CVS is somewhat less accurate. An overall error rate of 1.7%, including false positives and false negatives, is reported for CVS by Hogge, Schonberg and Golbus (1986), while amniocentesis has an error rate of less than 1%. Finally, while CVS can detect chromosomal and biochemical defects, it cannot diagnose neural tube defects. This relatively new procedure is the focus of much research attention. As more is learned about CVS, its safety and accuracy may improve.

PSYCHOLOGICAL ASPECTS

The Decision to Undergo Prenatal Diagnosis

Information and risk assessment. What factors are involved in a decision to undergo prenatal diagnosis? When a woman is faced with a choice of whether or not to have prenatal diagnosis, she has usually deemed herself to be at risk of delivering a diseased or disordered child. A woman's subjective assessment of risk can be confirmed objectively by a genetic counselor. Once her pregnancy is determined to be at risk, the woman must give informed consent to have diagnostic procedures carried out. In order to make a choice, the woman and her partner need access to information about the risks involved in the procedure, the possible outcomes of the procedure, the accuracy of the diagnosis and prognosis, and the options available in the event of a positive diagnosis (Donnai, 1987).

The risks involved with the various diagnostic techniques have been discussed. A woman considering prenatal diagnosis, amniocentesis and chorionic villus sampling in particular, must decide whether or not the information to be gained from such an assessment is worth the possible dangers to herself and her fetus inherent in the procedure (Kolker, 1989).

Usually, diagnostic testing of the fetus is performed to determine the presence or absence of a particular disease, for example, Tay-Sachs in Ashkenazi Jews, or DS in women over age 35. Women whose fetuses are determined to be at risk for a particular disease need to know the chances that their fetus will be affected, and the prognosis or degree of impairment of children with that disease.

The accuracy of the various methods of assessment may play a role in a woman's decision to have prenatal diagnosis. The woman considering prenatal diagnosis must be made aware of the precision of the testing instrument or technique, and the limits of confidence of both positive and negative diagnoses. Empirical validation of the importance of this information was provided by Faden et al. (1987). In this study, women were asked to report their willingness to abort a fetus during the fifth month of pregnancy if the probability that the fetus had a neural tube defect was one percent, 25 percent, 50 percent, 75 percent, 95 percent, or 100 percent. As the probability of a positive diagnosis increased from 25 to 95 percent, the number of women who indicated that they would abort the fetus increased linearly. However, when the diagnostic accuracy increased from 95 to 100 percent, there was a 50% increase in the number of women reporting that they would abort, which deviated from the linear trend. Because a difference in certainty of 5 percentage points can make quite a difference in women's management decisions, it is very important to provide women considering diagnostic procedures with precise information about accuracy.

Finally, knowledge about the possible courses of action once a positive diagnosis has been made will help a woman decide whether or not she wants to submit to the procedures. In most cases, there are only two options available in such a circumstance: abortion of the affected fetus, or birth of an abnormal child. This is not to say that a woman having prenatal diagnosis must decide beforehand what she would do in the event of a positive diagnosis and commit to a course of action. Rather, the woman ought to be aware of the kind of decision she may have to face once the results are known (Locke, 1981).

Because the decision to undergo prenatal diagnosis involves weighing many serious issues, one might expect that it would be made jointly by the woman and her partner. A recent investigation of men's reactions to prenatal diagnosis challenges this assumption (Sjogren, 1992). The men in this study were remarkably uninformed. Only one-third of the men interviewed were considered to have good knowledge about the risk of congenital disorders, while just over half were knowledgeable about the diagnostic method in question. Half of the men expressed satisfaction with the information they had received. Few men actively engaged in information gathering and decision making. Most men stated that the decision was ultimately up to their partner, and considered their own role in the process to be one of providing advice.

Advantages and Disadvantages. The issue of whether or not prenatal diagnosis ought to be performed has been raised in the literature. There are three main theoretical benefits of prenatal diagnosis that have been both advocated and criticized on ethical, technical, empirical, and theoretical grounds: b*alancing of risks, reassurance*, and *preparation*.

Rothman (1986) raises the issue of balancing of risks. For example, the use of amniocentesis to test fetal chromosomes for DS is generally advocated by medical professionals at maternal age 35, when the risk of miscarriage due to the amniocentesis procedure is roughly equivalent to the chances of having a child with the chromosomal abnormality. Rothman (1986) suggests that this is a faulty equation. The meaning of miscarriage cannot be uniformly equated with the meaning of bearing a child with DS, as the relative significance of these events will widely differ for each woman and each family. Therefore, a woman must personally assess the meaning of pregnancy loss and fetal abnormality when considering amniocentesis.

Prenatal diagnosis has also been advocated because of the reassurance a negative diagnosis can provide women who are concerned about the status of their fetus (e.g., Robinson & Henry, 1985). Because approximately 98% of the results obtained from prenatal diagnosis are negative (VanPutte, 1988), it can be argued that diagnostic procedures provide reassurance to the majority of women who have them. Marteau et al. (1989) provide empirical support for the practice of advising women to have prenatal diagnosis for the reassurance it can provide. Their study demonstrated that those who had prenatal diagnosis, with a negative result, were less anxious in the third trimester of pregnancy than those who did not have prenatal diagnosis. Fathers, too, express relief and anticipation of an untroubled continuation of pregnancy upon receiving a negative test result (Sjogren, 1992).

The opposing viewpoint, voiced by Rothman (1986), is that prenatal diagnosis is able to allay only those fears that it initially raises. This position, too, has received empirical support. Hunter, Tsoi, Pearce, Chudleigh, and Campbell, (1987) studied reactions to ultrasound in women with raised serum alpha-fetoprotein, compared with women undergoing routine ultrasound. Although both groups of women showed a reduction in anxiety after the scan (all scans displayed normal fetuses), the women with raised alpha-fetoprotein levels were significantly more anxious than the control women before the scan. Thus it appears that prenatal diagnosis may provide reassurance, but that it may also raise anxiety levels unnecessarily, in the event of false positive diagnoses. Additionally, some women take more reassurance from amniocentesis than it can objectively provide. That is, if it is determined that a woman's fetus does not have DS, she may mistakenly believe that her child will have no problems at all, a conclusion that cannot be provided by any prenatal test (Seeds & Azizkhan, 1990).

A third, debatable benefit of prenatal diagnosis is that it allows women to prepare themselves for the outcome. Adjustment to a handicapped infant will be stressful and will require emotional adaptation regardless of whether the parents learn of the child's problem prior to, or at the time of birth. It is possible that if the anomaly is learned of early, however, the woman (couple) will be able to go through a period of adjustment before the birth of the child, when there may be more energy available to devote to adjustment (Zuskar, 1987). It is possible that foreknowledge may make it easier for the parent(s) to accept the child at birth, because they have had a head start at the adjustment process.

The alternative viewpoint is that early detection of a fetal abnormality may actually impede adjustment. The main reason for this assertion is that the prognosis, chances for survival, or quality of life of children with many prenatally diagnosable conditions cannot be accurately predicted. Thus a clear and objective diagnosis may have no real meaning because the prognosis is uncertain (Rothman, 1986; Zuskar, 1987). Because each child is different, knowledge that one's baby has an extra chromosome, as in DS, is not adequate preparation for what the child will be like, nor for his or her precise neonatal needs. Instead, early detection may create a stressful continuation of pregnancy, and cause the parents-to-be to focus on the disability rather than on the individuality of the child (Rothman, 1986). Because anxiety during pregnancy has been associated with obstetric complications and neonatal difficulties, it is possible that the stress associated with foreknowledge of fetal status may serve only to jeopardize further the abnormal fetus (Zuskar, 1987).

Decisive Factors. Despite academic debate about the benefits of prenatal diagnosis, many women go through the decision-making process and choose for themselves either to submit to the procedures, or to wait until delivery day to discover the status of their child. What reasons are decisive for these women? Probably the most common reason for having prenatal diagnosis is medical encouragement (Rothman, 1986). Women who are determined to be at risk for the birth of an abnormal child, either because of maternal age (the most common reason; Alder & Kushnick, 1982), or because of historical information (Robinson & Henry, 1985), are typically encouraged by their physicians to have the procedures performed (Seeds & Azizkhan, 1990). Other reasons include spousal encouragement, and the desire not to raise a handicapped child.

Many women who would not consider selective abortion decide not to put themselves in the position of learning of fetal abnormality. For these women, the risks and the waiting involved in the process of amniocentesis are not worth the knowledge gained from the procedure. Rothman (1986) interviewed women who had made the choice not to proceed with prenatal testing, and asked them the decisive factors in their decision. Several of the reasons revolved around moral opposition to abortion. Others included faith that their child was going to be normal, or acceptance of whatever child is "given." In contrast to the women who chose to have amniocentesis, the women who decided against it were not particularly encouraged to have the procedure by medical staff, husbands, or friends. A final reason stated for choosing not to have amniocentesis is a history of miscarriage or infertility, because amniocentesis increases risk of miscarriage.

THE EXPERIENCE OF PRENATAL DIAGNOSIS

The Procedure

Once a woman has consented to prenatal testing, specific information about the procedure should be made available to her by the medical staff as soon as possible. The procedure should be offered at a time when accurate results are most likely (Donnai, 1987).

For the most part, the diagnostic procedures are physically painless. Emotional distress, rather than physical, is common among women undergoing amniocentesis, and is also reported by a significant minority of fathers (Sjogren, 1992). Some of this distress is due to the occurrence of obstetrical error during amniocentesis, which may result in multiple needle stabs, dry taps, or spilled samples. Yet, even when the procedure is performed smoothly, some women and their partners find the situation distressing because the risk of error and the possibility of miscarriage are omnipresent, and because the status of the fetus is yet unknown (Rothman, 1986; Sjogren, 1992).

In contrast to the negative psychological experience of amniocentesis in some cases, ultrasound generally has a positive effect on observers. The opportunity to view the fetus and to have its anatomy explained makes the procedure worthwhile to patients, and makes patients feel more confident, informed, involved, reassured, and relieved (Reading, Cox, & Campbell, 1988).

The Waiting Period

Most diagnostic techniques, with the exception of ultrasound, require some period of waiting before the results are known. During this period of uncertainty about the status of her fetus, the pregnant woman is reluctant to acknowledge the reality of her pregnancy (Rothman, 1986; Silvestre & Fresco, 1980). Heidrich and Cranly (1989) found that women awaiting amniocentesis to determine chromosomal constitution of the fetus had significantly lower maternal–fetal attachment scale scores than women awaiting ultrasound to determine fetal age and women not undergoing treatment, despite similar gestational ages. Fathers, too, appear weakly attached to the fetus at the time of pregnancy when amniocentesis is typically performed (Sjogren, 1992). Perhaps a pregnancy that may end in selective abortion is not fully experienced as real.

This time of ambivalence is experienced as stressful by many parents (Kolker, 1989; Sjogren, 1992). While some fathers are themselves very worried, others are able to attend to the mother's distress and provide emotional support (Sjogren, 1992).

THE OUTCOME OF PRENATAL DIAGNOSIS

Good Outcome

As previously indicated, the vast majority of diagnostic results are negative. With the receipt of negative results, the stress and anxiety expressed by parents waiting to hear the outcome of their tests often vanishes (Donnai, 1987; Sjogren, 1992). Relief, euphoria, confidence, and reassurance are common emotional reactions to a good outcome. Although it may be true that prenatal diagnosis augments anxiety during the waiting period (Rothman, 1986; Kolker, 1989), the receipt of negative results appears to prevent a third-trimester rise in anxiety levels normally observed in women with no knowledge of fetal status (Marteau et al., 1989).

Ultrasound has been shown to have a profound psychological impact on the mother's experience of her pregnancy (e.g., Hunter et al., 1987; Langer et al., 1988; Villeneuve, Laroche, Lippman, & Marrache, 1988). Viewing the image of the fetus serves to confirm the reality of the pregnancy, especially for women who have not yet felt fetal movement (Donnai, 1987; Villeneuve et al., 1988). The process also seems to encourage a maternal perception of the infant as a unique individual, separate from the mother (Villeneuve et al., 1988).

Langer et al. (1988) assessed the change in maternal perceptions following a single ultrasound exam. Child image and, to a lesser extent, body perception were markedly changed after the procedure. Mothers perceived their babies as being significantly more active, strong, beautiful, and familiar after the procedure, as compared with before. Women's postscan perceptions of their own bodies changed toward the pleasant, relaxed, strong, and fearless poles of an analog scale. Thus the results of this study indicate that a woman's perceptions of both herself and her fetus are altered in a very positive way as a result of one ultrasound scan. A study by Villeneuve et al. (1988) corroborates these results, and adds that mothers report fetal movement to be the most positive feature of the imaging.

Bad Outcome

Immediate reactions. In approximately 2% of cases, the outcome of prenatal diagnosis is positive, indicating a problem with the fetus (VanPutte, 1988). The psychological reactions many women have to a diagnosis of fetal abnormality are typically profound. Hunter et al. (1987) report state anxiety levels in women with raised alpha-fetoprotein to be significantly higher than women undergoing a routine ultrasound, and "notably higher than other obstetrically normal women reported in the literature" (p. 37).

Being confronted with an abnormal fetal diagnosis precipitates a meaningful crisis for a woman. Typically, a woman's reactions include an initial state of shock, disorientation, and disbelief. Feelings of fear, unreality, despair, sadness, disappointment, and failure are common (Jorgensen, Uddenberg, & Ursing, 1985; Korenromp, Iedema-Kuiper, van Spijker, Christiaens, & Bersema, 1992; Rothman, 1986; VanPutte, 1988). VanPutte (1988) emphasizes the feelings of loss that these women experience. Women differ in what they perceive as being lost. That is, for some women it is the state of pregnancy which is lost; for others it is the fantasized perfect child, or the potential for parenthood. Regardless of the object of her loss, the patient's grieving process is characteristic of a major loss. Rothman (1986) agrees that regardless of the woman's termination decision, she has lost something precious, and has the right to grieve.

During this difficult time, women are more likely to turn to their husbands for emotional support than they are to discuss their feelings with relatives or members of a professional staff (Heymans & Winter, 1975). Adler and Kushnick (1982) found that other family members were unlikely to become involved with the subsequent decisions, although they occasionally played supportive roles. Some women find support in their religious communities.

Ultimately, upon receiving a bad diagnosis, the woman is forced to confront the decision of whether or not to abort the affected fetus. In Kenen's (1981) analysis, this decision creates double approach–avoidance. The pregnant woman desires a child, and may be morally opposed to abortion, yet she may also recognize that an abortion would alleviate future suffering, not only of the child, but of the family. This double approach–avoidance conflict illustrates the weight of responsibility which is inevitably felt regardless of which decision is made. Because the parents are forced to choose either abortion or acceptance of a disabled child, they will feel ultimately responsible for the outcome, whichever they decide (Rothman, 1986).

Pregnancy termination. Given that both options available to a woman receiving a positive diagnosis are aversive, how does she decide? Some reasons
given by women deciding in favor of the abortion (the most common choice)
include negative past experiences with handicapped children and/or adults, an
awareness or perception of society's cruelty to the mentally and physically handicapped, judgments about the future quality of the child's life, the effects on the
family, and the drain on society (Adler & Kushnick, 1982; Rothman, 1986).

A main factor in the decision to terminate is the diagnosis of a fatal condition
(Jorgensen et al., 1985; Rothman, 1986). To a woman convinced that her child
will die at birth or shortly thereafter, continuation of the pregnancy to term may
seem pointless. The mother may in fact feel that she is minimizing the child's
suffering by terminating the pregnancy. Faden et al. (1987) studied attitudes
toward the abortion of defective fetuses in a group of pregnant women. Subjects
were asked whether or not they felt they would have an abortion if they knew
that their pregnancy would have a particular outcome. The women in this study
were more likely to predict that they would terminate a pregnancy if the child
were going to die at birth or shortly thereafter, than if it was going to survive but
be severely handicapped. In interpreting this finding, the authors speculate that
abortion may be viewed as less morally wrong if the baby will die anyway. This
interpretation is supported by Jorgensen and colleagues (1985), who report that
a majority of women claim to be morally opposed to abortion, but find it
acceptable in the case of a malformed fetus.

The choice of selective abortion over delivery of a handicapped infant is
rarely an easy decision. It is simply a choice between two tragic alternatives
(Kolker, 1989). Because the woman is making a conscious decision to terminate
a desired pregnancy, she will often experience very negative psychologic sequelae.
Part of what makes the experience of selective abortion so aversive are the
characteristics of the procedure. The most common diagnostic technique to
precede selective abortion is amniocentesis. Due to the nature of this technique,
by the time a woman finally learns of her fetus' diagnosis, she is well into her
second trimester, and has begun to show significant signs of being pregnant.

In the second trimester, there are a variety of procedural options for inducing
abortions (see Chapter 13). Although each has its unique advantages and disadvantages, each is unpleasant and none is ideal. If labor is induced, severe labor
pain and drug side effects are common (VanPutte, 1988). This pain is often
accompanied by sadness and disappointment, in stark contrast to the joy that
usually accompanies the birth of a child (Kolker, 1989; Rothman, 1986). One
advantage of having an induced-labor abortion is that it allows couples to see,
hold, and/or bury their fetus if they desire to do so (VanPutte, 1988). Viewing
the fetus afterward seems to make the situation a reality, and to confirm the
woman's belief that she made the right choice (Jorgensen et al., 1985; Rothman,

1986). Not all women will choose to see the premature baby after it is aborted, however.

Dilation and evacuation is emotionally less traumatic for those women who wish not to confront the fetus (Kolker, 1989). It does not require the pregnant woman to endure labor, and it has fewer complications than some labor-induction methods. Because this technique is more taxing to the physician, however, many are reluctant to perform it (Kolker, 1989). Jones et al. (1984) recommend surgical termination because it may result in fewer episodes of posttermination depression. Korenromp et al. (1992), however, recommend induction of labor because it offers the parents an opportunity to identify with the subject of their grief, which they cite as a positive factor in coping. Ultimately, the choice of the second-trimester termination method should be made by the parents.

To make the termination of a wanted pregnancy less emotionally painful, it is important for centers to provide appropriate settings and for staff to be sensitive to the unique situation. The placement of such a patient on a hospital maternity ward, where she would be surrounded by new mothers and healthy babies, for example, would be highly inappropriate (Kolker, 1989; Rothman, 1986; VanPutte, 1988). In a clinic setting, staff may be unaccustomed to dealing with selective terminations, and may be unprepared for the parents' emotional reactions of anger and sadness (Rothman, 1986). In any center, grief can be minimized by tailoring the setting characteristics and counseling approaches to the individual situation.

Psychologic sequelae of termination vary greatly, from gratitude that the available procedures allowed for the abortion, to long-term emotional difficulties. While there are some women who do not experience posttermination depression, but rather happiness that amniocentesis was available (Adler & Kushnick, 1982; Rothman, 1986), most women feel profound pain and grief, which has been likened in degree to that experienced by women losing a child perinatally (Jorgensen et al., 1985; Rothman, 1986). Because the object of her grief is not as well defined as that of a mother losing her child perinatally, however, the degree of distress felt by the woman is not generally recognized by the rest of society, including medical professionals and the woman's husband (Kolker, 1989). Feelings of guilt are common among women who terminate their pregnancies for a nonlethal fetal defect, but are are rarely expressed by women terminating for other reasons (Korenromp et al., 1992).

Adler and Kushnick (1982) succinctly describe the progression of emotions after selective abortion. For the first few hours after the termination, most women experience denial of the event. Several conflicting feelings follow:

> . . . sadness for losing the baby, relief that it was over, guilt for having gone through with the termination, bitterness as to why it should have happened to

them and not to others, and doubts as to their role of being able to reproduce satisfactorily. (p. 97)

This phase typically lasts for 2–3 months. Yet these feelings of inadequacy have been known to persist longer than a year in some cases, with the anniversary of the abortion or the expected date of birth being particularly difficult times. In this way, grief following selective abortion shares many attributes with grief reactions to perinatal and postnatal deaths.

Men's reactions to the termination appear to differ from women's. Korenromp et al. (1992) interviewed 40 women who underwent termination for genetic reasons, and 31 of their husbands. They found that men expressed strong feelings of helplessness and of being an outsider. Men felt pressure to remain strong, and were perceived as having repressed their feelings as a result of this pressure. Tensions between husband and wife were in several cases attributed to the man's repression of his emotions. Men were less likely to talk with others about the event, which wives tended to attribute to a lack of caring on the part of the husband. Actually, the men expressed greater fear of subsequent pregnancy than did the wives. Six months after the termination, Korenromp et al. (1992) found that the majority of their sample still suffered episodes of sadness and low spirits. Respondents identified the third and fourth months as the most difficult phase of grieving, during which time a subsample of individuals who had suffered serious psychological or social problems prior to this pregnancy required professional assistance to cope with the termination.

Acceptance of a disabled child. Finally, it is important to consider the alternative to selective abortion. Relatively few women receiving a positive diagnosis choose not to terminate. For this reason, little is known about the psychological reactions of those who knowingly give birth to an abnormal child. Literature on parents of non-prenatally diagnosed handicapped children reveals that these parents experience some reactions in common with parents learning of their baby's anomaly through prenatal diagnosis. In particular, they report the stages of shock, denial, sadness, anger, adaptation, and reorganization common to those receiving a prenatal diagnosis of fetal abnormality (Zuskar, 1987). An interesting, yet small population for future study are the women who choose to continue their pregnancy despite a positive prenatal diagnosis.

CLINICAL CARE

Throughout the process of prenatal diagnosis, there are many opportunities for psychological intervention. Decision making and crisis resolution are two areas in which women undergoing prenatal diagnosis, or even considering it, may profit from intervention.

As mentioned previously, a choice of whether or not to have prenatal diagnosis requires a substantial amount of information. Specifically, the woman needs access to information about the risks involved in the procedure, the possible outcomes of the procedure, the accuracy of the diagnosis and prognosis, and the options available in the event of a positive diagnosis (Donnai, 1987). All of this information may be difficult to assimilate, especially if the woman is already pregnant and pressured by time constraints (Jorgensen et al., 1985). Thus a pregnant woman may require professional assistance to assimilate all the information on which she must base her decision whether or not to undergo diagnostic testing.

Women who decide in favor of prenatal diagnosis (particularly amniocentesis) must wait two weeks, and sometimes up to four weeks, for the results. To reduce some of the uncertainty inherent in this time of waiting (Heidrich & Cranly, 1989; Rothman, 1986; Silvestre & Fresco, 1980), the woman should be given a precise indication of when the results will be available. Scheduling an appointment in advance for the discussion of the results may help, especially if the woman is told that she may bring a spouse, friend, or relative (Donnai, 1987). In addition, some women feel that an opportunity to talk with other "waiting" women would have helped them during this time. While a woman waiting for the results of her amniocentesis may publicly deny her pregnancy, she may need support from those close to her who are informed of the pregnancy. In the event that this social support is absent, supportive counseling may be a worthwhile option.

When the results of prenatal testing indicate an abnormal fetus, it is essential that information be provided to the woman in a detailed, yet sensitive way. The patient must be given a careful, complete, and accurate assessment of the diagnosis, as well as a simple and understandable prognosis of the particular disorder in the event that the child is carried to term. The patient needs to know what to expect on the day she gives birth, as to the condition of the child, and any special delivery circumstances that the condition warrants (Seeds & Azizkhan, 1990). Because a positive diagnosis is experienced as a crisis in many situations (Jorgensen et al., 1985; Rothman, 1986; VanPutte, 1988) these patients have special needs. Upon hearing the bad news, subjects in a study described by VanPutte (1988) reported the need for help with crisis resolution, the need for assistance in coming to terms with the reality of the event, a sense of urgency, and a need for and appreciation of the opportunity to speak with medical staff immediately after the diagnostic information was relayed to them. Thus women receiving bad diagnoses require continued support and information from health professionals, and some may require help with crisis resolution.

Although the majority of women receiving a positive diagnosis opt to abort, women should be warned against making that decision too hastily (Jorgensen et al., 1985; VanPutte, 1988). Patients need to take time for multiple contacts with medical professionals, and to think things through for themselves. Once the decision has been made, continued contact with the medical facility is essential. Some centers have integrated counseling services that extend beyond the period of selective termination, or that provide ongoing support and counseling to couples who choose to continue the pregnancy of an affected fetus (Williamson, 1994).

The majority of women who selectively abort an affected fetus retrospectively report satisfaction with their decision (VanPutte, 1988). However, a small percentage of women who have selective abortion go through an extended period of grieving, which has been observed to last up to three years (the ceiling on most longitudinal studies in this literature). The main problem confronting couples who are deeply hurt by the selective abortion is whether or not to attempt another pregnancy (Silvestre & Fresco, 1980). Any subsequent pregnancy can be a stressful time for women who have previously terminated, and for their husbands (Sjogren, 1992). Continuity of care provided by staff who are familiar with the woman's history is essential, because anxieties are evident even after the birth of a normal child (Donnai, 1987).

Like many women who opt for selective abortion, those bearing handicapped children often grieve for extended periods. A woman in this situation needs continuing information and emotional support from her counseling care givers.

In summary, the role of the psychological service provider throughout the process of prenatal diagnosis varies with each stage of the process. A woman whose pregnancy is determined to be at risk may require assistance from a nonjudgmental professional in order to assimilate the information and to make a decision. While the woman is waiting to hear the results of her test, she may require supportive counseling. Crisis management may be required in the event of a positive diagnosis, and continued support may be necessary for those who experience extended grieving for an aborted fetus.

SUMMARY

Throughout the entire process of prenatal diagnosis, from the decision-making point, through the procedure and waiting period, to the informing of outcomes and the subsequent decision-making, procedures and adjustment, a woman has several needs. Information is vital. A woman and her partner need all the information available about risks, procedures, and options. They also need emotional support. The hospital or clinic staff need to provide the couple everything necessary to make a decision, and then to support them in the decision, and in the hard times that may follow. In short, a practitioner must compliment his or her procedural knowledge with sensitivity to the parents' psychological reactions to the experience.

REFERENCES

Abramson, F. D. (1981). Policy decisions in prenatal diagnosis: The example of fetal alcoholism syndrome. In H. B. Holmes, B. B. Hoskins, & M. Gross (Eds.), *The custom-made child?* (pp. 89–94). Clifton, NJ: Humana Press.

Adler, B., & Kushnick, T. (1982). Genetic counseling in prenatally diagnosed trisomy 18 and 21: Psychosocial aspects. *Pediatrics, 69,* 94–99.

Ampola, M. G. (1981). Prenatal diagnosis. In H. B. Holmes, B. B. Hoskins, & M. Gross (Eds.), *The custom-made child?* (pp. 75–80). Clifton, NJ: Humana Press.

de Francisco, C. P., & Dreyfuss, G. (1981). Prenatal diagnosis: Psychiatric aspects. *Biological Psychiatry, 16,* 109–110.

Donnai, D. (1987). The management of the patient having fetal diagnosis. *Bailliere's Clinical Obstetrics and Gynaecology, 1,* 737–745.

Elias, S., & Simpson, J. L. (1986). Amniocentesis. In A. Milunsky (Ed.), *Genetic disorders and the fetus: Diagnosis, prevention, and treatment* (pp. 31–52). New York: Plenum Press.

Faden, R. R., Chwalow, A. J., Quaid, K., Chase, G. A., Lopes, C., Leonard, C. O., & Holtzman, N. A. (1987). Prenatal screening and pregnant women's attitudes toward the abortion of defective fetuses. *American Journal of Public Health, 77,* 288–290.

Heidrich, S. M., & Cranley, M. S. (1989). Effect of fetal movement, ultrasound scans, and amniocentesis on maternal–fetal attachment. *Nursing Research, 38,* 81–84.

Heymans, H., & Winter, S. T. (1975). Fears during pregnancy. *Israeli Journal of Medical Science, 111,* 1102–1105.

Hogge, W. A., Schonberg, S. A., & Golbus, M. S. (1986). Chorionic villus sampling: Experience of the first 1000 cases. *American Journal of Obstetrics and Gynecology, 154,* 1249–1252.

Hunter, M. S., Tsoi, M. M., Pearce, M., Chudleigh, P., & Campbell, S. (1987). Ultrasound scanning in women with raised serum alpha fetoprotein: Long term psychological effects. *Journal of Psychosomatic Obstetrics and Gynaecology, 6,* 25–31.

Jones, C. W., Penn, N. E., Schuchter, S., Stafford, C. A., Richards, T., Kernahan, C., Gutierrez, J., & Cherkin, P. (1984). Parental response to mid-trimester therapeutic abortion following amniocentesis. *Prenatal Diagnosis, 4,* 249–256.

Jorgensen, C., Uddenberg, N., & Ursing, I. (1985). Ultrasound diagnosis of fetal malformation in the second trimester. The psychological reactions of the women. *Journal of Psychosomatic Obstetrics and Gynaecology, 4,* 31–40.

Kenen, R. H. (1981). A look at prenatal diagnosis within the context of changing parental and reproductive norms. In H. B. Holmes, B. B. Hoskins, & M. Gross (Eds.), *The custom-made child?* (pp. 67–74). Clifton, NJ: Humana Press.

Kolker, A. (1989). Advances in prenatal diagnosis: Social-psychological and policy issues. *International Journal of Technology Assessment in Health Care, 5,* 601–617.

Korenromp, M. J., Iedema-Kuiper, H. R., van Spijker, H. G., Christiaens, G.C.M.L., & Bergsma, J. (1992). Termination of pregnancy on genetic grounds; coping with grieving. *Journal of Psychosomatic Obstetrics and Gynaecology, 13,* 93–105.

Langer, M., Ringler, M., & Reinold, E. (1988). Psychological effects of ultrasound examinations: Changes of body perception and child image in pregnancy. *Journal of Psychosomatic Obstetrics and Gynaecology, 8,* 199–208.

Locke, E. (1981). Antenatal diagnosis: The physician–patient relationship. In H. B. Holmes, B. B. Hoskins, & M. Gross (Eds.), *The custom-made child?* (pp. 81–88). Clifton, NJ: Humana Press.

Marteau, T. M., Johnston, M., Shaw, R. W., Michie, S., Kidd, J., & New, M. (1989). The impact of prenatal screening and diagnostic testing upon the cognitions, emotions and behaviour of pregnant women. *Journal of Psychosomatic Research, 33,* 7–16.

Milunsky, A. (1986). The prenatal diagnosis of neural tube and other congenital defects. In A. Milunsky (Ed.), *Genetic disorders and the fetus: Diagnosis, prevention, and treatment* (pp. 453–520). New York: Plenum Press.

Nicolaides, K. H., & Campbell, S. (1986). Diagnosis of fetal abnormalities by ultrasound. In A. Milunsky (Ed.), *Genetic disorders and the fetus: Diagnosis, prevention, and treatment* (pp. 521–570). New York: Plenum Press.

Nightingale, E. O., & Goodman, M. (1990). *Before birth: Prenatal testing for genetic disease.* Cambridge, MA: Harvard University Press.

Olds, S. B., London, M. L., & Ladewig, P. A. (1988). *Maternal-newborn nursing: A family-centered approach,* 3rd ed., (pp. 529–558). Menlo Park, CA: Addison-Wesley.

Reading, A. E., Cox, D. N., & Campbell, S. (1988). A controlled, prospective evaluation of the acceptability of ultrasound in prenatal care. *Journal of Psychosomatic Obstetrics and Gynaecology, 8,* 191–198.

Robinson, A., & Henry, G. P. (1985). Prenatal diagnosis by amniocentesis. *Annual Review of Medicine, 36,* 13–26.

Rothman, B. K. (1986). *The tentative pregnancy: Prenatal diagnosis and the future of motherhood.* New York: Viking.

Seeds, J. W., & Azizkhan, R. G. (1990). *Congenital malformations: Antenatal diagnosis, perinatal management and counseling* (pp. 1–66). Rockville, MD: Aspen Publishers.

Silvestre, D., & Fresco, N. (1980). Reactions to prenatal diagnosis: An analysis of 87 interviews. *American Journal of Orthopsychiatry, 50,* 610–617.

Sjogren, B. (1992). The expectant father and prenatal diagnosis. *Journal of Psychosomatic Obstetrics and Gynaecology, 13,* 197–208.

VanPutte, A. W. (1988). Perinatal bereavement crisis: Coping with negative outcomes from prenatal diagnosis. *Journal of Perinatal and Neonatal Nursing, 2*(2), 12–22.

Villeneuve, C., Laroche, C., Lippman, A., & Marrache, M. (1988). Psychological aspects of ultrasound imaging during pregnancy. *Canadian Journal of Psychiatry, 33,* 530–535.

Wald, N. J., Cucle, H. S., Densem, J. W., Mamchahal, K., Royston, P., Chard, T., Haddow, J. E., Knight, G. J., Palomaki, G. E., & Canick, J. A. (1988). Maternal serum screening for Down's syndrome in early pregnancy. *British Medical Journal, 297,* 883–887.

Williamson, R. A. (1994). Abnormalities of alpha-fetoprotein and other biochemical tests. In D. K. James, P. J. Steer, C. P. Weiner, & B. Gonik (Eds.), *High risk pregnancy: Management options* (pp. 643–659). Philadelphia: W. B. Saunders.

Zuskar, D. M. (1987). The psychological impact of prenatal diagnosis of fetal abnormality: Strategies for investigation and intervention. *Women & Health, 12,* 91–103.

11

Childbirth Preparation

Elizabeth F. Swanson-Hyland

Childbirth is experienced by approximately 85 to 90 percent of women. Although it is often considered painful, childbirth remains a source of great joy and pleasure for most women. Various techniques, such as education, have been employed to increase a woman's positive experience with labor and decrease its painful aspects. These techniques generally focus on reducing anxiety, providing factual information, and providing practical tools for coping with pain during labor (Hassid, 1978). However, it is not clear to what extent these goals are being met through current childbirth preparation methods nor is it clear which components of childbirth preparation may be responsible for beneficial effects.

Because many pregnant women obtain some form of childbirth preparation (Worthington, 1982), the efficacy of these preparation techniques will be examined. First, this chapter presents an overview of the stages of labor. Second, three different types of childbirth preparation and some of the potentially important outcomes of childbirth preparation will be examined. Third, methodological concerns about the research on the effectiveness of childbirth preparation will be discussed. Fourth, the efficacy of childbirth preparation as well as the components of childbirth preparation will be reviewed. Finally, the clinical implications of childbirth preparation and its efficacy will be discussed.

STAGES OF LABOR

The providing of information about the three stages of labor is considered important in minimizing the anxiety and discomfort of labor by most methods of childbirth preparation. Research conducted to examine the efficacy of childbirth preparation also focuses on the sense of pain associated with a particular stage of labor. For these reasons, the stages of labor will be reviewed.

The first stage of labor starts with the first uterine contractions and continues until the cervix is completely dilated to 10 cm. The contractions help thin the cervix until it becomes completely effaced, merging with the walls of the uterus, generally at a dilation of 2–3 cm. The mean duration of the first stage of labor is 9.7 hours for a nullipara and 8.0 hours for a multipara (O'Brien & Cefalo, 1991).

When the second stage begins, contractions become more powerful and there is an accompanying urge to push the baby out and down the birth canal. Women are advised to push only when experiencing a contraction so that the two forces, pushing and contracting, can work together and conserve the woman's energy. The second stage of labor ends when the baby emerges from the birth canal. This stage has a mean duration of 33 minutes for the first birth and 8.5 minutes for subsequent births (O'Brien & Cefalo, 1991).

The third stage of labor begins with the delivery of the baby and ends with the delivery of the placenta. After delivery of the baby, the uterus continues to contract to expel the placenta. The mean duration of the third stage of labor is 5 minutes for both nulliparas and multiparas (O'Brien & Cefalo, 1991). After the delivery of the placenta is complete, medication may be given to prevent excessive bleeding and stimulate the uterine muscles to contract. Also, any tears or incisions in the vagina and perineum are repaired. There is a great deal of variability in the length of labor from woman to woman. Different methods of childbirth preparation approach these stages of labor in different ways.

TYPES OF CHILDBIRTH PREPARATION

In this section the principal elements and rationale for three methods of childbirth preparation, the *Lamaze* (or psychoprophylactic) approach (Lamaze, 1970), the *Dick-Read* approach (Dick-Read, 1959), and *hypnosis* (Harmon, Hynan, & Tyre, 1990; Venn, 1986) will be presented. Other methods of childbirth preparation include the LeBoyer and the Bradley methods (Hassid, 1978). There is, however, a relatively poor research base for these methods and they will not be discussed.

Lamaze

Lamaze may be the most commonly used method of child birth preparation, being used to prepare as many as one-half of all women for delivery (Wideman

& Singer, 1984). The Lamaze approach, which promotes childbirth without pain, is highly structured and generally consists of six to eight classes held in the last trimester of pregnancy. This approach is based on Pavlov's principles of classical conditioning and the work of Platonov and Velvosky in Russia. Platonov and Velvosky viewed pain in childbirth as a social phenomenon that was unnecessary and useless (Lamaze, 1970). Platonov and Velvosky also assumed that the pain of childbirth is exacerbated when the woman interprets the bodily process of labor as "pain" and reacts accordingly (Calhoun, Selby, & Calhoun, 1980). It was further assumed that a woman can learn not to interpret contractions as "pain" and substitute another behavior for the pain behavior (Calhoun et al., 1980).

As taught in the United States, Lamaze classes involve instruction in several domains, including: a) the anatomy and physiology of pregnancy and labor; b) the physiological and psychological basis of painless childbirth; c) breathing techniques; d) conditioned relaxation; and e) social support (Lamaze, 1970; Wideman & Singer, 1984). More specifically, the instruction on anatomy and physiology consists of an explanation of pregnancy, fetal development, uterine contractions, stages of labor, as well as an explanation of the birth process (Lamaze, 1970). The role of the nervous system and classical conditioning in the experiencing of pain are also discussed, providing a framework for the discussion of the physiological and psychological basis for painless childbirth (Lamaze, 1970).

Controlled breathing is taught, to maintain a balanced level of carbon dioxide and oxygen during labor and delivery and to inhibit responding to stimuli or sensations from the uterus (Lamaze, 1970). Controlled, rhythmic breathing is used during much of the first stage of labor, and shallow, rapid breathing is used at the end of the first stage. During the second stage of labor, rapid breathing is believed to be most effective (Lamaze, 1970). The specific pattern of breathing can be altered as needed at any time during delivery and there are variations on these techniques that may be used.

Conditioned relaxation is also taught in Lamaze childbirth preparation. Women are taught relaxation techniques so that the stimulus of a contraction is a signal to begin relaxation. First, the woman assumes a comfortable position. She is next instructed to focus on a spot on the wall to enhance concentration on both breathing and relaxing. The next step is for the woman to take a deep breath and relax as she exhales. Finally, the coach instructs her selectively to tense one part of her body, for example, the right leg, accompanied by inhalation, and to relax her muscles along with exhalation.

Lamaze childbirth preparation also encourages a supportive spouse or friend to take part in the preparation and childbirth. The coach attends classes with the woman, oversees practice at home, and participates in the delivery. The coach may provide a light abdominal or lower-back massage, help the woman remember the relaxation and breathing techniques, and help with the timing and execution of the techniques during labor. In addition, the coach may provide reassurance, caring, and support for the mother (Wideman & Singer, 1984).

Dick-Read

The Dick-Read method of childbirth preparation promotes "childbirth without fear" (Dick-Read, 1959). Dick-Read argued that labor pain and discomfort occurred because women expected labor and delivery to be painful. He reasoned that because normal processes are not ordinarily painful and childbirth is a normal process, it should not be painful. A Fear–Tension–Pain Syndrome was proposed as the cause of pain experienced during childbirth. The Fear–Tension–Pain Syndrome is a cycle in which the fear of pain leads to excessive tension in the uterus which leads to the experience of pain which in turn leads to increased fear (Dick-Read, 1959).

Women are given instruction in four areas: *anatomy and physiology of labor and childbirth, correct breathing, relaxation,* and *general fitness exercises* (Dick-Read, 1959). Lectures on the anatomy and physiology of labor and childbirth include information on the anatomy of the uterus, the role of the nervous system, the growth and development of the fetus, the hygiene of pregnancy, and an explanation of labor (Dick-Read, 1959).

The second area of instruction in the Dick-Read method is correct breathing, which, he argued, was the foundation of good health. During the first stage of labor, as the contractions increase in intensity, the woman's respiration becomes deeper and more rapid. In the second stage of labor, when the woman is bearing down, she is taught to hold her breath when bearing down, and take two or three controlled deep breaths while waiting for the next contraction. When the baby crowns, the woman is instructed to pant with rapid and shallow breaths rather than hold her breath as before (Dick-Read, 1959).

The third and fourth areas of instruction are relaxation and exercise. The relaxation component is based on Jacobson's progressive relaxation technique (Jacobson, 1938). This method of relaxation entails tensing and relaxing various groups of muscles to facilitate whole-body relaxation. The exercise component is used to enhance the woman's general sense of well-being and also to enhance the mobility and flexibility of the pelvic muscles and joints.

These classes are generally unstructured and individual instructors make changes according to their own beliefs (Hassid, 1978). An undirected or nondirective agenda for teaching the techniques of coping with labor allows the woman the freedom to decide on the use or nonuse of the techniques.

The Lamaze and Dick-Read method differ primarily in the theoretical underpinnings of the method and not so much in the actual preparation. Some variability will be introduced by the instructors of the classes, although variability is likely to be greater in classes using the Dick-Read method than the Lamaze method. Although both methods strive to minimize pain during childbirth, the goal of the Lamaze method is to prevent the occurrence of pain, whereas the goal of the Dick-Read method is to reduce tension and fear in order to reduce pain. Additionally, both methods attempt to minimize the use of analgesics and anesthetics during labor. The Lamaze method recognizes that medication may be necessary during childbirth although the goal is to reduce or eliminate medication. The Dick-Read method is more explicit in its attempt to reduce medical interference.

Hypnosis

In addition to the Lamaze method and the Dick-Read method, hypnosis has also been used in childbirth preparation. Hypnosis in this context refers to a temporary mental state in which the woman experiences an increased susceptibility to suggestion which can, in turn, lead to sensory and physical changes (Macfarlane, 1977). During hypnosis, the woman is given the suggestions to feel the contractions during labor but not to experience them as painful. Suggestions are also given about increased relaxation during childbirth, enjoyment of childbirth, and postpartum well-being and healing. The women utilizing this preparation method practice hypnosis daily by listening to tapes with the aforementioned suggestions. When a woman is ready to go into labor, she is given either a posthypnotic suggestion before labor, as previously mentioned, or she may be in a hypnotized state throughout the entire labor and delivery.

Hypnosis has a long history in childbirth preparation. In the early 1900s, Russians were using hypnosis in childbirth, however, it proved to be unreliable and ineffective for large groups (Hassid, 1978; Lamaze, 1970). More recently it has been argued that hypnosis and Lamaze have many similarities (Venn, 1986). Both hypnosis and Lamaze use relaxation, controlled breathing, eye fixation, suggestion, a group setting, an authority figure, and reassurance to the woman that she can cope with the stresses of childbirth. Therefore, it has been argued that the two may function similarly (Venn, 1986).

METHODOLOGICAL CONCERNS

Studies of the efficacy of childbirth preparation programs suffer from a number of methodological problems. These problems include a lack of random assignment of subjects to groups or appropriate control groups, reliance on self-report data, poor descriptions of the preparation program, and little attention to the importance of the various components of that package. The consequence of these problems will be briefly discussed.

Often, women are not randomly assigned to receive or not receive childbirth preparation (Beck & Hall, 1978; Beck & Siegel, 1980). As a consequence, the women who choose to receive preparation may be different from women who do not choose to receive preparation, resulting in a referral bias. Women who receive childbirth preparation reportedly tend to have a higher level of prenatal care and prenatal monitoring than women who do not receive childbirth preparation (Wideman & Singer, 1984). In addition, the failure to use attention-placebo control groups make it difficult to determine if the effects of factors such as demand characteristics, that is, the subject responding the way she believes the experimenter wants her to respond, and attention may be responsible for the treatment effects (Beck & Hall, 1978; Beck & Siegel, 1980).

Several investigators have suggested that maternal self-report after delivery is unreliable (Fridh, Kopare, Gaston-Johansson, & Turner Norvell, 1988; Wideman & Singer, 1984). In contrast, other research has suggested that reports of pain during labor are stable and reliable for at least six months after childbirth (Cogan, Perkowski, & Anderson, 1988). A related issue is that pain fluctuates quite a bit during labor, and a global rating of pain will not capture pain levels at different stages of labor (Erskine, Morley, & Pearce, 1990). An approach which may be used in conjunction with self-report or in place of self-report is the use of observer ratings. Observer ratings of pain during childbirth have been found to be lower than self-reported ratings of pain (Brown, 1990). However, observer ratings and self-report ratings seem to be highly correlated (Broome & Koehler, 1986).

The specific content of the classes, the effectiveness and approach of the teacher, and specific supportive behaviors by the companion are not often detailed by researchers (Simkin & Enkin, 1989). These are important variables that need to be conceptualized clearly in future research. A related problem with this research is the issue of which components of the childbirth preparation methods are responsible for the positive outcomes. Much of this research is done on multicomponent preparations, making it difficult to identify factors responsible for the therapeutic effects (Beck & Siegel, 1980).

EFFICACY OF CHILDBIRTH PREPARATION

Beneficial effects of childbirth preparation may include reduced pain and discomfort, more positive subjective evaluations of the birthing process, and improved obstetrical outcome (Broome & Koehler, 1986; Calhoun et al., 1980; Hughey, McElin, & Young, 1978; Leventhal, Leventhal, Shacham, & Easterling, 1989; Lowe, 1989; Melzack, Taenzer, Feldman, & Kinch, 1981; Wideman & Singer, 1984). The evidence for these beneficial effects and the overall efficacy of the previously described methods of childbirth preparation will be reviewed followed by a review of the efficacy of the components of these methods.

Pain and Discomfort

Pain in childbirth has been variously described as sharp, cramping, pulling, aching, throbbing, stabbing, hot, shooting, heavy, tiring, exhausting, intense, unbearable, and tight (Brown, 1990; Melzack, 1984). It is clear that the pain of childbirth can be significant and that efforts at lessening the pain of childbirth are worthwhile.

Both anesthesia and analgesia are used to help control the pain of childbirth. Two types of anesthesia are fairly common during vaginal delivery. Epidural anesthesia involves injecting a local anesthetic agent into the space outside the spinal canal below the base of the spine, to numb the sensory nerves running to the lower half of the body (Cohen, Acker, & Friedman, 1989). This provides anesthesia for both labor and delivery. A pudendal block is a local anesthetic injected through the vagina (Chestnut & Gibbs, 1991), to numb the lower pelvis and perineum at the time of vaginal delivery. Nalbuphine and meperidine (Nubain, Demerol) are narcotic analgesics widely used during labor being injected intravenously or intramuscularly (Chestnut & Gibbs, 1991).

Research, including some controlled studies, has suggested that childbirth preparation may be useful in reducing pain and medication use during labor. Women who have received either the Lamaze or the Dick-Read method of childbirth preparation report less pain and discomfort during delivery than women who did not receive preparation (Calhoun et al., 1980; Leventhal, et al., 1989; Lowe, 1989; Melzack et al., 1981). Pain is not eliminated altogether, however (Melzack, 1984). In addition to decreased pain and discomfort, women who received childbirth preparation were rated as less tense and anxious by medical personnel than women who did not receive preparation. Furthermore, these women reported lower anxiety levels (Klusman, 1975; Zax, Sameroff, & Farnum, 1975) and used less general and local anesthesia (Hetherington, 1990; Timm, 1979).

Several studies have documented an association between childbirth preparation and decreased use of anesthesia and/or analgesia during labor (Broome & Koehler, 1986; Calhoun et al., 1980; Hughey et al., 1978; Scott & Rose, 1976; Worthington, 1982). Melzack and his colleagues (1981) reported, however, that 83% of a sample of 141 women who received Lamaze training requested epidural anesthesia despite their instructor's advice against it. Moreover, Patton, English, and Hambleton (1985) found no difference in the use of anesthesia and analgesia between Lamaze-prepared women and those with no preparation. Thus, conflicting results and poor methodology limit the conclusions that can be drawn regarding the influence of childbirth preparation on the use of anesthesia and analgesia.

Subjective Evaluations

In research on childbirth preparation programs, subjective evaluations from both the mother and father have been examined. Maternal evaluation has included women's attitudes toward pregnancy, labor and delivery, themselves, their husbands, and their children. Fathers' attitudes and feelings of control during delivery have also been assessed.

Research has suggested that women who receive childbirth preparation may have more positive recollections about the childbirth experience than women who have not received this preparation (Calhoun et al., 1980). In one study, women who received childbirth preparation exhibited more positive views toward pregnancy, labor and delivery, themselves, and their husbands and children than did women who had not received preparation (Broome & Koehler, 1986; Wideman & Singer, 1984). It should be noted, however, that the concept of satisfaction with childbirth is broadly defined and that a reliable and valid assessment instrument does not exist (Hodnett & Osborn, 1989). Without a consistent definition of "satisfaction with childbirth," caution must be exercised in the interpretation of these results.

Childbirth preparation may influence fathers' attitudes as well. Men who participate in childbirth preparation may view themselves as having greater control than men who do not have preparation (Wideman & Singer, 1984). In one study, fathers reported feeling more positive about their participation in childbirth and more positive toward their wives after childbirth preparation (Cronenwett & Newmark, 1974).

Obstetrical Outcomes

A number of studies have examined the relation of childbirth preparation and Apgar scores—scales rating a newborn's physical health status (Apgar, 1953). Babies of mothers who have received childbirth preparation had higher Apgar scores at both the 1-minute (Hetherington, 1990) and 5-minute ratings than babies of mothers who had not received training (Hughey et al., 1978). These findings, however, have not been substantiated, and may reflect the selection/ referral biases in nonrandomized trials, as noted above (Leventhal et al., 1989; Patton et al., 1985; Scott & Rose, 1976; Sturrock & Johnson, 1990).

With respect to other obstetrical outcomes, Lamaze-prepared women have been reported by some to have fewer complications, including fewer: cesarean sections, premature births, peritoneal lacerations, postpartum infections, preeclampsia, postpartum hemorrhage, and perinatal mortality (Hughey et al.,

1978; Timm 1979). Again, the findings regarding decreased obstetrical complications are not consistently supported, making it unclear if childbirth preparation is effective (Leventhal et al., 1989; Patton et al., 1985; Scott & Rose, 1976). Broome and Koehler (1986) have noted that the variability of the definition of complications as well as differences in physician practices are possible methodological problems. That is, physicians who encourage preparation may be less likely to use forceps or cesarean sections (Broome & Koehler, 1986).

Duration of labor as an outcome of childbirth preparation has also been studied. The results on this outcome are also equivocal (Broome & Koehler, 1986; Calhoun et al., 1980). Although some studies have suggested that women who receive childbirth preparation may have shorter labors, several other studies have found no relation between preparation and duration of labor (Leventhal et al., 1989; Patton et al., 1985; Scott & Rose, 1976; Timm 1979).

EFFICACY OF HYPNOSIS

Few studies have examined the effects of hypnosis on childbirth. A recent study (Harmon et al., 1990) divided subjects into high and low susceptibility to hypnosis. Subjects then received childbirth preparation combined with skill mastery. Half of the subjects received a hypnotic induction suggesting relaxation associated with labor and delivery, enjoyment of childbirth, numbness in the dominant arm that spreads to other areas of the body, and postpartum well-being and healing (4 groups total). Women who had been hypnotically prepared had shorter first stages of labor, used less medication, had more spontaneous deliveries, and had babies with higher Apgar scores than control subjects. Lower depression scores were reported by highly susceptible, hypnotically prepared women than women in the other groups. Another study compared hypnosis alone, Lamaze alone, and hypnosis plus Lamaze (Venn, 1986). No differences were found in self-ratings of pain, amount of medication, nurse ratings of pain, or duration of labor.

Research addressing the efficacy of childbirth preparation programs has measured variables such as pain and discomfort, subjective evaluations of the birthing process, and obstetrical outcomes. As mentioned previously, one problem with the research on the overall efficacy of the methods of childbirth preparation is the lack of controlled research. In contrast, research conducted to evaluate the efficacy of the various components of childbirth preparation methods has more often been appropriately controlled and is thus more useful.

EFFICACY OF COMPONENTS OF
CHILDBIRTH PREPARATION

Laboratory analog studies are often used to determine the utility of the components of childbirth preparation. That is, much of the research examining components of childbirth preparation is conducted with stressful procedures other than childbirth, for example, the cold pressor test. In the cold pressor test, an individual is asked to put her hand and forearm into ice water and hold it there as long as possible. Although a technique may be effective for coping with the pain of a cold pressor test, it may not be effective for coping with the pain of childbirth. It is also not clear to what extent the efficacy of various components of these methods generalizes to the efficacy of a preparation technique as a whole. Additionally, the mechanism of action for equally efficacious techniques may not be the same.

To address the issue of comparability of stressful procedures, Worthington (1982) conducted a study in which he compared subjects on tolerance, pain, and distress during both a cold pressor test and during labor. The subjects were either pregnant women who had received Lamaze training or pregnant women who had received parenting classes without Lamaze training. Worthington's results suggested that women who had greater tolerance and reported less pain and distress on the cold pressor test also exhibited greater tolerance and reported less pain and distress during labor than women who did not perform well on the cold pressor test. Based on these findings, the cold pressor test may be a valid means for assessing the effects of Lamaze training or its components on women's pain management during labor. More research is needed, however, before firm conclusions can be drawn about the utility of this laboratory analog paradigm and its relation to childbirth pain.

The factors of childbirth preparation that cause or contribute to the beneficial effects remain unclear. Furthermore, components of the preparation program that may be interfering with potential benefits are also unclear. Components of childbirth preparation that may account for the efficacy of preparation include information, both by itself and with modeling of relaxation and controlled breathing, controlled breathing, relaxation and visual focus, and social support. Much of the research on the effective components of childbirth preparation has been analog research. The research involves attempts to control or alleviate laboratory-induced pain or controlling pain in other painful medical procedures.

Information

Childbirth preparation may help in the formation of accurate expectations and create a sense of security so that anticipatory distress will be reduced (Leventhal et al., 1989). This is potentially important because inaccurate expectations about pain and discomfort have been associated with a higher intensity of labor pain (Fridh et al., 1988).

In a childbirth-preparation analog study, Manderino and Bzdek (1984) compared subjects who received videotaped information, videotaped modeling, both videotaped information and modeling, and an irrelevant control condition. The subjects who received both videotaped information and modeling reported significantly lower pain levels than the other three groups. Thus, sensory information accompanied by modeling may be one beneficial component of childbirth preparation and merits further research.

Controlled Breathing

Controlled breathing appears to reduce autonomic responsivity to painful stimuli (Harris, Katkin, Lick, & Haberfield, 1976). Controlled breathing also may serve as a distractor and thereby increase pain tolerance (Beck & Siegel, 1980). Worthington and Martin (1980) conducted a study comparing women who had received Lamaze training in controlled breathing and women who had not received training. Women who used the Lamaze training techniques demonstrated greater pain tolerance on a cold pressor test than women using deep slow breathing. However, studies testing changes in breathing in response to changes in the stimulus, as occurs with labor and delivery, have not been conducted (Wideman & Singer, 1984).

Attentional Focus

Wideman and Singer (1984) and Beck and Siegel (1980) failed to find data to support the use of attention focusing alone to influence anxiety or pain. When combined with relaxation training, Stevens and Heide (1977) reported increased pain endurance and decreased pain perception. Other studies (Beck & Siegel, 1980) have suggested that relaxation does not decrease pain, anxiety, or stress more than attention or placebo effects.

Social Support

The presence of a supportive and encouraging partner has also been addressed. Research has suggested that social support has a positive influence on childbirth. It results in fewer complications, shorter duration of labor, enhanced interaction by the mothers with their newborns, less medication, and less pain (Beck & Siegel, 1980; Broome & Koehler, 1986; Wideman & Singer, 1984). Copstick, Taylor, Hayes, and Morris (1986) reported that support and encouragement to use psychological methods of pain control were significantly related to the decreased use of epidural anesthesia. In a randomized study, Hodnett and Osborn

(1989) compared childbirth outcomes among prepared subjects who were supported by a lay midwife as well as a spouse or partner. Women receiving professional support were significantly less likely to receive anesthesia or analgesia and to have episiotomies than women receiving only the support of a spouse or partner.

Not all evidence has been supportive of the beneficial impact of social support. Melzack (1984) reported that pain scores were higher when the husband was present than when he was absent. The presence of a companion may also interfere with labor because of factors such as the quality of the relationship with the companion and the quality of supportive behavior displayed by the companion (Keirse, Enkin, & Lumley, 1989). Further research is needed on the influence of social support and pain control before conclusions can be drawn.

SUMMARY

The prevailing clinical impression is that the Lamaze and Dick-Read methods are beneficial, at least when compared with no preparation. Women who receive childbirth preparation appear to experience less painful deliveries and may exhibit fewer obstetric complications. These methods are not, however, receiving unequivocal empirical support. It is likely that discrepancies in effectiveness of childbirth preparation reflect many methodological inadequacies that characterize much of this research.

For these reasons, it is difficult to draw valid conclusions as to which method of childbirth preparation is most efficacious. A majority of the research has been done on the Lamaze method and it is also the most structured of the more popular methods of childbirth preparation. Clearly, more controlled research needs to be done on alternative methods of childbirth preparation, especially examining the overlap between hypnosis and Lamaze. Another problem that arises in the use of any of these childbirth preparation techniques is that, as labor progresses, fewer women use the coping techniques they have been taught. For example, by the beginning of the second stage, only one-third of the women were using any of the techniques taught during childbirth preparation (Copstick, Hayes, Taylor, & Morris, 1985).

IMPLICATIONS FOR CLINICAL PRACTICE

During childbirth preparation, the obstetrical staff, psychologists, and others might be able to enhance the utility of childbirth preparation by incorporating more sophisticated research methods and psychological principles. A number of methodological concerns have been raised about research on the utility of childbirth preparation. As future research begins to address these concerns, psychological principles in childbirth preparation will be more clearly defined and may also be more effectively incorporated into programs. For example, modeling may be useful for increasing the use of techniques taught during childbirth preparation. Women receiving childbirth preparation might benefit from viewing a videotape of a woman successfully using the techniques during actual labor and delivery. Research will be necessary to determine the utility of this approach and the extent to which it may already be used.

Although unequivocal evidence in support of childbirth preparation does not exist, there is evidence suggestive of beneficial effects. Because of the methodological limitations of much of the current research, further research is needed. This research should address the issues of the efficacy of childbirth preparation and the components of childbirth preparation that may be responsible for beneficial effects.

REFERENCES

Apgar, V. (1953). A proposal for a new method of evaluating the newborn infant. *Anesthesiology and Analgesia Current Researches, 32*, 260–267.

Beck, N. C., & Hall, D. (1978). Natural childbirth: A review and analysis. *Obstetrics and Gynecology, 52*, 371–379.

Beck, N. C., & Siegel, L. J. (1980). Preparation for childbirth and contemporary research on pain, anxiety, and stress reduction: A review and critique. *Psychosomatic Medicine, 42*, 429–447.

Broome, M. E., & Koehler, C. (1986). Childbirth education: A review of effects on the woman and her family. *Family and Community Health, 9*, 33–44.

Brown, S. (1990). Characteristics of labour pain. *Nursing Times, 86*, 53.

Calhoun, L. G., Selby, J. W., & Calhoun, M. L. (1980). The psychological value of prepared childbirth. In J. W. Selby, L. G. Calhoun, A. V. Vogel, & H. E. King (Eds.), *Psychology and human reproduction* (pp. 39–54). New York: Free Press.

Chestnut, D. H., & Gibbs, C. D. (1991). Obstetric anesthesia. In S. G. Gabbe, J. R. Niebyl, & J. L. Simpson (Eds.), *Obstetrics: Normal and problem pregnancies* (2nd ed.) (pp. 493–538). New York: Churchill Livingstone.

Cogan, R., Perkowski, S., & Anderson, D. A. (1988). Memories of labor and birth: Reliability of post partum questionnaire reports. *Perceptual and Motor Skills, 67*, 75–79.

Cohen, W. R., Acker, D. B., & Friedman, E. A. (1989). *Management of labor* (2nd ed.). Rockville, MD: Aspen Publishers.

Copstick, S. M., Hayes, R. W., Taylor, K. E., & Morris, N. F. (1985). A test of a common assumption regarding the use of antenatal training during labour. *Journal of Psychosomatic Research, 29*, 215–218.

Copstick, S. M., Taylor, K. E., Hayes, R., & Morris, N. (1986). Partner support and the use of coping techniques in labor. *Journal of Psychosomatic Research, 30*, 497–503.

Cronenwett, L., & Newmark, L. (1974). Fathers' response to childbirth. *Nursing Research,* *23*, 210–217.

Dick-Read, G. (1959). *Childbirth without fear* (2nd rev. ed.). New York: Harper & Brothers.

Erskine, A., Morley, S., & Pearce, S. (1990). Memory for pain: A review. *Pain, 41*, 255–265.

Fridh, G., Kopare, T., Gaston-Johansson, F., & Turner Norvell, K. (1988). Factors associated with more intense labor pain. *Research in Nursing and Health, 11*, 117–124.

Harmon, T. M., Hynan, M. T., & Tyre, T. E. (1990). Improved obstetric outcomes using hypnotic analgesia and skill mastery combined with childbirth education. *Journal of Consulting and Clinical Psychology, 58*, 525–530.

Harris, V. A., Katkin, E. S., Lick, J. R., & Haberfield, T. (1976). Paced respiration as a technique for the autonomic response to stress. *Psychophysiology, 13*, 386–391.

Hassid, P. (1978). *Textbook for childbirth educators*. New York: Harper & Row.

Hetherington, S. E. (1990). A controlled study of the effect of prepared childbirth classes on obstetric outcome. *Birth, 17*, 86–91.

Hodnett, E. D., & Osborn, R. W. (1989). Effects of continuous intrapartum professional support on childbirth outcomes. *Research in Nursing and Health, 12*, 289–297.

Hughey, M. J., McElin, T. W., & Young, T. (1978). Maternal and fetal outcomes of Lamaze-prepared patients. *Obstetrics and Gynecology, 51*, 643–647.

Jacobson, E. (1938). *Progressive relaxation*. Chicago: University of Chicago Press.

Keirse, M.J.N.C., Enkin, M., & Lumley, J. (1989). Social and professional support during childbirth. In I. Chalmers, M. W. Enkin, & M.J.N.C. Keirse (Eds.), *Effective care in pregnancy and childbirth*. Oxford: Oxford University Press.

Klusman, L. E. (1975). Reduction of pain in childbirth by the alleviation of anxiety during pregnancy. *Journal of Consulting and Clinical Psychology, 43*, 162–165.

Lamaze, F. (1970). *Painless childbirth: Psychoprophylactic method* (L. R. Celestin, Trans.). Chicago: Henry Regnery Company. (Original work published in 1956).

Leventhal, E. A., Leventhal, H., Shacham, S., & Easterling, D. V. (1989). Active coping reduces reports of pain from childbirth. *Journal of Consulting and Clinical Psychology, 57*, 365–371.

Lowe, N. K. (1989). Explaining the pain of active labor: The importance of maternal confidence. *Research in Nursing and Health, 12*, 237–245.

Macfarlane, A. (1977). *The psychology of childbirth*. Cambridge, MA.: Harvard University Press.

Manderino, M. A., & Bzdek, V. M. (1984). Effects of modeling and information on reactions to pain: A childbirth-preparation analogue. *Nursing Research, 33*, 9–14.

Melzack, R. (1984). The myth of painless childbirth (The John J. Bonica Lecture). *Pain, 19*, 321–337.

Melzack, R., Taenzer, P., Feldman, P., & Kinch, R. A. (1981). Labour is still painful after prepared childbirth training. *Canadian Medical Association Journal, 125*, 357–363.

O'Brien, W. F., & Cefalo, R. C. (1991). Labor and delivery. In S. G. Gabbe, J. R. Niebyl, & J. L. Simpson (Eds.), *Obstetrics: Normal and problem pregnancies* (2nd ed.) (pp.427–456). New York: Churchill Livingstone.

Patton, L. L., English, E. C., & Hambleton, J. D. (1985). Childbirth preparation and outcomes of labor and delivery in primiparous women. *Journal of Family Practice, 20*, 375–378.

Scott, J. R., & Rose, N. B. (1976). Effect of psychoprophylaxis (Lamaze preparation) on labor and delivery in primiparas. *New England Journal of Medicine, 294*, 1205–1207.

Simkin, P., & Enkin, M. (1989). Antenatal classes. In I. Chalmers, M. W. Enkin, & M.J.N.C. Keirse (Eds.), *Effective care in pregnancy and childbirth*. Oxford: Oxford University Press.

Stevens, R. J., & Heide, F. (1977). Analgesic characteristics of prepared childbirth techniques: Attention focusing and systematic relaxation. *Journal of Psychosomatic Research, 21*, 429–438.

Sturrock, W. A., & Johnson, J. A. (1990). The relationship between childbirth education classes and obstetric outcome. *Birth, 17*, 82–85.

Timm, M. (1979). Prenatal education evaluation. *Nursing Research, 28*, 338–342

Venn, J. (1986). Hypnosis and the Lamaze method: A reply to Wideman and Singer. *American Psychologist, 41*, 475–476.

Wideman, M. V., & Singer, J. E. (1984). The role of psychological mechanisms in preparation for childbirth. *American Psychologist, 39*, 1357–1371.

Worthington, E. (1982). Labor room and laboratory: Clinical validation of the cold pressor as a means of testing preparation for childbirth strategies. *Journal of Psychosomatic Research, 26*, 223–230.

Worthington, E., & Martin, G. A. (1980). A laboratory analysis of response to pain after training in three Lamaze techniques. *Journal of Psychosomatic Research, 24*, 109–116.

Zax, M., Sameroff, A. J., & Farnum, J. E. (1975). Childbirth education, maternal attitudes and delivery. *American Journal of Obstetrics and Gynecology, 123*, 185–190.

12

Pregnancy Loss Through Miscarriage or Stillbirth

Kerrie L. Cole

MEDICAL ASPECTS

Terminology

Pregnancy loss can occur in many forms, including elective abortion, miscarriage, stillbirth, ectopic pregnancy, and termination following prenatal diagnosis. A miscarriage, or spontaneous abortion, is an unintended termination of pregnancy before the twentieth week of gestation (Shapiro, 1988). Stillbirth, or fetal death, refers to death of the fetus between 20 weeks and delivery. Fetal death may be detected while the fetus is in the uterus, during labor, or (rarely) at delivery. The term "perinatal death" refers to both stillbirth and neonatal death, usually including deaths of babies up to one month old. This chapter will focus on the effects of miscarriage and stillbirth.

Approximately 15–20 percent of all recognized pregnancies are lost through stillbirth or spontaneous abortion. One in eighty pregnancies ends in stillbirth, while estimates of the incidence of spontaneous abortion range from 15% to 50% of all pregnancies, depending on the measurement method used. The higher rates, however, are associated with extremely sensitive early pregnancy detection, and most of these are "subclinical", or go unrecognized by women

(Sweeney, Meyer, Mills, Aarons, & LaPorte, 1989). Seventy-five percent of miscarriages occur before the twelfth week of gestation (Shapiro, 1988).

Causes and Risk Factors

Most miscarriages have no discernible cause. The most common known etiology is a chromosomal abnormality in the ovum that is too severe for the fetus to survive (Friedman & Gradstein, 1982). These chromosomal abnormalities are usually due to chance mutations, rather than abnormalities that also would affect subsequent pregnancies. Anatomical causes of miscarriage include uterine malformations, and cervical incompetence, that is, a cervix that does not stay closed for the duration of the pregnancy (Friedman & Gradstein, 1982).

A variety of factors have been found to be correlated with increased risk for spontaneous abortion. Radiation exposure (e.g., from X-rays), maternal age, maternal disease (e.g., rubella, mumps), and drug use (including alcohol) have all been associated with increased risk (Friedman & Gradstein, 1982; McBride, 1991). More controversial links exist between miscarriage and hormonal factors (specifically, progesterone), diethylstilbestrol (DES) exposure, and blood type incompatibility (Friedman & Gradstein, 1982).

Other factors that have been studied and have not been shown to increase the risk for miscarriage include the use of a spermicide containing nonoxynol–9 (Schlesselman, 1987), the use of an oral contraceptive or intrauterine device prior to pregnancy (Shapiro, 1988), previous gonorrhea or other venereal disease, previous elective abortion, horseback riding, exercise, and sexual intercourse (Friedman & Gradstein, 1982).

As with miscarriage, the etiology of stillbirth cannot always be determined. One of the most common causes of death is *abruptio placentae*, which is bleeding from the placenta which results in its complete or partial detachment from the uterine wall. Other etiologies include congenital malformations and intrauterine infections (Fretts, Boyd, Usher, & Usher, 1992).

The Medical Experience

The presenting symptoms of miscarriage and stillbirth are often the same. Vaginal bleeding is the most common symptom of a threatened abortion, but also may be indicative of other complications (Friedman & Gradstein, 1982). Many pregnancies with bleeding in the third trimester, however, carry to term normally. Persistent pelvic pain is another symptom of threatened abortion. The third major indication of threatened abortion is the absence of symptoms of pregnancy. This includes the absence or disappearance of morning sickness, fatigue, and breast tenderness. At more advanced gestational age (after 28 weeks), the absence of fetal movement for over twenty-four hours is an indication to contact the physician. In some cases the first sign of fetal death is the inability to detect a fetal heartbeat during a prenatal visit. With regard to the relative frequency of these signs and symptoms in miscarriage, Friedman (1989) found that 81% of the women who suffered a miscarriage had experienced vaginal bleeding as the first symptom, 12% experienced pain, and 3% lost the feeling of being pregnant. An additional 4.5% found that their pregnancy had not progressed during a routine examination.

As mentioned above, the presence of one of these symptoms does not necessarily mean pregnancy loss is inevitable. Some signs, such as the disappearance of a fetal heartbeat, are more conclusive than others, such as vaginal bleeding or persistent pelvic pain. It is usually possible to determine the probable outcome of early pregnancies using tests such as ultrasound or serial levels of the pregnancy-specific hormone, human chorionic gonadatrophin (HCG) (Friedman & Gradstein, 1982).

The latency between the first symptoms of a problem to the conclusion of the pregnancy is variable. Friedman (1989) found that 13% of miscarriages occurred within 24 hours, an additional 47% within one week, and 38% after one week.

The characteristics of the actual spontaneous abortion vary depending on the age of the fetus. Very early miscarriages may resemble a heavy menstrual flow, while later ones may either require surgical procedures or labor and delivery (Friedman & Gradstein, 1982). The miscarriage may occur before the woman has time to get to the hospital. When this happens, the woman is advised to collect the expelled material and take it to the hospital for the pathologist to examine (Friedman & Gradstein, 1982).

The experience of a stillbirth also varies depending on the gestational age of the fetus, and whether it is detected before labor, during labor, or at delivery. Stillbirths that occur before labor begins usually result in the mother going into labor spontaneously within two weeks if labor is not induced. Pregnancies not spontaneously terminating within four weeks after fetal death will be terminated by the physician, because of the small risk of developing a severe maternal blood-clotting disorder after prolonged fetal death (Friedman & Gradstein, 1982).

The decision about whether to induce labor artificially is made based on medical considerations and the preference of the woman. While most women prefer not to continue the pregnancy with the knowledge that the fetus is dead, some prefer to let labor progress naturally. The time before labor begins may be used to cope with the loss, and to make decisions about what to do during and after delivery. These decisions include whether or not to see the dead fetus and where to stay in the hospital (maternity versus general surgery, private room versus shared) after delivery.

In some cases, the death is not detected until the time of labor or delivery. In these situations, there is no warning for the parents or the staff. The physical pain of the delivery is combined with the shock at the news of the death.

After the miscarriage or stillbirth, some women are kept in the hospital for a short time, while others, especially those with an early miscarriage, may go home almost immediately. The physical changes the body goes through in returning to its nonpregnant state vary depending on the gestational age. Many women experience mild lower abdominal pain, resulting from uterine contractions, which control bleeding. These pains may last for a day or two. Lochia, or vaginal discharge from the site of placental implantation, begins at delivery and continues for up to six weeks. This discharge is initially bright red, later brown, and finally yellow-white. Women with second-trimester spontaneous abortions or stillbirths will begin lactating a few days after delivery (Friedman & Gradstein, 1982).

PSYCHOLOGICAL ASPECTS

Grief

A distinction is made in the grief literature between normal and pathological grief. The normal grief process has been described as having three phases: *shock*, *preoccupation with the deceased*, and *resolution* (Brown & Stoudemire, 1983). These have also been called nonreaction, full reaction, and resolution (Iles, 1989). Shock begins immediately after the loss, and lasts from one day to two weeks. The emotional symptoms of this stage include numbness, helplessness, anger, sadness, and a feeling of unreality or disbelief. Somatic symptoms include crying, chest tightness, nausea, and throat tightness (Brown & Stoudemire, 1983). In the second phase, the sense of unreality decreases and the full experience of sadness begins. This period is characterized by crying spells, insomnia, guilt, introversion, and fatigue. The most characteristic symptom of this phase is an intense preoccupation with the deceased, which may include vivid dreams and hallucinatory experiences. This phase may last from several weeks to several months (Iles, 1989). During the third phase, resolution, interest in activities is regained, and there is no longer preoccupation with the deceased. Crying spells and feelings of emptiness may continue, but are less intense (Brown & Stoudemire, 1983).

Pathological, or inappropriate, grief may be either delayed or distorted. Delayed grief is characterized by the lack of grief symptoms for a long period of time. Persons with delayed grief may be thought of by others as coping well, but intense symptoms are often experienced at a later time, such as at anniversary dates or after relatively minor losses. Persons with delayed grief also may have unusual somatic symptoms or physical symptoms of depression, such as sleep disturbance, weight loss, or restricted affect, but deny feelings of sadness (Brown & Stoudemire, 1983).

Distorted grief may take a variety of forms. These include deterioration of health, hostility, social isolation or alienation, severe depression, and economic decline (Lindemann, 1944). These symptoms usually occur in combination rather than alone (Brown & Stoudemire, 1983). Risk factors for pathological grief include ambivalence in the relationship, obsessional personality traits, multiple responsibilities, multiple losses, sudden bereavement, and previous unresolved losses (Condon, 1986).

PSYCHOLOGICAL IMPACT

The literature on the psychological impact of spontaneous abortion and stillbirth consists largely of general overviews. There are few studies, and those that do exist often lack control groups and standardized measures. Additionally, small numbers of subjects limit the generalizability of the findings.

The psychological sequelae of stillbirth were studied earlier than were the sequelae of miscarriage. Once stillbirth was perceived as not simply a physical experience, professionals began looking at psychological aspects of pregnancy loss earlier in gestation. Topics of research include normal reactions to pregnancy loss, pathological grief, management of grief, and the effect of pregnancy loss on subsequent pregnancies.

Normal Reactions to Pregnancy Loss

One of the earliest studies of stillbirth was an interview study conducted by Giles (1970). Forty women were interviewed shortly after loss through stillbirth or neonatal death. The most common reaction was numbness, which was described by over half of those interviewed. Other reactions included restlessness, sadness, guilt, and fatigue. These symptoms correspond closely to the first stage of grief previously described. Others have also found reactions which match descriptions of normal grief following perinatal death. Forrest, Standish, and Baum (1982) found that initial reactions included shock and numbness for the first day, followed by seeking an explanation for the death, and feelings of anger and guilt. Social relationships in the first few weeks were described as difficult. Wolff, Nielson, and Schiller (1970) described the reactions of all the mothers in their study as normal grief, except for two women with a premorbid history of psychiatric disorder.

Early studies of reaction to miscarriage also found symptoms of normal grief. One of the earliest studies to assess the impact of miscarriage did so indirectly (Simon, Rothman, Goff, & Senturia, 1969). In an investigation of the effects of elective abortion, women who aborted spontaneously were used as a control group. Unexpectedly, 13 of the 32 women in the miscarriage group reported depression, and 8 had subsequent psychiatric diagnoses, while none of the women who had an elective abortion had a psychiatric diagnosis.

In an interview study, Hamilton (1989) found tearfulness in almost all the women who miscarried, with irritability and tiredness also common. Some women also reported difficulty in sleeping and loss of appetite. These women were interviewed again six weeks later, with half still experiencing tearfulness, and over half reporting guilt.

A standardized measure was included in a study by Seibel and Graves (1980). They administered a self-report questionnaire while women were in the recovery room after dilation and curettage (D&C) for incomplete spontaneous abortions. This questionnaire included sixteen adjectives from the Multiple Affect Adjective Check List (MAACL; Zuckerman & Lubin, 1965). Adjectives checked ranged from "lucky" and "relieved" to "very unhappy." Almost 30% checked at least one positive adjective, while 44% checked at least one negative adjective. Thus there was considerable variation in response. It should be kept in mind that these women had undergone an operation and had been told of the potential operative risks. This may have contributed to the positive affect. No follow-up of these women was conducted.

A recent study compared women who had miscarried with pregnant women and a community sample of women who were not pregnant (Neugebauer et al., 1992). Women who had miscarried were interviewed at two weeks, six weeks, and six months after the loss, although not all women entered the study at the same time. They were also administered the Center for Epidemiological Studies–Depression (CES–D) scale (Radloff, 1977). Women who had miscarried scored significantly higher than the other groups on the CES–D scale, and a higher percentage of these women were classified as highly symptomatic, with scores greater than the mean for psychiatric populations.

Effects of Gestational Age on Reaction to Pregnancy Loss

A few researchers have addressed the effect of gestational age on the reaction to pregnancy loss. Peppers and Knapp (1980) compared grief scores of women who experienced loss through miscarriage, stillbirth, or neonatal death. These grief scores were based on severity of sixteen symptoms. No significant differences were found between groups either for retrospective report of the time of the loss or at the time of the assessment. The assessment was conducted from 6 months to 36 years after the loss, which was an important methodological flaw. Assessment closer in time to the pregnancy loss may have found group differences. Still, this study was important in drawing attention to the impact of miscarriage.

Other researchers have addressed the effect of gestational age. In one study (Theut et al., 1989), women in their eighth month of pregnancy after a previous pregnancy loss were given the Perinatal Bereavement Scale. This scale was designed to be specific to the perinatal loss situation, covering a variety of grief symptoms. Women who had previously experienced loss through miscarriage reported less grief than women who had experienced stillbirth or neonatal death. The same effect was found six weeks postnatally, although both groups reported fewer symptoms at that time. The major problem with this study was that, again, the comparison was made at a variable and sometimes prolonged interval after the original loss. The average time since the loss was not reported, although all losses had occurred within the previous two years.

In a study conducted 6 to 8 weeks after the loss (Goldbach, Dunn, Toedter, & Lasker, 1991), parents who had experienced either spontaneous abortion or ectopic pregnancy were compared with those who had experienced stillbirth or neonatal death on the Perinatal Grief Scale (Toedter, Lasker, & Alhadeff, 1988). The early-loss group reported less grief than did the late-loss group at the initial assessment, as well as at 12–15 month and 26–30 month follow-ups. Although the early-loss group did experience grief, it was not as intense or long-lasting as the late-loss group.

Pathological Grief

While some researchers have focused on normal reactions to pregnancy loss, others have studied pathological grief. These studies concentrate on the risk factors for pathological reactions. The few studies that have been conducted suggest that pathological reactions occur in from 13% (LaRoche et al., 1984) to 23% (LaRoche et al., 1982; Rowe et al., 1978) of women after perinatal death.

The findings on risk factors for pathological grief reactions have been mixed. Factors which have not been found to have a significant effect include age, educational level, socioeconomic status, religious faith, cause of death, previous abortions, previous perinatal loss, and history of infertility (LaRoche et al., 1982; LaRoche et al., 1984; Lasker & Toedter, 1991; Nicol, Tompkins, Campbell, & Syme, 1986; Rowe et al., 1978). Other factors were found to have an effect in at least one study, but no effect in at least one other study, so their significance is uncertain at this time. These include the presence of living children in the home, not having the opportunity to touch the baby, stressful events during the pregnancy, perceived lack of support from the husband or family, the suddenness of the loss, hospital disposal of the baby (instead of the family making the arrangements) and whether the pregnancy was planned (LaRoche et al., 1982; LaRoche et al., 1984; Lasker & Toedter, 1991; Nicol et al., 1986; Rowe et al., 1978). A history of depression before the pregnancy has been addressed in only one study, but was found to have a significant effect (Lasker & Toedter, 1991). The existence of a surviving twin was related to lower levels of grief in one study (LaRoche et al., 1984), but was related to pathological grief in another (Rowe et al., 1978).

A factor which has received considerable attention is the timing of the subsequent pregnancy, and again the reports in the literature are variable. Bourne and Lewis (1984) state that becoming pregnant again too soon interferes with the mourning processing and contributes to pathological mourning. This is supported by earlier research, which found that becoming pregnant less than 5 or 6 months after the loss is a risk factor for pathological mourning (Rowe et al., 1978). Other studies have found no effect for the timing of the subsequent pregnancy (Davis, Stewart, & Harmon, 1989; LaRoche et al., 1984). Davis and colleagues suggest that some grief feelings will be experienced by most couples after a subsequent pregnancy, regardless of when that pregnancy occurs. Phipps (1985–1986) interviewed couples after a subsequent viable pregnancy, and found that the pregnancy tended to be characterized by a degree of detachment, rising levels of anxiety over the course of the pregnancy, and especially negative feelings at the gestational age of the previous loss. Parents attached normally, however, to the children within a few days of delivery.

One study (Friedman & Gath, 1989) suggested that "pathological" reactions may be common in the short term. The Present State Examination (Wing, Cooper, & Sartorius, 1974) was administered one month following miscarriage. At that time, 48% of the group were classified as having a depressive illness severe enough to be called a psychiatric case. Three of these women attempted to harm themselves.

Unfortunately, the literature on risk factors for pathological grief has many methodological limitations. Sample sizes tend to be small (around 30 in most studies). Varying definitions of pathological grief are used, with some basing their decision on interviewer judgment and others using questionnaires. The timing of the assessment also varies greatly, from a few months after the loss up to three years. In addition, more must be known about the normal course of mourning after perinatal loss before conclusions about pathological reactions can be made.

INTERVENTIONS

While much remains unknown about reactions to pregnancy loss, the growing awareness that this can be a very distressing, and sometimes extremely disruptive, event has led to many articles advising how to manage the psychological sequelae of pregnancy loss. A few of these are based on experimental research, but most seem based on clinical experience.

The need for a change in management practice has been addressed by a few

researchers. Friedman (1989) interviewed 67 women one month after a spontaneous abortion. He found that 25% were dissatisfied with the care they received
before admission, and many were upset with the lack of information received at
discharge. These women also reported anger when the experience of the miscarriage was downplayed by the physician, who often said that it was just an early
pregnancy and that they could try again. Thus one important intervention for
medical staff is increased sensitivity to the effects that even early pregnancy loss
may have.

Hutti (1988) reviewed the literature on recommended interventions for pregnancy loss and neonatal death. She categorized 50 interventions into four groups:
a) *validation of the loss*, b) *education about grief*, c) *strategies used during hospitalization*, and d) *making the loss real*. Decisions about which of these strategies to use
should be based on the circumstances of the loss, including the gestational age
of the fetus, whether surgical procedures and/or hospitalization are necessary,
and the wishes of the couple.

Many strategies are recommended for validating the loss. One of the most
basic of these is acknowledging that feelings of loss and grief are normal. Similarly, one should not downplay or rationalize the experience by saying that it is
natural or that the woman will be able to have other babies. The care giver must
be willing to talk about the loss with the couple, and refer them to support
groups.

The couple also should be taught about the grief process. This should include
a discussion of symptoms of grief and the variability in reactions that may occur.
They should be told of the course of the grief process, which includes possible
recurrence of symptoms around the anniversary of the loss or of the due date.

Strategies used during hospitalization include repeatedly giving clear explanations, giving the couple choices regarding the unit in which to be hospitalized
(e.g., maternity or general surgery) and disposal of the fetal remains, and informing the woman of the signs and symptoms that she may experience after
discharge. Many of these strategies apply specifically to women who have experienced loss later in pregnancy.

"Making the loss real" applies much more to stillbirths than miscarriage,
because in miscarriage the fetal remains often cannot be identified. The strategies in this category include discussing the medical findings and autopsy results
in a direct yet sensitive manner, giving parents mementos such as footprints
and/or photographs, and allowing them to hold the baby if they wish. If the
parents do choose to see and hold the dead baby, it should be bathed and
wrapped in a baby blanket to demonstrate respect for it. The parents should be
prepared for what they will see, including the body temperature, color, size, and
any bruises or deformities. If parents choose not to see the baby at the time of
the loss, a photograph should be kept on file in case they change their mind
(Hutti, 1988).

The efficacy of structured interventions has been addressed in a few studies. In one study (Evans & Englebardt, 1990) newly bereaved couples were visited by a member of the referral team. The team member explained the program and let the couple decide if they wanted to participate. The intervention consisted of contact with a trained volunteer who had experienced a pregnancy loss at least one year earlier. The goal was to provide support, information, and an opportunity to express feelings. This program was evaluated after four years through questionnaires sent to those who did and did not decide to participate. Of those who participated, 96% were either satisfied or very satisfied with the volunteer. Of those who did not participate, 54% said they would participate if they had to do it over again. One obvious methodological flaw in this study was the lack of randomization, which may have resulted in significant selection bias. For example, patients electing to participate in the program may have had lower baseline levels of morbidity or better coping strategies than patients who deferred. Furthermore, self-reported adjustment did not differ greatly between those who did and did not participate, although statistical significance tests were not used.

In a no-treatment control study of the effect of counseling following perinatal death, Forrest, Standish, and Baum (1982) assessed women at 6 and 14 months after the loss. The supported group was treated with many of the above recommendations, including encouragement to see, hold, and name the dead baby; choice of maternity ward or another location; the offer of bereavement counseling 24 to 48 hours after the loss; and follow-up, including a discussion of the postmortem results. The care that the control group received varied, but was based on the normal hospital routine. Based on questionnaire data, fewer of the women in the supported group than the control group met the criteria for psychiatric disorder at six months, while there was no difference between the groups at 14 months.

Another important area of intervention concerns the timing of subsequent pregnancy. A recent study (Davis, Stewart, & Harmon, 1989) found that mothers were dissatisfied with doctor's advice on the timing of subsequent pregnancy, because it is a personal decision based on many factors. Instead of specific advice on timing, women expressed preference for receiving information on the possible physical and emotional consequences of when they timed their next pregnancy, in order to make an informed decision. Forrest, Standish and Baum (1982) found that none of the three women in the supported group who were pregnant at six months met the questionnaire cut-off for psychiatric disorder, while six of the eight pregnant women in the control group scored above the cut-off. At fourteen months, one of the two pregnant women in the supported group and one of the five women in the control group met the cut-off. While these data are by no means conclusive, this suggests that a structured intervention may help resolve the issue of subsequent pregnancies, either by aiding in the decision of timing or by aiding in resolution of grief.

The reader interested in more detailed advice on management of pregnancy loss is referred to Hutti (1988). Those interested in nursing interventions may benefit from the Perinatal Grief Checklist (Beckey, Price, Okersen, & Riley, 1985). Therapists involved in counseling those who have experienced perinatal loss are referred to a recent article that addressed the questions brought up in therapy (DeFrain, 1991). This article, based on a series of studies including over 800 family members, lists the most common questions and offers advice on how to address them.

SUMMARY

The psychological impact of miscarriage and stillbirth has been of increasing interest in the last ten years. Although much of the research is descriptive, there is a trend toward more standardized methods. The consensus of both the clinical lore and empirical research is that a pregnancy loss is not merely another physical condition, and may result in a prolonged period of grief. The awareness by health professionals of the possible sequelae, and the increasing popularity of structured intervention programs, may be helpful in preventing the grief from becoming pathological.

REFERENCES

Beckey, R. D., Price, R. A., Okerson, M., & Riley, K. W. (1985). Development of a perinatal grief checklist. *Journal of Obstetric Gynecologic and Neonatal Nursing*, 194–199.

Bourne, S., & Lewis, E. (1984). Pregnancy after stillbirth or neonatal death. *Lancet, 1*, 31–33.

Brown, J. T., & Stoudemire, A. (1983). Normal and pathological grief. *Journal of the American Medical Association, 250*, 378–382.

Condon, J. T. (1986). Management of established pathological grief reaction after stillbirth. *American Journal of Psychiatry, 143*, 987–992.

Davis, D. L., Stewart, M., & Harmon, R. J. (1989). Postponing pregnancy after perinatal death: Perspectives on doctor advice. *Journal of the American Academy of Child and Adolescent Psychiatry, 28*, 481–487.

DeFrain, J. (1991). Learning about grief from normal families: SIDS, stillbirth, and miscarriage. *Journal of Marital and Family Therapy, 17*, 215–232.

Evans, M. L., & Englebardt, S. P. (1990). Evaluation of a multidisciplinary perinatal bereavement program. *Neonatal Network, 8*, 31–35.

Forrest, G. C., Standish, E., & Baum, J. D. (1982). Support after perinatal death: A study of support and counseling after perinatal bereavement. *British Medical Journal, 285,* 1475–1479.

Fretts, R. C., Boyd, M. E., Usher, R. H., & Usher, H. A. (1992). The changing pattern of fetal death, 1961–1988. *Obstetrics and Gynecology, 79,* 35–39.

Friedman, R., & Gradstein, B. (1982). *Surviving pregnancy loss.* (pp. 29–56). Boston: Little, Brown.

Friedman, T. (1989). Women's experience of general practitioner management of miscarriage. *Journal of the Royal College of General Practitioners, 39,* 456–458.

Friedman, T., & Gath, D. (1989). The psychiatric consequences of spontaneous abortion. *British Journal of Psychiatry, 128,* 74–79.

Giles, P.F.H. (1970). Reactions of women to perinatal death. *Australia and New Zealand Journal of Obstetrics and Gynecology, 10,* 207–210.

Goldbach, K.R.C, Dunn, D. S., Toedter, L. J., & Lasker, J. N. (1991). The effects of gestational age and gender on grief after pregnancy loss. *American Journal of Orthopsychiatry, 61,* 461–467.

Hamilton, S. M. (1989). Should follow-up be provided after miscarriage? *British Journal of Obstetrics and Gynaecology, 96,* 743–745.

Hutti, M. H. (1988). A quick reference table of interventions to assist families to cope with pregnancy loss or neonatal death. *Birth, 15,* 33–35.

Iles, S. (1989). The loss of early pregnancy. *Baillière's Clinical Obstetrics and Gynecology, 3,* 769–790.

LaRoche, C., Fuller, N., Lalinec-Michaud, M., Copp, M., Engelsmann, F. & Vasilevsky, K. (1982). Grief reactions to perinatal death: An exploratory study. *Psychosomatics, 23,* 510–518.

LaRoche, C., Lalinec-Michaud, M., Engelsmann, F., Fuller, N., Copp, M., McQuade-Soldatos, L., & Azima, R. (1984). Grief reactions to perinatal death: A follow-up study. *Canadian Journal of Psychiatry, 29,* 14–19.

Laskar, J. N., & Toedter, L. J. (1991). Acute versus chronic grief: The case of pregnancy loss. *American Journal of Orthopsychiatry, 61,* 510–522.

Lindemann, E., (1944). Symptomatology and management of acute grief. *American Journal of Psychiatry, 101,* 141–148.

McBride, W. Z. (1991). Spontaneous abortion. *American Family Physician, 43,* 175–182.

Neugebauer, R., Kline, J., O'Connor, P., Shrout, P., Johnson, J., Skodol, A., Wicks, J., & Susser, M. (1992). Depressive symptoms in women in the six months after miscarriage. *American Journal of Obstetrics and Gynecology, 166,* 104–109.

Nicol, M. T., Tompkins, J. R., Campbell, N. A., & Syme, G. J. (1986). Maternal grieving response after perinatal death. *Medical Journal of Australia, 144,* 287–289.

Peppers, L. G., & Knapp, R. J. (1980). Maternal reactions to involuntary fetal/infant death. *Psychiatry, 43,* 155–159.

Phipps, S. (1985–1986). The subsequent pregnancy after stillbirth: Anticipatory parenthood in the face of uncertainty. *International Journal of Psychiatry in Medicine, 15,* 243–263.

Radloff, L. S. (1977). The CES-D Scale: A self-report depression scale for research in the general population. *Applied Psychological Measures, 1,* 385–401.

Rowe, J., Clyman, R., Green, C., Mikkelsen, C., Haight, J., & Ataide, L. (1978). Follow-up of families who experience a perinatal death. *Pediatrics, 62,* 166–170.

Schlesselman, J. J. (1987). Proof of cause and effect in epidemiologic studies: Criteria for judgement. *Preventive Medicine, 16*, 195–210.

Seibel, M., & Graves, W. L. (1980). The psychological impact of spontaneous abortions. *Journal of Reproductive Medicine, 25*, 161–165.

Shapiro, C. (1988). *Infertility and pregnancy loss.* (pp. 148–164). San Francisco: Jossey-Bass.

Simon, N. M., Rothman, D., Goff, J. T., & Senturia, A. (1969). Psychiatric sequelae of abortion. *Archives of General Psychiatry, 15*, 378–389.

Sweeney, A. M., Meyer, M. R., Mills, J. L., Aarons, J. H., & LaPorte, R. E. (1989). Evaluation of recruitment strategies for prospective studies of spontaneous abortion. *Journal of Occupational Medicine, 31*, 980–985.

Theut, S. K., Pedersen, F. A., Zaslow, M. J., Cain, R. L., Rabinovich, B. A., & Morihisa, J. M. (1989). Perinatal loss and parental bereavement. *American Journal of Psychiatry, 146*, 635–639.

Toedter, L. J., Lasker, J. N., & Alhadeff, J. M. (1988). The Perinatal Grief Scale: Development and initial validation. *American Journal of Orthopsychiatry, 58*, 435–448.

Wing, J. K., Cooper, J. E., & Sartorius, N. (1974). *The measurement and classification of psychiatric symptoms.* London: Cambridge University Press.

Wolff, J. R., Nielson, P. E., & Schiller, P. (1970). The emotional reaction to a stillbirth. *American Journal of Obstetrics and Gynecology, 108*, 73–77.

Zuckerman, M., & Lubin, B. (1965). Multiple Affect Adjective Check List. San Diego: Educational and Industrial Testing Service.

13

Abortion

Elizabeth A. Weerts Whitmore

A woman's desire for children is generally greatly exceeded by her childbearing potential. A sexually active and fertile woman is capable of producing children for more than a thirty-year period, and therefore must actively limit her reproduction to desired levels through contraception. Each year in the United States alone, more than three million women fail to achieve their birth control goals (Alan Guttmacher Institute, 1990). It is not surprising, therefore, that the majority of women not desiring a pregnancy await the arrival of their menstrual period each month with anticipation, anxiety, and concern. If it does not arrive and pregnancy is confirmed, the woman faces an extremely difficult and controversial decision—whether or not to abort the pregnancy. Although modern abortions are relatively simple medical procedures, facing an unwanted pregnancy in a technologically advanced, legally permissive society places the woman in the difficult position of having sanctioned power over the determination of potential life. For most women, the intense distress of the unwanted pregnancy and of having to undergo the abortion procedure will dissipate rapidly following the completion of the abortion procedure (Payne, Kravitz, Notman, & Anderson, 1976). For some, however, the physical, emotional, moral, and social consequences of the decision may bear heavily upon her for the rest of her life.

The abortion issue has been present for as long as there have been unwanted pregnancies. Over time, the debate has continued to center on whether the termination of unborn life is legally, ethically, and morally justified. Throughout history, societies have recognized that the survival of the species depends on laws or restrictions that protect life. The type of abortion regulations that exist in

207

society usually reflect other basic religious or moral values of the society (Sachdev, 1985; Smith, 1982). As of 1989, approximately 1.6 million abortions were being performed each year in the United States alone, with approximately 30% of pregnancies ending in abortion (National Abortion Federation, 1989a). Clearly, there is a strong desire among women to control their own fertility in a safe and effective manner, regardless of the heated arguments and restrictive laws dissuading these practices.

The 1973 United States Supreme Court decision, *Roe v. Wade*, brought about a dramatic change in the status of abortion in this country. In this decision, the Supreme Court declared that a woman has a constitutionally protected right to obtain a first-trimester abortion based on her right of privacy. The court allowed states to regulate abortion during the second trimester, but only for the purpose of protecting a woman's health. The recent 1992 Supreme Court ruling regarding abortion, *Planned Parenthood of Southeastern Pennsylvania v. Casey*, upheld the constitutionality of a woman's right to obtain an abortion, but also affirmed the states' ability to regulate abortion, provided that these regulations do not place an "undue burden" on the woman. They rejected the previous trimester framework approach for restricting abortion, holding instead that the viability of the fetus marks the earliest point at which the states may constitutionally ban nontherapeutic abortion.

Research on the nonmedical aspects of abortion conducted before the Court's original 1973 decision has questionable contemporary validity, because it was conducted during the time period when abortion was illegal. Therefore, when analyzing the literature on the psychosocial aspects of abortion, it is important to consider the temporal and societal context in which this research was conducted.

CHARACTERISTICS OF WOMEN OBTAINING ABORTIONS

The problem of an unwanted pregnancy is not specific to certain populations. Heterosexually active women of all ages, religions, socioeconomic classes, backgrounds, and situations have similar probabilities of facing this problem at some point in their lives. In addition, there are a variety of reasons why a woman would choose to abort her child (Torres & Forrest, 1988). For these reasons, there is no typical prototype of the woman seeking an abortion. Statistics about abortion do, however, reveal some similarities in demographics among abortion seekers.

According to several sources (Alan Guttmacher Institute, 1990; National Center for Health Statistics: Kochanek, 1991) most of the women obtaining abortions are young, unmarried, and less than 10 weeks into their pregnancy. The majority of women are under the age of 25, and consistent with age norms, 79%

of them are unmarried. The distribution of abortions by race is highly dispro-
portionate. Although nearly 70% of all women who obtain abortions are Cauca-
sian (National Abortion Federation, 1989a), women of minority races have higher
abortion ratios (abortions per 1,000 live births) (Grimes, 1985; Henshaw &
Silverman, 1988). Women of all religions and of varied socioeconomic status
obtain abortions at approximately equal levels (National Abortion Federation,
1989a), with the exception of Jews and evangelical Christians, who make up
only a small percentage of those seeking abortions (Henshaw & Silverman,
1988).

Characteristics associated with above-average likelihood of abortion are current school enrollment, employment, Medicaid coverage, intention to have no
more children, and residence in a metropolitan community (Henshaw &
Silverman, 1988). Women who seek second-trimester abortions generally fall
into two groups: 1) women who are younger, less educated, and therefore less
aware of their pregnancy state; or 2) women who are older, more educated, and
are aborting their fetus as the result of an amniocentesis test or an earlier false
negative pregnancy test (National Abortion Federation, 1990; Smith, 1982). It is
particularly notable that half of all abortion patients surveyed in 1987 by the
Alan Guttmacher Institute reported practicing contraception during the month
in which they conceived. Only nine percent had never used birth control, and
these women tended to be young, poor, African-American, Hispanic, and less
educated (Henshaw & Silverman, 1988).

THE DECISION TO OBTAIN AN ABORTION

The Alan Guttmacher Institute, an independent nonprofit data-collection agency,
has periodically surveyed U.S. abortion providers to obtain data about abortions
performed each year. The most recent survey, in 1987, revealed that the most
common reasons given for women wanting an abortion were the inability to
afford and/or the unreadiness to start or expand their families due to existing
responsibilities. Both reasons were cited by 21% of the women as being the most
important factor affecting their decision (Torres & Forrest, 1988). In addition,
16% of respondents were most concerned about the changes in their lives brought
about by pregnancy and bearing a child and 12% were concerned with being a
single parent or with bringing a baby into a troubled relationship. Twenty
percent of women sought an abortion due to the health status of their fetus or of
themselves. The younger the woman, the more likely she was to be concerned
with the effect of a baby on her life and her lack of maturity regarding motherhood. Race and poverty status were not related to reasons given.

It is notable that most women report having more than one reason for obtaining an abortion, attesting to the complexity of this decision. Several authors have

discussed the dominance of the feeling of ambivalence surrounding the decision to abort a fetus (Adler, 1975; Smith, 1982). A significant concern about the effect of this ambivalence is that more than one-fifth of women report having their decision influenced by the wishes of others. Parental wishes affected the abortion decision of one-quarter of women under the age of 18, as did the desires of husbands on the decisions of married women (Torres & Forrest, 1988). Shaw, Funderburk, and Franklin (1979) suggest that the influence of significant others is important as a source of support in the abortion decision, but they failed to consider the possible deleterious psychological effects of coercion by others during the decision process (Bracken, Klerman, & Bracken, 1978).

ABORTION METHODS AND PROCEDURES

Abortion is usually defined as "the expulsion of a fetus before it is mature enough to live on its own" (National Abortion Federation, 1989b). Legally induced abortions are terminations of pregnancy that are brought about as the result of a medical or surgical procedure. A limited discussion of the most commonly used abortion methods is presented here. The reader is referred to several other sources for more detailed discussions of these procedures (Hern, 1984; Smith, 1982; Stubblefield, 1991).

Menstrual Extraction

Menstrual extraction (ME), the removal of the contents of the uterus up to 45 days from the day of the last menstrual period, does not necessarily require the confirmation of pregnancy. However, the practice of performing procedures on women who have not received a diagnosis of pregnancy is controversial among abortion practitioners (Hern, 1984). This procedure involves the aspiration of the contents of the uterus using negative pressure from a syringe. Little or no dilation of the cervix is needed at this early stage because the tube utilized is small enough to pass through the opening of the cervix (Shephard & Shephard, 1990). The advantages to this technique are that it can be performed more easily, earlier, and with less cost and risk than other methods. In addition, only a small amount of analgesic or anesthetic is needed (Smith, 1982). This procedure takes about 5 to 10 minutes to complete. Disadvantages include cramping, nausea, bleeding, pain, and the possibility of undergoing a medical procedure that may have been unnecessary (Hern, 1984). Because this method has a failure rate of 2.5%, it is important to verify that the woman is no longer pregnant once the woman reaches the point at which she is able to receive an accurate pregnancy test (Shephard & Shephard, 1990).

First-Trimester Vacuum Aspiration or Suction Curettage

The standard method for abortion between 7 and 14 weeks of pregnancy (dated from the first day of the last menstrual period) is vacuum aspiration or suction curettage (Moore, 1990). These procedures are usually performed in a doctor's office or outpatient clinic using a local anesthetic (paracervical block). The first part of the procedure involves dilation of the cervix, which can be accomplished in one of two ways. The first method involves the insertion and removal of graduated dilators, increasing the size of the rod until the cervix opening is less than 1 mm in diameter than the estimated length of gestation as measured in menstrual weeks (Stubblefield, 1991). A second method is the use of an osmotic dilator such as a seaweed root (*Laminaria*), a newer synthetic substitute (Dilapan), or a magnesium sulfate sponge (Lamicel). These small dilators, when inserted into the cervix, absorb the moisture of the cervix and swell, slowly dilating the cervix over the next few hours (Stubblefield, 1991). In either case, the physician inserts a small tube (cannula) that is attached to an aspirator machine into the opening of the cervix. The machine then suctions out the contents of the uterus, and the physician does a final check or clearing of the inside walls of the uterus using a small spoon-like instrument (curette) to be certain that there is no remaining tissue. This entire procedure takes about 15 minutes to complete. Women will typically experience some postabortal bleeding and cramping (Hern, 1984).

Prior to the introduction of the vacuum aspiration method into the United States, the most common first-trimester procedure was dilation and curettage (D & C). This procedure involves the scraping of the uterus, but it is rarely used today for a first-trimester procedure as the result of the superior safety of the vacuum aspiration method (Alan Guttmacher Institute, 1990).

Second-Trimester Pregnancy Abortions

Dilation and evacuation. Dilation and evacuation (D & E) is the most commonly performed procedure when a pregnancy termination is desired after the 13th week of pregnancy (as dated from the last menstrual period). The procedure usually takes place in a hospital or an outpatient surgical center under a local or general anesthetic. The cervix is gradually dilated using one of the standard procedures, but the osmotic dilators are generally left in place overnight. On the next day, the uterine membranes are broken and the uterine evacuation is completed. The D & E is a combination of the suction technique described earlier and the use of surgical instruments to remove larger parts of the fetal tissue and to empty the uterus. This procedure requires more time (generally 15 to 40 minutes) and may be more painful. The woman is given analgesic medication to control pain, and she may be lightly sedated (Stubblefield,

1991). Antibiotics are also prescribed to guard against any infections that may arise as a result of the procedure, and medication to contract the uterus is also administered.

   Instillation or induction of labor. Because D & E procedures become progressively more difficult as gestational age increases, labor-induction techniques are favored for procedures performed more than 20 weeks since the last menstrual period (Stubblefield, 1991). These techniques can be performed when pregnancy termination is desired after the 17th week of pregnancy (as dated from the last menstrual period), but they are responsible for only 3% of all abortions in the United States (National Abortion Federation, 1989b). This procedure involves the injection or instillation of abortifacient agents, such as prostaglandins, urea, or saline solution into the uterine cavity that cause uterine contractions which are similar to labor contractions. These contractions cause the dilation of the cervix and the expulsion of the fetus, usually within 8 to 26 hours following the injection (Stubblefield, 1991). This procedure is done using a local anesthetic and it requires overnight hospitalization.

Follow-Up Care

The woman is usually monitored for about an hour following the abortion. It is important that she remain in the clinic until her blood pressure, heart rate, and bleeding are stable and normal. It is critical that she return for a follow-up appointment within 2 to 6 weeks to ensure that the abortion is complete and to attend to any infections or complications that may have developed (Hern, 1984). Some women may require special services: a blood count to check for anemia, an injection of RhoGAM (if Rh negative blood), or counseling (Denney, 1983). The woman will be given a phone number to call in case of emergency, and she will be asked to abstain from intercourse until the follow-up appointment, as the uterus and cervix generally take several weeks to involute (return to normal size).

SAFETY AND THE RISKS OF ABORTION

Although abortion is one of the safest medical procedures available (Moore, 1990), there are potentially serious risks. Women often tend to weigh the risks of having an abortion against the risks of not having one, but this comparison may make the risks of the abortion procedure seem less consequential than they really are (Denney, 1984). The overall risk of death as the result of complications from abortion is 25 times less likely, however, than that of carrying a child to term and experiencing childbirth (Moore, 1990; Smith, 1982). The risk of death and complications increases with the length of the pregnancy, in part due to the increased use of anesthesics during second-trimester abortions (Moore, 1990; Shephard & Shephard, 1990). Abortion-related deaths are most often associated with anesthesia and are not due to the abortion procedure itself (Moore, 1990). According to the National Abortion Federation (1988), only 1 in 200,000 women obtaining legal abortions will die as a consequence of the procedure.

Abortions performed before the 13th week of pregnancy, which account for 90% of all abortions, have a 1–4% complication rate (Smith, 1982). The complication rates for second-trimester abortions are slightly higher (Cates, Schultz, Grimes, & Tyler, 1977). The major types of complications include: injury to the uterus and surrounding structures, infections, incomplete abortions, and excessive bleeding. In addition, life-threatening problems may arise if the woman has an unrecognized ectopic pregnancy, since this would not have been terminated by the abortion. For this reason, it is important for the woman to have a follow-up pregnancy test to make sure that the pregnancy was terminated. Women who have two or more abortions may be at increased risk for subsequent miscarriage or pregnancy complications, but the literature is inconclusive about these risks (see reviews by Hern, 1984; Stubblefield, 1991).

PSYCHOLOGICAL AFTERMATH

Although a substantial amount of research has been published on the sequelae of abortion, the research methodology has generally been faulty and limited in scope and time frame. The fact that most abortions are currently being performed in strongly supportive settings makes it difficult to generalize from previous research mainly conducted in a society that had more restrictive legislation and more negative public attitudes toward abortion. There is a serious need for prospective, controlled studies which evaluate the short- and long-term emotional and psychological effects of having undergone an abortion. Two excellent, early reviews (Kummer, 1963; Simon & Senturia, 1966) noted that the widespread presumption of the negative effects of the abortion experience on the psychological well-being of the woman was based on impression, not statistical comparisons. Kummer's (1963) investigation led him to conclude that postabortion psychiatric illness was so rare that its existence was probably a myth.

Several investigators since that time have reached similar conclusions (Athanasiou, Oppel, Michelson, Unger, & Yager, 1973; Greer, Lal, Lewis, Belsey, & Beard, 1976; Osofsky & Osofsky, 1972). Former U.S. Surgeon General C. Everett Koop, after reviewing the medical and psychological health effects of abortion (see Congressional Record, 1989; Committee on Government Operations, 1989), declared that "the available scientific evidence about the psychological sequelae of abortion simply cannot support either the preconceived beliefs of those pro-life or of those pro-choice." There are, however, no high-quality studies showing that there is evidence of widespread negative impact as the result of abortion (Moore, 1990).

Studies of Outcome

An expert panel on the psychological and emotional responses of women to abortion was recently convened by the American Psychological Association (Adler, David, Major, Roth, Russo, & Wyatt, 1990). This panel's review of the methodologically sound studies in this area indicated that "distress is generally greatest before the abortion and that the incidence of severe negative responses is low" (p. 41). In addition, a recent extensive review of 58 empirical studies conducted on abortion from 1966 to 1988 indicates that the mean incidence of psychological disturbance in women following an abortion is about 15 percent (Rogers, Stoms, & Phifer, 1989).

The most typical response of a woman who chooses to have a legal abortion is that of relief (Adler, 1975; Burnell & Norfleet, 1987; Lazarus, 1985; Osofsky & Osofsky, 1972). Lazarus (1985), for example, reported that 76% of women receiving first-trimester abortions felt relief two weeks following the procedure. The most common negative reaction, guilt, was experienced by 17% of the women. Adler's (1975) factor analysis of three-month postabortion emotional responses revealed three independent factors: negative socially based emotions (shame, guilt, fear of disapproval), negative internally based emotions (regret, anxiety, depression, doubt, anger), and positive emotions (relief, happiness). The positive factor explained most of the variation in affect and was experienced most strongly of the three factors, reflecting a domination of feelings of happiness over feelings of sadness following the abortion.

Women generally report satisfaction with their decision to abort. Osofsky and Osofsky's (1972) study of 250 women receiving abortions revealed that 79% were happy with their decision immediately after the abortion. Smith (1973) reported that 94% of women were satisfied with their decision to abort at one-year follow-up. Burnell and Norfleet's (1987) retrospective reporting of women's responses to abortion indicated that while 45% reported satisfaction with their decision to abort, negative responses (guilt, regret) were reported by less than 20% of those responding.

Only two studies have compared women terminating their pregnancies with women giving birth. Both attest to the lack of adverse psychological effects following abortion. Athanasiou and colleagues (1973) compared three groups of 38 women each: those obtaining early abortion by suction, those obtaining late abortion by saline injection, and those giving birth. No significant differences were seen among groups on measures of self-esteem, social integration, or the psychopathology scores on the MMPI clinical scales when measured more than a year after the abortion or delivery. Similarly, Zabin, Hirsch, and Emerson (1989) demonstrated more positive psychological outcomes in adolescents receiving an abortion as compared with those who received negative pregnancy tests and to those who carried their pregnancies to term.

When negative reactions to abortion have been observed, they are usually mild, transient, and associated with feelings of regret, depression, anger, and guilt (Alan Guttmacher Institute, 1990; Smith, 1973). Negative feelings are usually transient, peaking immediately before the procedure and dropping dramatically afterward (Freeman, Rickels, Huggins, Garcia & Polin, 1980; Payne et al., 1976). In contrast to the majority of evidence on outcome, McAll and Wilson (1987) cite incidence rates of 7–41% of negative psychological sequelae to abortion and they argue that the presence of positive responses to abortion do not negate the deleterious outcomes sometimes seen in women who have aborted their pregnancies.

Kumar and Robson (1978) examined the impact of abortion on later desired pregnancies. They found that women who had previously obtained legal abortions were significantly more likely than other women to become clinically anxious and depressed during their first wanted pregnancy. Peppers (1987–1988) found the postabortion grief process to be symptomatically similar, but more quickly resolved, than that which occurs with involuntary fetal loss. He found the length of pregnancy to predict positively the intensity of the grief reaction. In addition, the results of Cohen and Roth's (1984) examination of the coping styles of abortion seekers demonstrated that abortion patients are similar to other stressed populations in their stress–response patterns.

Given the consistency of the conclusions of many researchers, it now appears that there is little evidence to suggest that obtaining a legal, first-trimester abortion is any more psychologically dangerous than undergoing any other stressful life event.

PREDICTION OF OUTCOME

Although abortion does not appear to be a psychological hazard for most women, approximately 10% of women may experience some negative reactions (Lemkau, 1988). For this reason, it may be useful to identify predictors of women who may be at high risk for negative consequences following abortion. Researchers examining the predictors of psychological outcome of abortion suggest that several variables may contribute to the distress following an abortion. Former Surgeon General C. Everett Koop concluded, from his recent review of the medical and psychological health effects of abortion, that some women are at a greater risk than others for experiencing emotional distress following an abortion. According to Koop, "It appears likely that certain factors combine to make deciding to have an abortion and coping with its aftermath more difficult for some women than for others. These factors include strongly held personal values, an ambivalence about abortion, excessive pressure from others, the termination of an originally desired conception, a decision made late into the second trimester, or the lack of partner or family support" (Congressional Record, 1989, p. E908).

Personal Variables

Preabortion psychological status has been found to be predictive of postabortion outcome in several studies. Rizzardo, Magni, Desideri, Cosentino, and Salmaso (1992) demonstrated that women who were high in extraversion and low in neuroticism not only experienced an initial low level of distress at the time of the abortion, but also showed a general psychological improvement three months after the abortion. Payne, Kravitz, Notman, and Anderson (1976) analyzed the relation between psychological outcome and several variables in the six-month period following abortion. Their data suggest that women with a previous history of serious emotional problems, conflictual relationships, and ambivalence toward abortion are most vulnerable to experiencing postabortion psychological conflicts. Similar results were previously obtained by a number of other researchers (Athanasiou et al., 1973; Belsey, Greer, Lal, Lewis, & Beard, 1977; and Greer et al., 1976).

The coping style of the woman prior to and during her abortion may also be a potentially important predictor variable. Cohen and Roth (1984) reported that improved psychological adjustment to the abortion was achieved by women who actively confront problems as compared with women who utilize avoidant coping styles. Major, Mueller, and Hildebrandt (1985) examined the cognitive predictors of coping with an abortion in 247 women undergoing vacuum aspiration first-trimester abortions. They found the expectation of coping ability, attribution of blame, and meaningfulness of the pregnancy to be significantly related to physical, affective, and cognitive outcome. Women who had low coping expectations and who blamed their pregnancy on their character had significantly more adverse psychological reactions than those with high coping expectations and with low character blame. In addition, those who found their pregnancy highly meaningful and who had a greater desire for the pregnancy coped worse immediately after the abortion than those who found less meaning in the pregnancy.

Difficulty in making the decision to terminate a pregnancy has been implicated as a predictive factor of adverse psychological reactions. Adler (1975) asked women to rate how difficult it was for them to decide to have the abortion on a 5-point Likert-type scale. She found that "the more difficulty a woman had in deciding whether or not to have the abortion, the more strongly she experienced the internally based emotions afterwards." Also, Osofsky and Osofsky (1972) reported a significant relation between the difficulty of the decision and the guilt experienced about having the abortion.

Negative outcomes may also be predicted by previous attitudes toward abortion (Adler, 1975; Payne, Kravitz, Norman, & Anderson, 1976). Blackburne-Stover, Belenky, and Gilligan (1982), however, suggest that cognitive maturation associated with moral development affects how women recall their decision to abort. Osofsky and Osofsky (1972) indicated that conservative religious views about abortion had a negative psychological impact. Women who identified themselves as Catholic in their study experienced more psychological stress.

Social Variables

Several researchers have demonstrated that the amount of social support a woman receives for her abortion is positively reflected in her psychological outcome. Schusterman (1979) found intimacy and involvement with the male partner to be a significant predictor of emotional outcome following abortion. Bracken, Phil, Hachamovitch, and Grossman (1974) analyzed the importance of the level of support of significant others for the decision to abort as a predictor of outcome in a sample of 489 women. They found that partner support was a significant predictor of positive outcome for older women, whereas parental support was an important predictor for younger women. Moseley, Follingstad, Harley, and Heckel (1981) reported that greater pre- and postabortion distress was related to making the abortion decision alone, having negative feelings toward their partner, and experiencing less support from their partners and parents. Finally, Belsey et al. (1977) revealed that having poor support from families and friends resulted in greater disturbance three months after the abortion.

In contrast to the findings of studies of perceived social support, Major et al.'s (1985) study of *actual* social support revealed a worse coping pattern for women who were accompanied to an abortion clinic than for women who came alone. Women who came for the abortion with a partner were significantly more depressed and had significantly more physical complaints than did unaccompanied women. These effects were still seen even after the effects of age and coping expectations were controlled, but they were not present at a 3-week follow-up. These authors concluded that these results may have been an artifact of more depressed women needing to bring a companion with them to the clinic. It is also possible that the effects of social support are related to the amount of support a woman *perceives*, rather than the amount she objectively receives.

Finally, it is important that the degree of social support a woman receives is not confused with the degree of influence others have on her attitudes, motivations, or decisions. Bracken et al. (1978) suggest that a woman's adjustment and reactions after an abortion are directly related to the degree to which she acted upon her own desires and motives. While it is clear that the difficulty in making the decision is related to the amount of guilt experienced after the abortion (Bracken et al., 1974), it appears that women who are most vulnerable to negative outcome following abortion are those who are pressured or persuaded by others to have the abortion (Bracken et al., 1978).

CLINICAL IMPLICATIONS: COUNSELING FOLLOWING ABORTION

Experiencing an unwanted pregnancy is a stressful event. When this stress is compounded by the stresses of making a decision regarding abortion and undergoing a medical procedure, many women need counseling or psychotherapy to help them resolve and cope with some of these issues. Although the data indicate that a woman's reactions to abortion are more likely to be positive than negative, counselors and psychotherapists need to be alert to the possibility that psychotherapy or counseling focused on abortion issues may be beneficial to a subset of women.

Psychotherapy and counseling in this context has centered on four main aspects of the abortion experience: 1) *helping the woman through the decision-making process*; 2) *helping the woman deal with feelings of ambivalence and anxiety* regarding the decision and the procedure; 3) *helping a woman cope with any negative reactions* (e.g., grief, regret) she may have over the loss of the future of her child; and 4) *providing the woman with information* about the abortion procedures, the psychological aftermath, and contraception. In addition to counseling the woman before, during, and shortly after the abortion, the woman may need help dealing with the abortion decision and experience at several later points in her life, in part due to the "anniversary reactions" experienced by many (Smith, 1977). Anniversary reactions to the abortion experience are depressive episodes which occur around the anniversary of the date of the abortion or the anniversary of the date that the child would have been born.

Because women with unplanned pregnancies are often in a state of crisis, they may need short-term crisis-centered therapy to help them address their immediate needs and to help them make decisions. Counseling provided prior to the abortion to help the woman explore ambivalent feelings and alternatives to abortion will be the most beneficial in the long run. An excellent model for postabortion support groups, which is aimed at clarifying feelings, reducing isolation, facilitating appropriate mourning, increasing self-esteem, and bringing closure to the abortion experience, is provided by Lodl, McGettigan, and Bucy (1984–1985). In addition, an innovative program of group counseling for male partners of women undergoing abortion has been developed (Gordon & Kilpatrick, 1977).

A number of women receiving counseling for depression have unresolved grief issues over a prior abortion and counseling for their grief is likely to be helpful in most cases. Counselors may find that taking a cognitive approach to therapy early on will help them establish a firm basis for dealing with affect-laden issues (Gould, 1980; Joy, 1985). This approach would include identifying the woman's rationale for choosing to abort her fetus early, delineating factors which contributed to that decision, and utilizing coping strategies and outside sources of support. In cases where a woman is experiencing considerable guilt over having "killed" her fetus, several authors have proposed Gestaltian techniques such as the use of the "Empty Chair" technique (Fagan & Shepherd, 1970), which allows the client to explain reasons for her decision to the fetus and explore the option of forgiveness (Buckles, 1982; Joy, 1985). Alternatively, it is important for the clinician to remember that the issues surrounding the loss of a fetus through abortion are significantly different from other perinatal losses (Leon, 1987). Because abortion involves a conscious decision and because feelings following an abortion may also be positive, it should not be assumed that the bereavement pattern will be the same for both groups.

An essential component of abortion counseling is that of providing support for the woman through active listening. Counselors must be clear, however, about their individual perspectives on abortion in this context. Ideally, the counselor should serve as a "mirror" or "sounding board" for the client, helping her identify areas of conflict or problematic issues, rather than attempting to influence or guide the woman's decision-making or coping processes. The counselor may also help the woman explore various alternatives to abortion, as well as help her identify what factors are contributing to her decision and to her distress. It is important that the woman not be pushed into making such a consequential and irreversible decision. Therapists can be utilized as important screeners and identifiers of abortion candidates who are not comfortable with their decision and these women can be given further consultations, information, and counseling before they complete the procedure. In addition, counselors or psychotherapists are useful in identifying the small percentage of patients who do experience adverse psychological reactions to the abortion.

The ideal program of counseling for women undergoing abortion is probably one which provides a variety of services and treatment modalities. Unfortunately, this ideal is limited by the fact that there are relatively few services such as these available for women. Surprisingly little information on abortion counseling and psychotherapy has been provided in the literature. There is some evidence to suggest, however, that counseling before, during, and after legal abortion may have a positive effect (Burnell, Dworsky, & Harrington, 1972; Dauber, Zalar, & Goldstein, 1972). Professionals seeking detailed information about how to provide abortion counseling may make use of one of several training manuals now available (Baker, 1981; Beresford, 1977).

CONCLUSIONS

A review of the literature on the psychological impact of abortion reveals several deficiencies in this area including: 1) lack of psychological assessment of the prepregnant state of the woman; 2) inadequate follow-up periods; 3) lack of comparison or control groups; 4) absence of investigation of the relationship between medical and psychological outcome; and 5) inadequate assessment instruments or techniques which may not adequately reflect the woman's psychological state. Future research needs to address these deficiencies in order for more specific conclusions to be drawn.

Despite the methodological problems with these studies, however, the aggregation of research in this area demonstrates consistency in the finding that negative psychological outcomes following abortion are rare and that abortion is perceived by most women as a relieving, positive experience. A small minority of women experience negative feelings, usually centered on guilt and grief over their loss, and these women may require supportive counseling. The low incidence of negative reactions such as grief, sadness, and depression following abortion, however, has led Payne et al. (1976) to the conclusion that "abortion is not experienced as a major loss to most women."

Women who have more social support, less difficulty making the abortion decision, high coping expectations, and stable psychological traits have better psychological adjustment and outcome following abortion. In contrast, woman who have emotional or psychiatric problems, self-blame, ambivalence toward the abortion, conservative religious views, low coping expectations, difficulty in making the abortion decision, and less social support show poorer outcome. These latter factors may be, in part, what contribute to delay in seeking abortion and may be responsible for subjecting women to the greater stress and risk of second-trimester procedures (Adler et al., 1990). Hopefully, further research will lead us to more accurate and informative predictions of the psychological and emotional sequelae of abortion.

REFERENCES

Adler, N. (1975). Emotional responses of women following therapeutic abortion. *American Journal of Orthopsychiatry, 45*, 446–454.

Adler, N. E., David, H. P., Major, B. N., Roth, S. H., Russo, N. F., & Wyatt, G. E. (1990). Psychological responses after abortion. *Science, 248*, 41–44.

Alan Guttmacher Institute (1990). *Abortion and women's health: A turning point for America?* New York: Author.

Athanasiou, R., Oppel, W., Michelson, L., Unger, T., & Yager, M. (1973). Psychiatric sequelae to term birth and induced early and late abortion: A longitudinal study. *Family Planning Perspectives, 5*, 227–231.

Baker, A. (1981). *Problem pregnancy counseling*. Granite City, IL: Hope Clinic for Women.

Belsey, E., Greer, H., Lal, S., Lewis, S., & Beard, R. (1977). Predictive factors in emotional response to abortion: King's termination study IV. *Social Science Medicine, 11*, 71–82.

Beresford, T. (1977). *Short-term relationship counseling*. Baltimore: Planned Parenthood Association of Maryland.

Blackburne-Stover, G., Belenky, M., & Gilligan, C. (1982). Moral development and reconstructive memory: Recalling a decision to terminate an unplanned pregnancy. *Developmental Psychology, 18*, 862–870.

Bracken, M., Klerman, L., & Bracken, M. (1978). Abortion, adoption or motherhood: An empirical study of decision-making during pregnancy. *American Journal of Obstetrics and Gynecology, 130*, 251–262.

Bracken, M., Phil, M., Hachamovitch, M., & Grossman, G. (1974). The decision to abort and psychological sequelae. *Journal of Nervous and Mental Disease, 158*, 154–162.

Buckles, N. B. (1982). Abortion: A technique for working through grief. *Journal of the American College Health Association, 30*, 181–182.

Burnell, G. M., Dworsky, W. A., & Harrington, R. L. (1972). Post-abortion group therapy. *American Journal of Psychiatry, 129*, 220–223.

Burnell, G. M., & Norfleet, M. A. (1987). Women's self-reported responses to abortion. *Journal of Psychology, 12*, 71–76.

Cates, W., Schultz, K. F., Grimes, D. A., & Tyler, C. (1977). Abortion methods: Morbidity, costs and emotional impact. 1. The effect of delay and method choice on the risk of abortion morbidity. *Family Planning Perspectives, 9*, 266–268.

Cohen, L., & Roth, S. (1984). Coping with abortion. *Journal of Human Stress, 10*(3), 140–145.

Congressional Record, 135(33). (Mar. 21, 1989), p. E908.

Dauber, B., Zalar, M., & Goldstein, P. J. (1972). Abortion counseling and behavioral change. *Family Planning Perspectives, 4*, 23–27.

Denney, M. K. (1983). *A matter of choice: An essential guide to every aspect of abortion*. New York: Simon & Schuster.

Fagan, J., & Shephard, I. L. (Eds.). (1970). *Gestalt therapy now: Theory, techniques, applications*. Palo Alto, CA: Science and Behavior Books.

Freeman, E., Rickels, K., Huggins, G., Garcia, C., & Polin, J. (1980). Emotional distress patterns among women having first or repeat abortions. *Obstetrics and Gynecology, 55*, 630–636.

Gordon, R. H., & Kilpatrick, C. A. (1977). A program of group counseling for men who accompany women seeking legal abortions. *Community Mental Health Journal, 13*, 291–295.

Gould, N. B. (1980). Post-abortion depressive reactions in college women. *Journal of the American College Health Association, 28*, 316–321.

Greer, M. S., Lal, S., Lewis, S. C., Belsey, E., & Beard, R. (1976). Psychosocial consequences of therapeutic abortion: King's Termination Study III. *British Journal of Psychiatry, 128*, 74–79.

Grimes, D. A. (1985). Provision of abortion services in the United States. In the Ciba Foundation Symposium 115, *Abortion: Medical progress and social implications*. London: Pitman.

Henshaw, S. K., & Silverman, J. (1988). The characteristics and prior contraceptive use of U.S. abortion patients. *Family Planning Perspectives, 20*, 158–166.

Hern, W. M. (1984). *Abortion practice*. Philadelphia: J. B. Lippincott.

Joy, S. S. (1985). Abortion: An issue to grieve? *Journal of Counseling and Development, 63*, 375–376.

Kochanek, K. D. (1991). Induced terminations of pregnancy: Reporting States, 1988. *Monthly Vital Statistics Report, 39(12) Supplement*. Hyattsville, MD: National Center for Health Statistics, U.S. Department of Health and Human Services, Centers for Disease Control.

Kumar, R., & Robson, K. (1978). Previous induced abortion and ante-natal depression in primiparae: Preliminary report of a survey of mental health of pregnancy. *Psychological Medicine, 8*, 711–715.

Kummer, J. (1963). Post-abortion psychiatric illness: A myth? *American Journal of Psychiatry, 119*, 980–983.

Lazarus, A. (1985). Psychiatric sequelae of legalized elective first trimester abortion. *Journal of Psychosomatic Obstetrics and Gynaecology, 4*, 141–150.

Lemkau, J. P. (1988). Emotional sequelae of abortion: Implications for clinical practice. *Psychology of Women Quarterly, 12*, 461–472.

Leon, I. G. (1987). Short-term psychotherapy for perinatal loss. *Psychotherapy, 24*, 186–195.

Lodl, K., McGettigan, A., & Bucy, J. (1984–1985). Women's responses to abortion: Implications for post-abortion support groups. *Journal of Social Work and Human Sexuality, 3*, 119–132.

Major, B., Mueller, P., & Hildebrandt, K. (1985). Attributions, expectations, and coping with abortion. *Journal of Personality and Social Psychology, 48*, 585–599.

McAll, K., & Wilson, W. (1987). Ritual mourning for unresolved grief after abortion. *Southern Medical Journal, 80*, 817–821.

Moore, K. G. (Ed.) (1990). *Public health policy implications of abortion: A government relations handbook for health professionals*. Washington, DC: American College of Obstetricians and Gynecologists.

Moseley, D. T., Follingstad, D. R., Harley, H., & Heckel, R. (1981). Psychological factors that predict reaction to abortion. *Journal of Clinical Psychology, 37*, 276–279.

National Abortion Federation (1988). *Safety of abortion*. Washington, DC: Author.

National Abortion Federation (1989a). *Women who have abortions*. Washington, DC: Author.

National Abortion Federation (1989b). *What is abortion?* Washington, DC: Author.

National Abortion Federation (1990). *Abortion after twelve weeks*. Washington, DC: Author.

Osofsky, J., & Osofsky, H. (1972). The psychological reaction of patients to legalized abortion. *American Journal of Orthopsychiatry, 42*, 48–60.

Payne, E. C., Kravitz, A. R., Norman, M. T., & Anderson, J. (1976). Outcome following therapeutic abortion. *Archives of General Psychiatry, 33*, 725–733.

Peppers, L. (1987–1988). Grief and elective abortion: Breaking the emotional bond? *Omega, 18*, 1–12.

Planned Parenthood of Southeastern Pennsylvania v. Casey. (1992). Nos. 91-744 and 91-902 (U.S. Supreme Court, June 29, 1992).

Rizzardo, R., Magni, G., Desideri, A., Cosentino, M., & Salmaso, P. (1992). Personality and psychological distress before and after legal abortion: A prospective study. *Journal of Psychosomatic Obstetrics and Gynaecology, 13*, 75–91.

Roe v. Wade. (1973). 410 *United States Reporter* 113.

Rogers, J. L., Stoms, G. B., & Phifer, J.L. (1989). Psychological impact of abortion: Methodological and outcomes summary of empirical research between 1966 and 1988. *Health Care Women International, 10*, 347–376.

Sachdev, P. (1985). *Perspectives on abortion*. Metuchen, NJ: Scarecrow Press.

Schusterman, L. R. (1979). Predicting the psychological consequences of abortion. *Social Science and Medicine, 13A*, 683–689.

Shaw, P. C., Funderburk, C., & Franklin, B. J. (1979). An investigation of the abortion decision process. *Psychology, A Quarterly Journal of Human Behavior, 16*, 11–19.

Shephard, B. D., & Shephard, C. A. (1990). *The complete guide to women's health, 2nd revised edition*. New York: Plume/Penguin Books.

Simon, N., & Senturia, A. (1966). Psychiatric sequelae of abortion. *Archives of General Psychiatry, 15*, 378.

Smith, E. D. (1982). *Abortion: Health care perspectives*. Norwalk, CT: Appleton–Century–Crofts.

Smith, E. M. (1973). A follow-up study of women who request abortion. *American Journal of Orthopsychiatry, 43*, 574–585.

Smith, E. M. (1977). Counseling for women who seek abortion. In R. Kalmar (Ed.), *Abortion, emotional implications* (pp. 75–83). Dubuque, IA: Kendall/Hunt.

Stubblefield, P.G. (1991). Pregnancy termination. In S. G. Gabbe, J. R. Niebyl, & J. L. Simpson (Eds.), *Obstetrics: Normal and problem pregnancies (2nd Edition)* (pp. 1303–1330). New York: Churchill-Livingstone.

Torres, A., & Forrest J. (1988). Why do women have abortions? *Family Planning Perspectives, 20*, 169–176.

Zabin, L. S., Hirsch, M. B., & Emerson, M. R. (1989). When urban adolescents choose abortion: Effects on education, psychological status and subsequent pregnancy. *Family Planning Perspectives, 21*, 248–255.

14

High-Risk Pregnancy

Laura L. Gorman

Every pregnancy has risks associated with it (Freeman & Pescar, 1982). Although the majority of pregnancies follow a normal course and result in the birth of a healthy baby, the risk of complications during pregnancy, labor, or delivery which result in adverse outcomes for the neonate or woman varies among individuals. A number of factors, such as the genetic constitution of the parents, maternal disease prior to and during pregnancy, psychological states during pregnancy, demographic characteristics, and health behaviors can contribute to increased risk for complications.

The purpose of this chapter is to examine the psychological aspects associated with high-risk pregnancy which may be of importance to medical personnel, including obstetricians, nurses, health and clinical psychologists, counselors, and social workers, involved in the care of women during their pregnancies. First, assessment procedures and identification methods for high-risk pregnancy will be examined. Second, the psychological reactions in women identified as having high-risk pregnancies will be discussed. Next, the literature examining the relation between psychological states during pregnancy, such as stress and anxiety, and pregnancy complications or adverse outcomes for the neonate will be reviewed. The fourth issue to be examined is the relation between health behaviors during pregnancy, such as smoking and alcohol or drug abuse, and the increased risk of adverse outcomes for the fetus or newborn. Finally, the clinical implications with regard to the psychological issues in high-risk pregnancy will be discussed.

ASSESSMENT OF RISK

High-risk pregnancy is defined as any pregnancy in which there is a factor—maternal or fetal—that potentially acts adversely to affect the outcome of pregnancy (Queenan, 1985). Perinatology or maternal–fetal medicine, a subspecialty of obstetrics, focuses specifically on identification and management of the high-risk pregnancy. Perinatologists work closely with the obstetrician and pediatrician to provide medical care to the fetus and pregnant woman in an effort to improve the likelihood of a favorable outcome. Although the majority of pregnancies have favorable outcomes, high-risk pregnancies need to be closely monitored and managed in order to reduce the probability of complications.

In the United States, the overall incidence of pregnancies classified as high-risk is 10–20% (Kemp & Pond, 1986). The incidence rates can be even higher in certain groups of women, such as adolescents and women from low socioeconomic backgrounds. Although the percentage of pregnancies categorized as high-risk is a cause of concern, competent management on the part of the physician and the cooperation of the pregnant woman can result in the birth of healthy infants from these high-risk pregnancies.

There are a number of factors that have been associated with increased risk to the infant during pregnancy or labor and delivery. Maternal demographic factors, maternal disease, and specific factors associated with the prepregnancy, prenatal, intrapartum, and postpartum periods have been identified as placing the fetus or neonate at increased risk (Blackburn, 1986). Some are preexisting, as is the case with genetic factors or chronic maternal disease, while other factors develop during pregnancy. A list of factors which may contribute to adverse outcomes in the neonate is presented in Table 14.1

The primary purpose of risk assessment during pregnancy is to identify the actual or potential presence of characteristics that may significantly influence the infant's or woman's well-being (Blackburn, 1986). By identifying early in the prenatal period individual factors or a combination of factors that are associated with increased risk, the woman's physician can implement appropriate treatment to prevent or minimize the negative effects on maternal–infant health. Recent technological advances in prenatal and neonatal care, such as amniocentesis, chorionic villus sampling, ultrasound, and electronic fetal monitoring, have aided in reducing and eliminating some of the adverse outcomes that result from a number of risk factors listed in Table 14.1

As the term "risk" implies, the designation of high-risk pregnancy signifies only the existence of a factor or factors, whether they are genetic, maternal, environmental, or fetal, that increase the probability of an adverse outcome for the infant or woman. Some pregnancies designated as high-risk do not result in complications for the mother or infant (a false positive). Conversely, some pregnancies without any identified risk factors do result in maternal–infant health

TABLE 14.1 Pregnancy Risk Factors

Maternal Demographic Factors
  maternal age (below 16 or above 35)
  over or underweight (by 20% or greater)
  low SES
  race (black)
Maternal Disease
  sickle-cell disease
  idiopathic thrombocytopenic pupura
  systemic lupus erythematosus
  cardiac disease
  renal disease
  diabetes mellitus
  hyperthyroidism
  hypothyroidism
  acute hepatitis
  asthma
  epilepsy
  hypertension
  cytomegalovirus
  herpes simplex
  rubella
  Group B streptococcus
  toxoplasmosis
  tuberculosis
  urinary tract disease
Prepregnancy Factors
  poor nutrition
  history of reproductive problems
    (previous preterm, stillborn, neonatal
    death, low birth weight infant)
  familial history of chromosomal
    disorders
  short interpregnancy intervals
  parity greater than four
  uterine malformations
Prenatal Factors
  pregnancy-induced hypertension
    (toxemia, preeclampsia, eclampsia)
  infection (e.g., HIV)
  no or late prenatal care
  substance abuse (smoking, alcohol,
    drugs)
  exposure to environmental or occupa-
    tional hazards

Prenatal Factors (cont.)
  decreased or increase amniotic fluid
    (oligohydramnios, hydramnios)
  isoimmunization
  poor or excessive weight gain
  anemia
  bleeding
Intrapartum Factors
  premature or prolonged (over 24 hours)
    rupture of the membrane
  premature labor (prior to 37 weeks)
  prolonged labor (over 24 hours for
    primiparas, 12 hours for multiparas;
    second stage over 3 hours)
  precipitous labor (less than 3 hours)
  placental abnormality (*placenta previa,
    abruptio placenta*)
  abnormal position (breech, face,
    shoulder, transverse)
  operative delivery (forceps, vacuum
    extractor, cesarian section)
  use of anesthesia, depressant drugs
  fetal distress (abnormal heart rate or
    pattern, meconium-stained fluid,
    abnormal fetal blood gases from scalp
    sample)
  prolapsed umbilical cord, cord abnor-
    malities
  multiple pregnancy
  postterm pregnancy (greater than 42
    weeks)
Neonatal Factors
  Apgar score of less than 5 (at 1 or 5
    minutes)
  birth weight <2500 or >4000 grams
  congenital anomalies, genetic or
    chromosomal syndrome, birth trauma
  infant medical problems (respiratory
    distress, sepsis, hypoglycemia,
    hypocalcemia, seizures, congestive
    heart failure, necrotizing enterocolitis,
    intraventricular hemorrhage, acidosis)

problems (a false negative). Because intervention and prevention efforts during the prenatal period can be successful in reducing the risk of adverse outcomes in the fetus or neonate, the cases in which risk factors are not identified may be the most troubling and unfortunate. Therefore, efforts should be taken to reduce their occurrence by implementing standard risk assessments for all pregnancies. However, false positives may also be problematic because of anxiety and stress the woman may experience knowing there is the possibility of complications developing during pregnancy, labor, or delivery.

The actual assessment of risk during pregnancy should include three health dimensions (Kemp & Pond, 1986). These include the appraisal of physiologic, psychologic, and environmental factors which may contribute to increased risk for poor maternal–infant health. Physiologic assessment would include knowing the woman's past obstetric history (e.g., previous miscarriages, bleeding during pregnancy, preeclampsia) and current obstetric complications (e.g., positive results on prenatal diagnostic procedures, gestational diabetes). It is also important to obtain past individual and family medical history, as well as information concerning family genetic disorders.

Assessment of psychological factors during pregnancy is also important. Stress or anxiety during pregnancy can result from the woman worrying about the health of the fetus and the fear of giving birth to a disabled child, or from outside influences associated with her career, finances, or interpersonal and family relationships. As will be discussed in the next section, stress and anxiety during pregnancy have been associated with adverse neonatal outcomes such as low birth weight and intrapartum complications. Therefore, identifying women who are extremely anxious or who have experienced numerous stressful life events during their pregnancy should not be overlooked as an important component in the risk-assessment process.

Consideration should also be given to the psychological reactions a women may experience when she becomes aware that her pregnancy carries the "high-risk" label. Increased anxiety due to the possibility of negative outcomes for the infant may interact with preexisting risk factors to make matters worse. Assessment of the woman's perception about the status of the pregnancy, her coping abilities, and her social support should be conducted (Kemp & Pond, 1986). Education and supportive interventions might then be implemented to help the woman adjust and make informed decisions regarding her pregnancy.

Environmental risk assessment should include determining the woman's socioeconomic status, personal health habits (e.g., nutrition, smoking, alcohol or other drug use), extent of prenatal care, and exposure to teratogens such as pesticides or other chemicals linked to pregnancy complications (Kemp & Pond, 1986). Examination of these and other environmental factors can help the physician identify a pregnancy at risk for poor maternal–infant outcomes, so that direction and guidance can be provided to the women to modify her behavior or pursue professional treatment interventions.

A variety of risk-scoring systems have been developed and are available for prenatal risk assessment. Three frequently used instruments are the Maternal–Child Health Care Index (Nesibitt & Aubry, 1969) and Labor Index (Aubry & Pennington, 1973), the Antepartum Fetal Risk Score (Goodwin, Dunne, & Thomas, 1969), and the Problem Oriented Perinatal Risk Assessment System (POPRAS) (Hobel, Youkeles, & Forsythe, 1979). These three instruments assess maternal and pregnancy factors. The POPRAS also assesses neonatal risk as does the widely used Apgar score. Although other obstetric risk-scoring systems are available for use (Knox, Sadler, Pattison, Mantell, & Mullins, 1993), no one particular assessment tool has been identified as ideal (Aumann & Baird, 1986).

In summary, assessment of risk is a very important component in the proper management of a woman's pregnancy. Careful consideration should be given to physiologic, psychologic, and environmental factors which may contribute to increased risk to the neonate and woman. It has also been suggested that reassessment of risk factors should be conducted as the pregnancy progresses to identify any changes in the woman's risk status (Aumann & Baird, 1986). Upon identification of a high-risk pregnancy, the woman's physician can implement intervention procedures in an effort to reduce or eliminate the possibility of adverse maternal–infant outcomes. These interventions may involve transferring the woman's pregnancy care to a regional health care center for more specialized obstetric care, or in the case of a woman with alcohol or drug-abuse problems, making a referral to another professional trained to treat these problems.

PSYCHOLOGICAL RESPONSES TO HIGH-RISK PREGNANCY

The woman's psychological responses to high-risk pregnancy have received little systematic investigation (Kemp & Page, 1987). High-risk pregnancy is usually a fairly stressful event for the woman. Determining whether women with high-risk pregnancies experience different feelings or emotions than low-risk women is of interest for a number of reasons, including the type of interventions that might be helpful for these women (Johnson & Murphy, 1986). Numerous reports have indicated that emotional and psychological reactions usually experienced in normal pregnancies are intensified or prolonged in high-risk pregnancies (Freeman & Pescar, 1982; Johnson & Murphy, 1986; Penticuff, 1982; Wohlreich, 1986). Therefore, before addressing the psychological responses that may occur in women with high-risk pregnancies, a brief overview of the psychological changes occurring during normal pregnancy is necessary.

Pregnancy has been described as a developmental crisis that can strain the individual woman and her family, but it can also be an event involving interpersonal growth and increased maturity (Wohlreich, 1986). The feelings and emotions the woman may experience are quite varied. Ambivalence toward or rejection of the pregnancy occurs in 50–60% of women after the pregnancy is confirmed (Selby, 1980). This ambivalence or rejection does not appear to be related to whether or not the pregnancy was planned. When ambivalence is present, acceptance of the pregnancy is a gradual process. Ambivalence found in the initial stages of the pregnancy is usually resolved by the third trimester (Selby, 1980). Quickening (maternal perception of fetal movement) in the second trimester has been reported to relieve many fears a woman may have about miscarriage and allows the normal process of attachment to begin (Leifer, 1980).

Definitive statements about mood states in pregnancy are difficult to make because different investigators use different indices of mood disturbances (e.g., symptomatology vs. syndromal indicators), compare heterogeneous samples of women (e.g., differences in demographic characteristics such as age, marital status, or socioeconomic level), and assess women at different times during the pregnancy (Tunis & Golbus, 1991). Keeping this in mind, Selby (1980) reviewed a number of studies and found that many women report increases in anxiety, depression, crying, and lability of mood during the nine months of pregnancy. Anxiety levels in an uncomplicated pregnancy have been shown to be lowest during the second trimester and highest during the third trimester. The woman's concerns about her competence as a mother and worries about the baby's health may be partially responsible for the increase in anxiety as labor and delivery approach (Wohlreich, 1986).

In a more recent study of 128 women, no significant group changes were found in anxiety, tension, or depression during pregnancy (Elliott, Rugg, Watson, & Brough, 1983). However, the investigators did report significant variation in the amount of change that occurred in women from late pregnancy to the puerperium. They concluded that making generalizations about childbearing women should be avoided and individual differences should be emphasized.

For women with high-risk pregnancies, ambivalence or doubt that is characteristically resolved by the third trimester in uncomplicated pregnancies may still be present. If the current risk is due to a history of obstetric or infertility problems, the woman cannot be sure that her current pregnancy will go to term without adverse outcomes. In this situation, ambivalence and doubt may continue until the end of the pregnancy. Wolhreich (1986) suggests that ambivalence can interfere with the normal process of attachment to the infant. However, evidence of abnormal maternal–fetus attachment in high-risk pregnancies was not found in a study by Kemp and Page (1987). They found both that women with normal pregnancies and those with high-risk pregnancies developed feelings of attachment to the fetus during pregnancy. A possible explanation involving denial of adverse outcomes on the part of women with high-risk pregnancies was discounted by the investigators because the high-risk women were asked to express in writing the reasons for their high-risk status. In summary, even though feelings of ambivalence toward the pregnancy may exist in women with high-risk pregnancies, it does not appear to interfere with the development of feelings of attachment toward the fetus.

Anxiety over concerns such as the health of the fetus or the woman's competence as a mother is commonly found in women at some point during normal pregnancy. For high-risk women, levels of anxiety may be intensified and occur at times when anxiety is usually low (i.e., during the second trimester). Mercer and Ferketich (1988) conducted one of the few controlled studies examining the differences in psychological responses during pregnancy between women identified as being at low or high risk. In this study, high-risk women were recruited from referral hospitals where they had been hospitalized for their condition. Pregnancy risk was assessed using a version of Hobel and colleagues' (1979) instrument, updated to reflect current diagnostic procedures and interventions. Low-risk women were attending a low-risk antepartum clinic, had no chronic disease, and were responsive to routine management of mild symptoms of pregnancy-induced disease if this occurred. All women were between the 24th and 34th week of gestation, and the low- and high-risk groups did not differ in socioeconomic status, race, or marital status.

Results from this study indicated that high-risk women reported greater negative life events stress and anxiety than low-risk women. Further analysis using negative life events, pregnancy risk score, perceived social support, received social support, social network size, self-esteem, and sense of mastery as predictor variables indicated that only negative life events and lower self-esteem predicted anxiety in the high-risk group. The failure of received social support or social network size to predict anxiety in high-risk women was contrary to the investigators' prediction. They suggested that in times of crisis a different type of support may be indicated.

Although the Mercer and Ferketich study examined differences in level of anxiety between low- and high-risk women during the third trimester, high levels of anxiety have also been reported at other times during the high-risk pregnancy. Diagnostic procedures, such as amniocentesis, which are performed to confirm or clarify risks to the fetus, usually take place during the first or second trimester and have been associated with increased anxiety. Phipps and Zinn (1986) compared anxiety levels in pregnant women undergoing amniocentesis and in women who were not having the procedure. Assessments of anxiety were conducted at three times for the women undergoing amniocentesis: 1) after genetic counselling; 2) after amniocentesis; and 3) one week after receiving the results. Assessments for the other women took place at comparable gestational stages in their pregnancies. The findings indicated that women undergoing amniocentesis had significantly higher anxiety levels after the procedure was completed, but before the results were known than women not having the procedure. The waiting period between the actual procedure and communication of the results may extend up to three weeks in amniocentesis. Thus prenatal diagnostic tests during the first or second trimester and the necessary prenatal care which follows from these tests may produce increased anxiety at times during the high-risk pregnancy when anxiety levels are usually at their lowest levels in a low-risk pregnancy.

Depressed mood is common in normal pregnancy. However, the level of depressive symptoms in high-risk women is significantly higher than in low-risk women during the third trimester (Mercer & Ferketich, 1988). Mercer and Ferketich also found that a higher percentage of high-risk women showed evidence of clinical depression as measured with the Center for Epidemiologic Studies depression scale (CES-D; Radloff, 1977). In this study, 51% of the high-risk women compared to 24% of the low-risk women, had scores on the CES-D indicative of clinical depression. Hierarchical regression analysis revealed that negative life events, pregnancy risk score, low self-esteem, and a low sense of control predicted level of depression in the high-risk women.

Feelings of low self-esteem have also been reported to exist at higher levels in women with high-risk pregnancies compared with women having low-risk pregnancies; however, the available data are not conclusive. Kemp and Page (1987) found that women experiencing a high-risk pregnancy had lower self-esteem than women having a normal pregnancy. The investigators caution against interpreting the results as an indication that high-risk status causes lower levels of self-esteem because the relation between risk status and self-esteem is correlational. It is equally probable that the high-risk women had lower self-esteem prior to their high-risk status. In contrast to these findings, Mercer and Ferketich (1988) did not find any differences between low- and high-risk women in self-esteem in their sample.

Psychological reactions such as anger, guilt, fear, and denial have also been reported in women identified as having high-risk pregnancies (Johnson & Murphy, 1986). However, these reports are not based on systematic investigations. Some high-risk women experience anger, not infrequently directed at other women with normal pregnancies. They may often ask the question "Why me?" Feelings of guilt may exist if the woman feels she is responsible for the complication. This may occur when the woman exposes herself and the fetus to teratogens that could have been avoided, such as toxic chemicals, tobacco, or alcohol. High-risk women who are not experiencing anxiety or expressing concern over the potential risks to the infant may be exhibiting denial in response to the existence of the possibility of a negative outcome. Although this may be adaptive in some respects (e.g., lower anxiety levels), it may be maladaptive if the woman does not obtain special prenatal care which may reduce the possibility of a negative outcome. Johnson and Murphy (1986) recommend that health care providers be aware of the possibility of denial and help the pregnant woman exhibiting denial overcome this psychological response. Doing so may make the woman more likely to endorse and be compliant with medical procedures.

To summarize, there is empirical evidence indicating that some women identified as having a high-risk pregnancy experience higher levels of anxiety and depression than low-risk women. There is equivocal evidence supporting the finding that women with high-risk pregnancies have lower self-esteem. It does not appear that high-risk women, in general, have difficulty forming attachments to the fetus, even though ambivalence toward the pregnancy may not be resolved in a high-risk pregnancy as it usually is in normal pregnancy. Other emotional reactions, such as anger, guilt, and fear, may exist and occur at higher intensities in women experiencing a high-risk compared to low-risk pregnancy, but this has not been empirically validated.

PSYCHOLOGICAL FACTORS CONTRIBUTING TO INCREASED RISK

Psychological variables such as stress or anxiety increasingly have been acknowledged as important contributors to health outcomes with respect to cardiovascular disease, gastrointestinal disease, and other medical disorders (Selye, 1976). The effects of stress and anxiety have also been examined in the context of pregnancy outcomes in attempts to ascertain whether these psychological factors are causally related to increased risk of poor pregnancy outcomes. Differences among investigators in the conceptualization and measurement of "stress" are common and contribute to some of the variation in outcomes across studies. Among researchers, "stress" is sometimes defined as a stimulus (e.g., a life event or life change) or as a response (e.g., anxiety). Frequently studies include measures of both life changes or life events and anxiety and examine the relation of both to the outcome of interest (e.g., low birth weight, antepartum complications, etc.). In the next section, the relation between stress, defined as life change, life events, or anxiety, and negative pregnancy outcomes, will be examined.

A number of studies have investigated the relation between life stress or anxiety and complications during pregnancy, labor, or delivery. Because of methodological problems in some of the studies, inconsistencies have resulted in the literature making it difficult to compare findings across studies. These problems include using different methods to measure life stress and anxiety and assessing these variables at different times during the pregnancy. Another methodological factor that contributes to the variability in findings across studies is the reliance on retrospective reporting of life events and anxiety experienced during pregnancy. The use of retrospective reports can be problematic because the woman may under- or overreport life events that occurred during pregnancy. In the case of underreporting, a relation between stress and complications during pregnancy or labor and delivery that actually exists may not be apparent in the statistical analysis. Retrospective overreporting of life events that occurred during pregnancy may result if the woman tries to find explanations for the negative outcome in the neonate. This may lead to apparent relations between negative life events and negative outcomes that are not actually significant (Brown, Sklair, Harris, & Birley, 1973).

Another methodological problem which may contribute to some of the inconsistency in the literature is the variation among studies regarding the definition of an adverse outcome for the infant. Depending on the study, adverse outcomes have included low birth weight (less than 2500 g), prematurity, antepartum complications including preeclampsia and threatened abortion, and intrapartum complications, or conditions which pose a risk to the neonate during labor and delivery, such as prolonged labor or fetal respiratory distress. In addition to the heterogeneity existing in the types of outcomes used as dependent variables, wide variation exists in the severity of antepartum and intrapartum complications. For example, in one of the earlier studies, intrapartum complications ranged from a neonate with a bruised nose to a stillborn infant (Davids & DeVault, 1962).

In a review by Levin and DeFrank (1988), the results of 26 studies published through 1986 investigating the relation between maternal psychosocial stress and pregnancy outcomes were examined. Pregnancy outcomes were divided into four general categories, low birth weight, prematurity, antepartum complications, and intrapartum complications. The reviewers then summarized the findings regarding the link between maternal life change stress or anxiety and each of the outcomes.

With respect to low birth weight, three of the four studies reviewed showed nonsignificant associations between stress and low birth weight. However, these three studies had methodological flaws, such as small sample sizes and skewed distributions of anxiety and life change stress scores, which may have affected the results. In the most recently conducted study reviewed by Levin and DeFrank, a significant relation was found between the number of major life events and low birth weight and between state anxiety and low birth weight (Newton & Hunt, 1984), although this association did not remain significant after controlling for cigarette smoking.

Two studies, published since Levin and DeFrank's review, have shown that life events stress is significantly related to low birth weight. Both of these studies were prospective and controlled for biomedical risk factors (e.g., cigarette smoking, maternal height, history of medical disorders such as diabetes or heart disease, or high blood pressure) and demographic variables that have been associated with low birth weight. Reeb, Graham, Zyzanski, and Kitson (1987) found that stressful life events occurring during pregnancy were predictive of low birth weight. Eighty-five percent of the mothers having low birth weight infants experienced one or more stressful life events during pregnancy compared to 55% of the mothers having infants with normal birth weights. In the second prospective study of 100 women, Pagel, Smilkstein, Regen, and Montano (1990) found that higher levels of life events before and during pregnancy were associated with lower birth weight after controlling for biomedical risk factors and lifestyles (which included smoking and drinking).

Although the evidence from the studies conducted over the past 35 years do not unequivocally support the association between life change stress or anxiety and low birth weight, the more recent and better-designed studies suggest that life change stress and anxiety during pregnancy are significantly related to birth weight.

The association between prematurity, a significant health risk to the infant, and stress has also been investigated. Levin and DeFrank (1988) found that prematurity (defined as birth at less than 37 weeks gestation in most studies) was a consistent correlate of maternal stress. In four of the five studies they reviewed, significant associations were found between high levels of life change and premature birth. It should be noted, however, that in three of the four studies showing a significant relation between life events and premature birth, retrospective reporting may have inflated the women's reporting of events occurring during pregnancy. Results from the only prospective study in the review showed that life change in the final trimester contributed most to premature birth (Newton & Hunt, 1984).

In a more recent prospective study of 100 women, Pagel et al. (1990) found a significant relation between anxiety and prematurity. The investigators reported that higher levels of anxiety were predictive of lower gestational age. However, further analysis indicated that neither anxiety nor life events significantly accounted for any of the variance in gestational length when biomedical risks and demographic factors were controlled.

In summary, there appears to be support for the relation between life change stress or anxiety and prematurity. Empirical evidence from numerous studies has shown that high levels of stress are deleteriously related to gestational length (Levin & DeFrank, 1988). Whether there is a directional or causative association between stress and shorter gestational age is unknown since the relation does not remain significant when biomedical risk factors are considered.

Antepartum complications or those complications occurring during pregnancy have also been associated with stress and anxiety during pregnancy. Just as stress can contribute to hypertension in nonpregnant women, it may also contribute to hypertension during pregnancy which, if severe enough, can be a significant risk factor. Although there is no research to confirm the association between stress and this specific antepartum complication, there is evidence supporting an association between stress and complications during pregnancy in general. Levin and DeFrank's review of nine studies suggests that higher levels of either anxiety or life change stress increased the woman's risk of reporting one or more complications during pregnancy. Because most of the studies assessed stress and antepartum complications concurrently, it is not possible to determine whether high levels of anxiety and stress precede the antepartum complication or whether the increased anxiety and stress are the consequence of knowing one's infant is at risk.

Intrapartum complications, or those which occur during labor and delivery, have also been shown to be related to maternal stress and anxiety. Recent studies utilizing prospective designs and statistical control of biomedical risk factors and demographic factors (Pagel et al., 1990; Williamson, LeFevre, & Hector, 1989) have supported the association between stressors in the woman's life and complications during labor or delivery.

Williamson and colleagues (1989) found that women reporting an increase in stressful life events between mid-pregnancy and near the end of pregnancy had significantly higher ratings of poor outcomes than did women who did not experience increased stress. Approximately nine percent of the women who experienced increased stressful life events had infants who died, were put into intensive care units, had Apgar scores less than seven at five minutes, or weighed less than 2,500 grams compared to almost four percent of the women who did not experience a change in life stress. In the other prospective study, anxiety assessed between the 21st and 36th week of pregnancy was significantly predictive of depressed five-minute Apgar scores (Pagel et al., 1990).

Overall, the results of the studies published more recently, which are methodologically more sound than many of the earlier studies, suggest that life change stress and anxiety can be independent risk factors with regard to some pregnancy outcomes. Recent studies that have controlled for biomedical risk factors have found that life change stress has been associated with low birth weight and intrapartum complications. However, support for the relation between life change stress and antepartum complications and preterm birth has not been as forthcoming in studies that have controlled for biomedical risk factors. Thus, there is not clear evidence that high levels of stress during pregnancy independently contribute to all negative pregnancy outcomes.

Possible underlying neurobiological mechanisms that might be involved in the relation between stress and adverse pregnancy outcomes are not clearly understood in humans. However, Istvan (1986) outlined two neuroendocrine mechanisms receiving empirical support from research studies involving primates and ewes that may have potential relevance to humans. The first involves the sympathetic adrenomedullary activation response that occurs in primates following exposure to stressors. Myers (1977; Myers & Myers, 1979) argues that neuroendocrines, such as epinephrine and norepinephrine, released as part of the stress response to stressful activites, tend to reduce uterine blood flow in pregnant rhesus monkeys, resulting in fetal hypoxia, an adverse effect on the fetus. Although direct experimental examination of this association in women during pregnancy is not possible (for ethical reasons), the relation between life stress and neuroendocrine response in nonpregnant humans has been supported. Calloway and Dolan (1989) found that depressed patients with life events and difficulties showed increased urinary free cortisol compared to patients without events or difficulties.

The second neuroendocrine mechanism has its underpinnings in research with ewes where, as in humans, it is believed that parturition involves complex interactions between neuroendocrine and ovarian hormones. It has been proposed that the onset of labor is signaled by a substance contained in fetal urine. Although the nature of the substance in humans is not known for certain, in ewes, a rise in fetal cortisol production is critical to the onset of labor. Istvan (1986) speculates that maternal exposure to stress could be linked to ovarian hormone and neuroendocrine secretion that is associated with the onset of labor, potentially before the fetus reaches full gestational age. It must be pointed out that caution is necessary in interpreting and applying these findings from primates and ewes to humans, as there may be important differences in reproductive endocrinology (Istvan, 1986).

Because of the apparent association between stress and pregnancy complications and adverse outcomes, important moderator variables such as social support and coping styles are beginning to be investigated as factors that may reduce the negative effects of stress during pregnancy (Mercer & Ferketich, 1988; Norbeck & Tilden, 1983). Although the role of stress is receiving increased attention as a risk factor during pregnancy, it has not yet been incorporated systematically into any risk-scoring system. Based on the findings supporting the association between stress and complications during pregnancy, labor, and delivery, it would seem appropriate to assess the amount of stress present during pregnancy and acknowledge stress as a risk factor just as maternal disease, abnormal bleeding, drug and alcohol use, and other factors are assessed as risk factors. Pagel et al. (1990) suggest that greater specificity in the identification of women at high risk may be obtained by incorporating psychosocial factors, such as stress or anxiety, into risk-assessment protocols.

HEALTH BEHAVIORS AND THE ROLE OF PSYCHOLOGY

In recent years there has been increasing awareness regarding the importance of initiating and maintaining good health habits. Good nutrition, regular exercise, and avoiding substances, such as tobacco, alcohol, and other drugs, are often included in the advice given to patients by health care providers. Compliance with this type of medical advice during pregnancy is critical because the health of the fetus is affected by the woman's nutritional intake and exposure to these potentially teratogenic substances. Factors such as poor nutrition and substance abuse have been associated with increased risk for complications during pregnancy and negative outcomes for the infant. The following section will specifically address the effects of smoking and alcohol and drug abuse during pregnancy on the infant and the need for interventions to help the dependent woman reduce and eliminate her substance use during pregnancy.

Smoking

Despite public health campaigns aimed at educating people about the health risks associated with the use of tobacco, estimates regarding the percentage of adult females of childbearing age (15–44 years) who smoke range from 29–33% (Adams, Gfroerer, & Rouse, 1989; Khalsa & Gfroerer, 1991; Luoto, 1983). Hickner, Westenberg, and Dittenbir (1984) found that 22–28% of pregnant women smoke. In their survey of 66 pregnant women smokers, they found that 18% stopped smoking completely during pregnancy and 24% reduced their smoking by at least one-half pack per day during pregnancy. Fifty-eight percent of the women continued to smoke the same number of cigarettes they smoked before becoming pregnant or increased the number of cigarettes they smoked. Cnattingius (1989) reported that only 22% of the 673 women smoking at the time of conception had quit four to six weeks into the pregnancy. The results of these studies suggest that although pregnancy might be considered an ideal time for a woman to quit smoking, many women do not quit.

The effects of smoking during pregnancy have been reported in over 1,000 individual articles (Abel, 1984). Smoking has been associated with infertility, spontaneous abortion, low birth weight, placental anomalies, premature rupture of the membranes, stillbirth, fetal malformation, and reduced maximal intellectual attainment in children exposed *in utero* (Abel, 1984). Although the causal mechanism is not known, there is some suggestion that fetal hypoxia or decreased oxygenation in the placenta may be the underlying factor (Abel, 1984).

Because the risk to the fetus or neonate could be reduced or eliminated if the mother quits smoking, it seems appropriate that active intervention measures be implemented to help the woman quit smoking during pregnancy. Educating the woman about the risks associated with smoking should take place at her first prenatal visit. For some women, information about the adverse outcomes associated with smoking during pregnancy is sufficient motivation to quit smoking, but this may be true for only 20% of pregnant women smokers (Cnattingius,

1989). For the remaining 80% of women who don't stop smoking during pregnancy, smoking-cessation programs may be more effective.

Smoking-cessation programs with pregnant women have received little attention in the risk-reduction literature (Kabela & Andrasik, 1988). The studies examining the effectiveness of these programs have used small samples and lack control groups and thus have limited generalizability. One of the few studies done in the United States investigating the efficacy of smoking-cessation programs found that 4 of the 11 women quit smoking, 5 reduced the number of cigarettes smoked, and 2 showed no change or an increase in the number of cigarettes smoked following an intervention involving training in self-monitoring, deep-muscle relaxation, aversive smoking, and coping skills (Danaher, Shisslak, Thompson, & Ford, 1978).

Another study utilized a self-help approach and resulted in less successful outcomes (Aaronson, Ershoff, & Danaher, 1985). In addition to providing the women with booklets detailing specific strategies to stop smoking, the cessation program educated the women about health risks associated with smoking. The women were asked to call the health center three times a week and listen to taped messages encouraging them to adhere to the information presented in the booklets. At the end of the 8-week program, 28.5% of the women stopped smoking and 71.5% significantly reduced the number of cigarettes smoked from 17 cigarettes per day to 11 cigarettes per day.

Although the percentage of women who stopped smoking following the 8-week program is larger than the percentage of women who were able to stop smoking "on their own" in the study by Cnattingius (1989), the majority of women smokers continued to smoke during pregnancy. In order to decrease the risk of low birth weight and other pregnancy complications in infants of mothers who smoke, it appears that further research is needed to identify effective interventions to help women stop smoking during pregnancy. One program designed to train obstetric and family practice residents in giving smoking-cessation advice involved educating the woman about the adverse effects of smoking on the fetus and provision of a rationale to stop smoking, followed by a commitment from the woman to stop smoking and enrolling in a smoking-cessation program (Secker-Walker et al., 1992). Although the cessation success rates have not been evaluated, 54% of the women in the intervention group, compared to 14% of women in a control group who were advised to stop smoking and given a book on how to do so, agreed to stop smoking.

A study by Sexton and Hobel (1984) attests to the importance and implications of effective anti-smoking campaigns for pregnant women. In their randomized controlled study, a smoking intervention for women during pregnancy resulted in increased smoking-cessation rates and also increased infants' birth weights. Rantakallio (1978) found that women who quit smoking during the third trimester of pregnancy generally give birth to infants who more closely resemble infants of women who don't smoke, compared with women who continue to smoke. Encouraging women to reduce the number of cigarettes they smoke can benefit the unborn child since there is evidence of a dose-response relation between the number of cigarettes smoked and the degree of birth weight reduction (Rantakallio, 1979).

Further investigation that identifies efficacious components of smoking-cessation programs is greatly needed, as simply providing advice and information about the effects of smoking on pregnancy outcomes does not result in success for many women. It is possible that health and clinical psychologists may be able to intervene specifically to help pregnant women, perhaps with cognitive–behavioral techniques or relaxation training to cope with stress and negative emotional states that have been associated with smoking treatment failures (Tunstall, Ginsberg, & Hall, 1985).

Alcohol

As with smoking, alcohol abuse during pregnancy can result in negative outcomes for the neonate and is a significant risk factor. In 1981, the Surgeon General issued an advisory recommending abstinence from alcohol during pregnancy. Prevalence rates of alcohol abuse among pregnant women vary depending on the samples used and how abuse is defined in terms of the amount of alcohol consumed. In one epidemiologic study, Sokol, Miller, and Reed (1980) reported that 1.7% of pregnant women abused alcohol during pregnancy. Plant (1984) reported that 80.5% of 1,008 pregnant women interviewed drank some amount of alcohol within the first 12 weeks of pregnancy.

Many serious consequences are associated with alcohol abuse during pregnancy. Compared with nonalcoholic women, alcoholic women are at increased risk for a number of intrapartum complications such as precipitous delivery, heavy meconium, or placental anomalies, lower birth weights, congenital abnormalities, and giving birth to babies with fetal alcohol syndrome (Barrison & Wright, 1984; Sokol et al., 1980). Because of the risks associated with alcohol abuse during pregnancy, it is essential that health care providers attempt to identify alcohol-dependent women and help them to reduce or eliminate their consumption of alcohol during pregnancy. The use of an easily administered alcohol screening instrument such as the T-ACE (Sokol, Martier, & Ager, 1989) could be helpful in identiying women whose alcohol consumption is sufficient enough to potentially damage the fetus. Even modest reductions in alcohol intake can reduce the risk of negative outcomes to the fetus (Little, Young, Streissguth, & Uhl, 1984; Rosett, Ouellette, Weiner, & Owens, 1978).

Providing the pregnant woman with information about the risks associated with alcohol abuse during pregnancy is the first step in helping the woman reduce her alcohol consumption. There is evidence suggesting that supportive counseling for the woman may also be a means of reducing risk to the fetus or neonate by helping the woman reduce the amount of alcohol she drinks. (Rosett et al., 1978).

For the alcohol-dependent woman, it may be necessary to refer her to a substance abuse treatment program as an adjunct to the prenatal care provided. Jessup and Green (1987) have identified five steps to follow in the process of treating the pregnant alcohol-dependent woman. These include the following: 1) statement of the problem; 2) statement of the indicators of alcohol abuse or dependence; 3) explanation of the possible effects on the fetus and the benefits of abstinence; 4) expression of concern and a willingness to support recovery efforts; and 5) a referral for treatment of the drinking problem. It should be noted that locating alcohol treatment centers that are willing to accept pregnant women into their programs is often difficult. For those programs that do accept pregnant women, the specific needs of pregnant women are frequently not adequately addressed (e.g., nutritional counseling), or program interventions lack sensitivity to gender-related interpersonal group techniques (such as confrontation) that may alienate some women. Ideally, alcohol treatment programs for pregnant women would be part of a comprehensive, multidisciplinary approach to prenatal care which is sensitive to all the needs of the woman. However, resources for these types of programs are not widely available.

Drug Abuse

Illicit drug use, including marijuana, cocaine, amphetamines, and heroin, among pregnant women is associated with a number of adverse pregnancy outcomes. Some of these include preterm delivery, *abruptio placentae*, intrauterine growth retardation, low birth weight, physical anomalies, neurobehavioral and neurophysiological abnormalities, neonatal cerebrovascular accidents, neonatal drug withdrawal symptoms, and an increased risk for respiratory dysfunction, including Sudden Infant Death Syndrome (SIDS) (Bandstra & Burkett, 1991; Fried, 1991; Suguihara & Bancalari, 1991).

Estimates of prevalence rates of illicit drug use vary depending on the location surveyed (e.g., rural, urban, or inner-city areas) and how the information is obtained (e.g., anonymous drug screens at prenatal visits, self-report, or drug testing for exposure in the neonate). In a study examining substance abuse in a sample of pregnant women from rural areas attending the University of Missouri clinics for care (Sloan, Gay, Snyder, & Bales, 1992), 11% of urine samples obtained anonymously tested positive for screened substances which included cocaine, marijuana, amphetamines, barbituates, opiates, phencyclidine, and benzodiazepines (ethanol and nicotine were excluded in the 11%). Specifically, 9.4% of the samples tested positive for marijuana and 0.6% tested positive separately for cocaine, barbituates, or benzodiazepines. Although 11% of the samples tested positive for the illicit substances, only 8.3% reported illicit drug use during pregnancy. The discrepancy between toxicologic evidence and women's self-report of illicit substance use has been found in other studies as well. Christmas et al. (1992) found that only 41% of women testing positive for recent use of alcohol or other drugs admitted to current use.

In comparison to the rates found among pregnant women living in rural areas, Chasnoff, Landress, and Barrett (1990) found higher rates of drug use in women in urbanized Pinellas County, Florida. The overall rate of drug use in these women receiving prenatal care at both public and private hospitals and clinics was 13.3%, with 12% of the anonymous urine screens testing positive for marijuana, 3.4% testing positive for cocaine, and 0.3% for opiates. Other studies examining illicit drug use among lower SES women from inner-city areas have found even higher rates of drug use, ranging from 17% to 27% (Frank et al., 1988; Zuckerman et al., 1989). The possibility that these rates are underestimates of the true prevalence of drug use among women, because of the rapid metabolism of some drugs (e.g., less than one week following recent use for cocaine metabolites), is a source of further concern for prenatal care providers.

Because of the significant number of women using illicit substances during pregnancy and the adverse effects that can result for the mother and the neonate, identifying women in need of intervention for this problem is critical. Although performing routine drug screens in prenatal visits may identify drug-abusing women who do not report their drug use, ethical considerations prevent widespread use of this approach (Colmorgen, Johnson, Zazzarino, & Durinzi, 1992). Drug screening without informed consent in pregnant women is not only illegal, but may also deter some women from engaging in the critical prenatal care that they need (Chavkin, Allen, & Oberman, 1991). Recently there has been significant discussion regarding fetal and maternal rights and prenatal care provider responsibilities for drug-abusing women (Chavkin et al., 1991; Finnegan, 1991; Horowitz, 1991). This controversial topic involves many issues too broad to cover in detail in this chapter, but includes questions regarding the duty of care providers to disclose a women's substance abuse that may be putting the health of her fetus at risk, whether statutes concerning "child" abuse extend to the fetus, and a woman's right to refuse treatment vs. court-ordered treatment. Because of the unresolved nature of these issues in state legislatures, relying on routine drug screens to detect substance abuse in pregnant women is not a viable method to ascertain drug abuse as a risk factor, especially for women who do not give consent. Instead, obtain a detailed description of the woman's lifestyle that may put her at risk for substance abuse—e.g., having a partner who abuses drugs (Bresnahan, Zuckerman, & Cabral, 1992) or having a history of drug use or a combination of no prenatal care and cigarette use (McCalla, Minkoff, Feldman, Glass, & Valencia, 1992)—and develop a nonjudgmental, supportive relationship in which she does not fear punishment for her problem. This may lead to identification of drug use.

Following identification of illicit substance abuse in a pregnant woman, a multidisciplinary approach to prenatal care may be the most promising and beneficial. As with alcohol treatment centers, programs sensitive to the specific needs of pregnant women are insufficient in number and inadequate in structure. Ideally, comprehensive services that include professionals specifically trained in high-risk pregnancy and substance abuse are needed to provide treatment for these women. Finnegan (1991) has outlined a detailed model of treatment for drug dependence in pregnancy that includes the following components from a variety of disciplines: comprehensive prenatal care, HIV counseling and testing, nutritional counseling, prenatal testing, psychiatric evaluation, drug abuse treatment, life-skills management (e.g., problem solving, coping mechanisms, social skills training, and cognitive restructuring), survival management (e.g., provision of housing, clothing, food, and vocational assistance), and community liaisons (e.g., indigenous workers that might provide transportation to doctor appointments or distribute prevention and educational material).

Although these services may be made available to drug-abusing women, compliance and follow through is a separate consideration. Poland, Giblin, Waller, and Bayer (1991) found that low-income women cited the following reasons for missing prenatal appointments: no transportation (19%); prenatal care not seen as important (14%); no insurance (12%); and lack of child-care services (9%). Making services accessible and convenient for the woman may help to increase compliance with the specialized prenatal care these women need. Provision of transportation and child-care services is becoming more widely incorporated as a means to get women to their appointments.

In summary, it is very important for health care providers to encourage and assist the woman to initiate and maintain positive health behaviors during pregnancy. Adherence to guidelines regarding nutrition, exercise, and eliminating the woman's exposure to substances such as tobacco, alcohol, and other drugs is important in reducing the risk of negative outcomes. Particular emphasis should be put on the use of multidisciplinary approaches in helping the high-risk pregnant woman initiate and maintain good health habits during pregnancy.

IMPLICATIONS FOR CLINICAL CARE

The psychological aspects associated with high-risk pregnancy that have been discussed in this chapter have important implications for clinical care. First of all, thorough assessment of risk factors (i.e., genetic, medical, psychosocial, and health behaviors) early in pregnancy is very important. Although risk assessment should always be conducted at the first prenatal visit, continuous monitoring for changes in risk status should occur throughout the nine months of pregnancy.

As has been discussed previously, increased levels of stress or anxiety experienced by the woman while she is pregnant has been associated with complications occurring during pregnancy, labor, and delivery. Assessment of the source and level of the woman's distress should be conducted to evaluate whether a referral for specialized interventions is appropriate. Because the use of psychotropic medications to treat clinical depression, anxiety, or other psychiatric disorders may put the infant at even greater risk, psychologists may be able to provide psychological interventions (e.g., relaxation training, cognitive–behavioral techniques) to help alleviate the emotional distress the woman may be experiencing and provide her with adaptive coping skills.

For women who have been identified as having a high-risk pregnancy the same approach may be used for non–substance-abusing reasons. Clinical care workers should be aware of the possible psychological reactions (e.g., anxiety, depression, guilt, anger, fear) that may develop in the woman. Interventions, such as support groups or individual counseling, may be appropriate to help reduce the anxiety, depression, anger, guilt, or fear the high-risk woman may feel throughout the pregnancy and during diagnostic evaluations and other special prenatal care. Current research efforts continue to address the differences between low- and high-risk women with respect to these emotional states during pregnancy so that persons involved in the prenatal care of the high-risk woman will be better able to understand and deal effectively with the feelings she may be experiencing.

Finally, the importance of educating and assisting pregnant women to initiate good health behaviors is critically important to efforts aimed at reducing risk to the mother and neonate. A combination of education, support, and the use of specialized interventions for serious abuse or dependence on nicotine, alcohol, and illicit drugs should be used to help decrease adverse outcomes associated with poor health behaviors during pregnancy.

SUMMARY

In sum, there is a growing body of literature supporting an integrated, biopsychosocial model in high-risk pregnancy. The interaction between biomedical, psychological, and sociobehavioral risk factors during pregnancy should be emphasized and attended to in the assessment of risk. Additional research is needed to investigate the interaction of these factors so that assessment procedures and interventions can be designed to reduce the likelihood of negative outcomes in high-risk pregnancies. Obstetricians, perinatologists, nurses, health and clinical psychologists, social workers, and counselors may be able to reduce the probability of negative outcomes to the neonate in high-risk pregnancies by implementing appropriate medical procedures, education, support, and psychological interventions.

REFERENCES

Aaronson, N. K., Ershoff, D. H., & Danaher, B. G. (1985). Smoking cessation in pregnancy: A self-help approach. *Addictive Behaviors, 10*, 103–108.

Abel, E. L. (1984). Smoking and pregnancy. *Journal of Psychoactive Drugs, 16*, 327–338.

Adams, E., Gfroerer, J. C., & Rouse, B. A. (1989). Epidemiology of substance abuse including alcohol and cigarette smoking. *Annals of the New York Academy of Sciences, 562*, 14–20.

Aubry, R. H., & Pennington, J. C. (1973). Identification and evaluation of high-risk pregnancy: The perinatal concept. *Clinical Obstetrics and Gynecology, 16*, 3–27.

Aumann, G.M.E., & Baird, M. M. (1986). Screening for the high-risk pregnancy. In R. A. Knuppel, & J. E. Drukker (Eds.), *High-risk pregnancy: A team approach* (pp. 3–23). Philadelphia: W. B. Saunders.

Bandstra, E. S., & Burkett, G. (1991). Maternal-fetal and neonatal effects of in utero cocaine exposure. *Seminars in Perinatology, 15*, 288–301.

Barrison, I. G., & Wright, J. T. (1984). Moderate drinking during pregnancy and foetal outcome. *Alcohol and Alcoholism, 19*, 167–172.

Blackburn, S. T. (1986). Assessment of risk: Perinatal, family, and environmental perspectives. *Physical and Occupational Therapy in Pediatrics, 6*, 105–120.

Bresnahan, K., Zuckerman, B., & Cabral, H. (1992). Psychosocial correlates of drug and heavy alcohol use among pregnant women at risk for drug use. *Obstetrics and Gynecology, 80*, 976–980.

Brown, G. W., Sklair, F., Harris, T. O., & Birley, J. L. (1973). Life-events and psychiatric disorders: Part 1: Some methodological issues. *Psychological Medicine, 3*, 74–87.

Calloway, P., & Dolan, R. (1989). Endocrine changes and clinical profiles in depression. In G. W. Brown, & T. O. Harris (Eds.), *Life events and illness* (pp.139–160). New York: Guilford Press.

Chasnoff, I. J., Landress, H. J., & Barrett, M. E. (1990). The prevalence of illicit-drug or alcohol use during pregnancy and discrepancies in mandatory reporting in Pinellas County, Florida. *New England Journal of Medicine, 322*, 1202–1206.

Chavkin, W., Allen, M. H., & Oberman, M. (1991). Drug abuse and pregnancy: Some questions on public policy, clinical management, and maternal and fetal rights. *Birth, 18*, 107–112.

Christmas, J. T., Knisely, J. S., Dawson, K. S., Dinsmoor, M. J., Weber, S. E., & Schnoll, S. H. (1992). Comparison of questionnaire screening and urine toxicology for detection of pregnancy complicated by substance abuse. *Obstetrics and Gynecology, 80*, 750–754.

Cnattingius, S. (1989). Smoking habits in early pregnancy. *Addictive Behaviors, 14*, 453–457.

Colmorgen, G.H.C., Johnson, C., Zazzarino, M. A., & Durinzi, K. (1992). Routine urine drug screening at the first prenatal visit. *American Journal of Obstetrics and Gynecology, 166,* 588–590.

Danaher, B. G., Shisslak, C. M., Thompson, C. B., & Ford, J. D. (1978). A smoking cessation program for pregnant women: An exploratory study. *American Journal of Public Health, 68,* 896–898.

Davids, A., & DeVault, S. (1962). Maternal anxiety during pregnancy and childbirth abnormalities. *Psychosomatic Medicine, 24,* 464–470.

Elliott, S. A., Rugg, A. J., Watson, J. P., & Brough, D. I. (1983). Mood changes during pregnancy and after the birth of a child. *British Journal of Clinical Psychology, 22,* 295–308.

Finnegan, L. P. (1991). Perinatal substance abuse: Comments and perspectives. *Seminars in Perinatology, 15,* 331–339.

Frank, D. A., Zuckerman, B. S., Amaro, H., Aboagye, K., Bauchner, H., Cabral, H., Fried, L., Hingson, R., Kayne, H., Levenson, S. M., Parker, S., Reece, H., & Vinci, R. (1988). Cocaine use during pregnancy: Prevalence and correlates. *Pediatrics, 82,* 888–895.

Freeman, R. K., & Pescar, S. C. (1982). *Safe delivery: Protecting your baby during high risk pregnancy.* New York: Facts on File.

Fried, P. A. (1991). Marijuana use during pregnancy: Consequences for the offspring. *Seminars in Perinatology, 15,* 280–287.

Goodwin, J. W., Dunne, J. T., & Thomas, B. W. (1969). Antepartum assessment of the fetus at risk. *Canadian Medical Association Journal, 101,* 57.

Hickner, J., Westenberg, C., & Dittenbir, M. (1984). Effect of pregnancy on smoking behavior: A baseline study. *Journal of Family Practice, 18,* 241–244.

Hobel, C. J., Youkeles, L., & Forsythe, A. (1979). Prenatal and intrapartum high-risk screening: Risk factors assessed. *American Journal of Obstetrics and Gynecology, 135,* 1051–1056.

Horowitz, R. M. (1991). Drug use in pregnancy: To test, to tell—legal implications for the physician. *Seminars in Perinatology, 15,* 324–330.

Istvan, J. (1986). Stress, anxiety, and birth outcomes: A critical review of the evidence. *Psychological Bulletin, 100,* 331–348.

Jessup, M., & Green, J. R. (1987). Treatment of the pregnant alcohol-dependent woman. *Journal of Psychoactive Drugs, 19,* 193–203.

Johnson, T. M., & Murphy, J. M. (1986). Psychosocial implications of high-risk pregnancy. In R. A. Knuppel, & J. E. Drukker (Eds.), *High-risk pregnancy: A team approach* (pp. 173–186). Philadelphia: W. B. Saunders.

Kabela, E., & Andrasik, F. (1988). Behavioral and biochemical effects of gradual reductions in cigarette yields in pregnant and nonpregnant smokers. *Addictive Behavior, 13,* 231–243.

Kemp, V. H., & Page, C. (1987). Maternal self-esteem and prenatal attachment in high-risk pregnancy. *Maternal–Child Nursing Journal, 16,* 195–206.

Kemp, V. H., & Pond, E. F. (1986). Health assessment in high-risk pregnancies. *Family and Community Health, 8,* 10–17.

Khalsa, J. H., & Gfroerer, J. (1991). Epidemiology and health consequences of drug abuse among pregnant women. *Seminars in Perinatology, 15,* 265–270.

Knox, A. J., Sadler, L., Pattison, N. S., Mantell, C. D., & Mullins, P. (1993). An obstetric scoring system: Its development and application in obstetric management. *Obstetrics and Gynecology, 81*, 195–199.

Leifer, M. (1980). *Psychological effects of motherhood: A study of first pregnancy*. New York: Praeger.

Levin, J. S., & DeFrank, R. S. (1988). Maternal stress and pregnancy outcomes: A review of the psychosocial literature. *Journal of Psychosomatics, Obstetrics, and Gynaecology, 9*, 3–16.

Little, R. E., Young, A., Streissguth, A. P., & Uhl, C. N. (1984). Preventing fetal alcohol effects: Effectiveness of a demonstration project. In R. Porter, M. O'Connor, & J. Whelan (Eds.), *Mechanisms of alcohol damage in utero* (pp. 254–274). London: Pittman.

Luoto, J. (1983). Reducing the health consequences of smoking: A progress report. *Public Health Report, 98*, 34–39.

McCalla, S., Minkoff, H. L., Feldman, J., Glass, L., & Valencia, G. (1992). Predictors of cocaine use in pregnancy. *Obstetrics and Gynecology, 79*, 641–644.

Mercer, R. T., & Ferketich, S. L. (1988). Stress and social support as predictors of anxiety and depression during pregnancy. *Advances in Nursing Science, 10*, 26–39.

Myers, R. E. (1977). Production of fetal asphyxia by maternal psychological stress. *Pavlovian Journal of Biological Science, 12*, 51–62.

Myers, R. E., & Myers, S. E. (1979). Use of sedative, analgesic, and anesthetic drugs during labor and delivery. Bane or boon? *American Journal of Obstetrics and Gynecology, 133*, 83–104.

Nesibitt, R. E., & Aubry, R. H. (1969). High-risk obstetrics: II. Value of semiobjective grading system on identifying the vulnerable group. *American Journal of Obstetrics and Gynecology, 103*, 972–985.

Newton, R. W., & Hunt, L. P. (1984). Psychosocial stress in pregnancy and its relation to low birth weight. *British Medical Journal, 288*, 1191–1194.

Norbeck, J. S., & Tilden, V. P. (1983). Life stress, social support, and emotional disequilibrium in complications of pregnancy: A prospective, multivariate study. *Journal of Health and Social Behavior, 24*, 30–46.

Pagel, M. D., Smilkstein, G., Regen, H., & Montano, D. (1990). Psychosocial influences on new born outcomes: A controlled prospective study. *Social Science Medicine, 30*, 597–604.

Penticuff, J. H. (1982). Psychological implications in high-risk pregnancy. *Nursing Clinics of North America, 17*, 69–78.

Phipps, S., & Zinn, A. B. (1986). Psychological response to amniocentesis: I. Mood state and adaptation to pregnancy. *American Journal of Medical Genetics, 25*, 131–142.

Plant, M. L. (1984). Drinking amongst pregnant women: Some initial results from a prospective study. *Alcohol and Alcoholism, 19*, 153–157.

Poland, M. L., Giblin, P. T., Waller, J. B., & Bayer, I. S. (1991). Development of a paraprofessional home visiting program for low-income mothers and infants. *American Journal of Preventive Medicine, 7*, 204–207.

Queenan, J. T. (Ed.) (1985). *Management of high-risk pregnancy*. Oradell, NJ: Medical Economics Company.

Radloff, L. (1977). The CES-D scale: A self-report depression scale for research in the general population. *Journal of Applied Psychological Measurement, 1*, 385–401.

Rantakallio, P. (1978). Relationship of maternal smoking to morbidity and mortality of the child up to the age of five. *Acta Paediatrica Scandinavica, 67*, 621–631.

Rantakallio, P. (1979). Social background of mothers who smoke during pregnancy and influence of these factors on offspring. *Social Science and Medicine, 13A*, 423–449.

Reeb, K. G., Graham, A. V., Zyzanski, S. J., & Kitson, G. C. (1987). Predicting low birth weight and complicated labor in urban black women: A biopsychosocial perspective. *Social Science Medicine, 25*, 1321–1327.

Rosett, H. L., Ouellette, E. M., Weiner, L., & Owens, E. (1978). Therapy of heavy drinking during pregnancy. *Obstetrics and Gynecology, 51*, 41–46.

Secker-Walker, R. H., Solomon, L. J., Flynn, B. S., LePage, S. S., Crammond, J. E., Worden, J. K., & Mead, P. B. (1992). Training obstetric and family practice residents to give smoking cessation advice during prenatal care. *American Journal of Obstetrics and Gynecology, 166*, 1356–1363.

Selby, J. W. (1980). Psychological changes in pregnancy. In J. W. Selby, L. G. Calhoun, A. V. Vogel, & E. King (Eds.), *Psychology and human reproduction.* (pp. 3–36). New York: Free Press.

Selye, H. (1976). *Stress in health and disease.* Boston: Butterworths.

Sexton, M., & Hobel, R. (1984). A clinical trial of change in maternal smoking and its effects on birthweight. *Journal of the American Mecical Association, 251*, 911–915.

Sloan, L. B., Gay, J. W., Snyder, S. W., & Bales, W. R. (1992). Substance abuse during pregnancy in a rural population. *Obstetrics and Gynecology, 79*, 245–248.

Sokol, R. J., Martier, S. S., & Ager, J. W. (1989). The T-ACE questions: Practical prenatal detection of risk-drinking. *American Journal of Obstetrics and Gynecology, 160*, 863–870.

Sokol, R. J., Miller, S. I., & Reed, G. (1980). Alcohol abuse during pregnancy: An epidemiologic study. *Alcoholism: Clinical and Experimental Research, 4*, 135–145.

Suguihara, C., & Bancalari, E. (1991). Substance abuse during pregnancy: Effects on respiratory function in the infant. *Seminars in Perinatology, 15*, 302–309.

Tunis, S. L., & Golbus, M. S. (1991). Assessing mood states in pregnancy: Survey of the literature. *Obstetrical and Gynecological Survey, 46*, 340–345.

Tunstall, C. D., Ginsberg, D., & Hall, S. M. (1985). Quitting smoking. *International Journal of the Addictions, 20*, 1089–1112.

Williamson, H. A., LeFevre, M., & Hector, M. (1989). Association between life stress and serious perinatal complications. *Journal of Family Practice, 29*, 489–496.

Wohlreich, M. M. (1986). Psychiatric aspects of high-risk pregnancy. *Psychiatric Clinics of North America, 10*, 53–68.

Zuckerman, B. S., Frank, D. A., Hingson, R., Amaro, H., Levenson, S. M., Kayne, H., Parker, S., Vinci, R., Aboagye, K., Fried, L. E., Cabral, H., Timper, R., & Bauchner, H. (1989). Effects of maternal marijuana and cocaine use on fetal growth. *New England Journal of Medicine, 320*, 762–768.

15

Adolescent Pregnancy

Robin M. MacFarlane

Pregnancy is an important part of womens' lives both physically and psychologically. Adolescents who become pregnant present their own set of physical, psychological, and sociological considerations. Although there is consensus that adolescent pregnancy involves great cost to society and some degree of risk to young women's well-being, there is widespread disagreement regarding the most appropriate way to manage this problem. Many attempts to prevent early pregnancy, counsel pregnant adolescents, and provide assistance to adolescent mothers have been thwarted by political and religious groups that may be well-meaning but are often misinformed. Educators, family planning counselors, and other professionals dealing with adolescent health care must be familiar with research that will enable them to provide sound information and guidance to help adolescents make informed decisions.

The problems of adolescent pregnancy and childbearing are intimately related to the timing, sequence, and circumstances surrounding adolescents' decisions about sexual behavior, as well as society's ability to adapt to the needs of adolescents (Hayes, 1987). A young woman must decide whether to begin having intercourse, whether to use contraception, and whether to use contraception consistently. If a pregnancy occurs, she must confirm the pregnancy, and then decide whether to deliver or seek an abortion. If she chooses to deliver, she must decide whether to raise the child alone or within her family of origin, or to give up the child for adoption. If an adolescent chooses to raise the child, she is then confronted with the task of parenthood. This chapter will review some of the

248

research bearing on societal and psychological factors that influence adolescents' decisions at each of these junctures.

FACTORS ASSOCIATED WITH THE INCIDENCE OF ADOLESCENT PREGNANCY

Sociocultural Factors

Since 1970, adolescent birthrates have declined in the United States and in virtually all other industrialized countries (Alan Guttmacher Institute, 1981; 1988). However, the proportional rate of adolescent births remains highest in the United States. Among girls younger than 15, the birthrate is five times higher in the United States than in all other developed countries for which data are available (Alan Guttmacher Institute, 1981; 1988; Hayes, 1987). Jones (1986) and other investigators from the Alan Guttmacher Institute (1981; 1988) sought to uncover the reasons underlying the differential birthrates of the United States and other countries. In a collaborative cross-cultural study, investigators compared the United States with Canada, England, France, The Netherlands, and Sweden across several variables thought to influence the rate of adolescent pregnancy, most notably, racial heterogeneity, rate of abortion, incidence of sexual activity, general economic conditions, societal attitude toward sexuality, and contraceptive availability and use (Jones, 1986). The results give useful clues about the sociocultural determinants of adolescent pregnancy.

First, the United States is more racially heterogenous than most other countries, and the rate of pregnancy in minority groups aged 15 to 19 (19%) is higher than the rate among white adolescents of the same age (9%) (Dryfoos, 1982). However, when American minorities were excluded from Jones' (1986) analysis, the adolescent birth rate in the United States was still proportionally higher than in every other country. Therefore, high adolescent pregnancy rates in the United States cannot be accounted for only by racial heterogeneity. Second, the proportion of pregnant American teenagers who had abortions in 1981 (about 45%) was similar to the modal proportion for countries other than the U.S. (about 43%), indicating that abortion was not more common in other countries, and could not account for their lower birth rates. Third, it was found that American teenagers did not initiate sexual activity at an earlier age than did foreign teenagers, and that American teenagers were no more sexually active than teenagers in other countries. Taken together, these data indicate that the higher incidence of adolescent births in the United States may be partially accounted for by race, but cannot be accounted for by rate of abortion, or rate of sexual activity among American youth (Jones, 1986).

One difference between the United States and the comparison countries is the amount of poverty. It is generally believed that the poverty existing in America is essentially unknown in Canada and in Western Europe. Therefore, the relatively high rate of poverty in the United States may play a role in perpetuating adolescent pregnancy (Jones, 1986).

Another difference between the United States and the comparison countries is the societal attitude toward adolescent sexuality and contraception. The general American attitude is that sex among teenagers can be romantic, but at the same time, it is sinful, dirty, and not an acceptable part of adolescent life (Adler, Katz, & Jackson, 1985). In contrast, the European attitude is less ambivalent and condemning, and tends to be more "matter of fact" about sex among the young. For example, of the countries in the collaborative study, only the United States had developed government-sponsored programs designed to discourage adolescents from becoming sexually active. Contraceptives, particularly oral contraceptives, were notably more available in foreign countries. In all countries studied except the United States, teenagers reported having easy access to family planning clinics. Furthermore, adolescents who were given contraceptives did not have to obtain parental consent, were assured of confidentiality, and often were not charged a fee. Recent reports of contraceptive availability in Sweden (Wallace & Veinonen, 1989) and Finland (Sirpa, 1989) are consistent with results reported in the collaborative study. It is noteworthy that countries in which contraceptives were easily available did not have a higher rate of adolescent sexual activity than the United States. Other studies corroborate the notion that higher availabilty of contraceptives is not associated with higher rates of adolescent sexual activity (Furstenberg & Brooks-Gunn, 1985; Hayes, 1987; Jones, 1986; Kirby, 1984; Zabin, Hirsch, Smith, Street, & Hardy, 1986; Zelnik & Kim, 1982).

Psychological Factors

Although sociocultural factors are important correlates of adolescent pregnancy, it is undeniable that many young women are exposed to similar sociocultural environments and do not become pregnant. Psychological and attitudinal factors also are implicated.

Studies suggest that pregnant adolescents differ from nonpregnant adolescents in that they have lower educational motivation (Furstenberg, 1976) and they tend to be more impulsive and act-out more often (Coddington, 1979; Hart & Hilton, 1988; Meyerowitz & Malev, 1973). Although these differences exist, they are not strong predictors of adolescent pregnancy. Pregnant adolescents, when compared with control groups of nonpregnant peers, show almost no psychological differences (Quay, 1981; Troutman, 1988). It is likely that pregnant adolescents are too heterogenous to show predictable differences when compared with nonpregnant adolescents. Therefore, it may be useful to delineate subgroups of pregnant adolescents that are somewhat psychologically or attitudinally homogenous (Quay, 1981; Rosen, Campbell, & Arima, 1961; Semmens & Lammers, 1968). Delineation of subgroups manifesting meaningful psychological homogeneity could have implications for preventive interventions that would target specific groups.

One of the more clinically relevant classifications was proposed by Semmens and Lammers (1968). Adolescents' stated and inferred reasons for becoming pregnant were compiled into three categories: intentional, accidental, and uniformed (or misinformed). This classification seems quite useful because counseling sexually active adolescents often involves discussing the underlying reasons for having sex, identifying the extent to which the adolescent is willing to use contraceptives and, in some cases, identifying reasons for wishing to become pregnant (Greydanus, 1983).

Adolescents who report that they intended to become pregnant may have several motives (Phoenix, 1989; Semmens & Lammers, 1968). Quay (1981) described two subtypes of adolescents who intend to conceive. The first subtype tends to be influenced by a culture that accepts and may even reward early pregnancy. In interviews with African-American adolescent mothers in a poor section of the Washington, D.C., area, Dash (1989) found that their pregnancies were almost always intended and desired. In this group, early pregnancies were common, and were often modeled by mothers, aunts, and peers (Dash, 1989; Moore & Erickson, 1985). The second subtype of adolescents intending to conceive are often motivated to gain respect as an adult, to have someone to nurture and love, or to manipulate others, such as a boyfriend (Quay, 1981). Of this group, "intentional" does not necessarily mean "desired" (Kriepe, 1983). What may, in fact, be desired is maturity or love, and pregnancy is viewed (consciously or unconsciously) as a means to that end (Kriepe, 1983).

Although intentional adolescent pregnancies undoubtedly exist, the issue of intendedness is methodologically complicated, because reports of intentionality are usually collected after the pregnancy has occurred (Hayes, 1987). An unintended, unwanted conception may be increasingly perceived as "desired" and "intended" as the pregnancy continues (Hayes, 1987). It is likely that such an attribution is commonly made among adolescents who choose to deliver and parent their infants, because even though an adolescent may not have wanted to conceive, continuing to believe that a pregnancy was not intended may imply that the child is not desired (Kriepe, 1983).

The second and most common category of pregnant adolescents is composed of those who report that their pregnancy was accidental (Phoenix, 1989; Semmens & Lammers, 1968). According to Semmens and Lammers (1968), adolescents who accidentally conceive understand the proper way to contracept, but use contraception haphazardly or take risks and do not use contraception at all. True contraceptive failure accounts for a very small proportion of accidental pregnancy (Kriepe, 1983).

In the third category of pregnant adolescents—those who are considered to be uninformed (or misinformed)—pregnancy is thought to have been avoidable if proper contraceptive information had been provided. Research from other developed countries shows that even young sexually active teenagers can successfully avoid pregnancy if they are given appropriate information rather than being expected to seek information on their own (Jones, 1986; Sirpa, 1989; Wallace & Veinonen, 1989). If adolescents lack accurate information, they cannot be expected to use contraception reliably. Futhermore, even among adolescents who are somewhat knowledgeable, the extent of their sophistication may not be substantial. Adolescents are not often likely to question the extent of their knowledge, and are more likely to act on their subjective (and innaccurate) beliefs about the probability of becoming pregnant rather than seek appropriate information (Morrison, 1985; Philliber, Namerow, Kaye, & Kunkes, 1986). Most adolescents, even those who are fairly sophisticated, may benefit from appropriate information about contraception.

Implications for Prevention

Several findings from the cross-cultural study and from the studies of psychological factors have implications for the prevention of adolescent pregnancy, but most factors, such as American poverty, are not realistically changeable. However, two direct and readily implimented changes are recommended: more extensive education about sexuality and contraception, and an increase in the ease with which adolesents can obtain contraception (Hayes, 1987; Jones, 1986; Sirpa, 1989; Wallace & Veinonen, 1989). In addition, programs designed to enhance adolescents' life options may give young women the incentive to delay pregnancy (Dryfoos, 1983).

Programs designed to provide education about sexuality and contraception not only provide information, but also provide a basis for adolescents to reflect more intelligently on their attitudes toward sexuality (Hayes, 1987). For example, many adolescents delay the use of contraception for about six months after they begin having intercourse, either because they do not have accurate knowledge about reproduction or contraception, or because they cannot accept that they are engaging in something they have been taught was "wrong" (Zelnik, Kantner, & Ford, 1981). Educational interventions might ameliorate these circumstances. A careful study of a comprehensive school-based program in Baltimore showed that providing education about sexuality and contraception was associated with postponement of first intercourse and higher contraceptive use (Zabin et al., 1986). This finding is corroborated by studies indicating that adolescents who have had sex education are no more likely, and sometimes even less likely, to initiate sexual activity than those adolescents who have not had sex education (Furstenberg & Brooks-Gunn, 1985; Jones, 1986; Kirby, 1984; Zelnik & Kim, 1982).

Three types of community-based programs in the United States have been designed to increase contraceptive availability (Dryfoos, 1983; Hayes, 1987). First, family planning clinics provide reasonably priced contraceptives, among other services. It has been found that clinics are used more frequently if they advertise and provide outreach services, such as community education programs (Hofferth, 1987b). Second, school-based clinics, like family planning clinics, are not explicitly designed to provide contraception, although they do offer those services, along with sex education. Third, condom-distribution programs, usually arranged by family planning providers and public health organizations, choose locations ranging from emergency rooms to video arcades, and simply make condoms available (Hayes, 1987). These programs are often targeted toward young men. Although it is difficult to control for extraneous variables in community studies, some evidence suggests that condom-distribution programs may be associated with more condom use and lower adolescent birth rates in targeted areas (Dryfoos, 1985). It deserves restating that there is no evidence suggesting that heightened contraceptive availability increases adolescent sexual activity.

Programs that enhance life options have been designed to target psychological factors that may aid in the prevention of adolescent pregnancy (Dryfoos, 1983). These programs are based on the assumption that some adolescent pregnancies can be prevented if young women are instilled with a sense of self-worth and can understand the value of delaying motherhood in order to obtain educational and career opportunities (Hayes, 1987). Examples of these programs are role model and mentoring programs, programs to improve school performance, and youth employment programs (Dryfoos, 1983). Theoretically, these programs seem useful in preventing adolescent pregnancy, but studies have not been conducted to evaluate their efficacy.

DETERMINANTS OF CHILDBEARING: A SEQUENCE OF DECISIONS

Should a young woman conceive, her response to the pregnancy is influenced by the sociocultural and psychological factors discussed previously. An adolescent must somehow weigh and consider those factors and decide the outcome of her pregnancy. Understandably, pregnant adolescents are apt to have significant difficulty with this process. The role of the professional is to provide nonjudgmental, objective information about the options available to pregnant young women. It is also important for professionals to be knowledgeable about factors that may influence a pregnant adolescent's decision regarding the outcome of her pregnancy, and about the potential consequences of her choice. Psychological aspects of the decisions pregnant adolescents must make about abortion, delivery, adoption, and marriage will be discussed in this section. In the section to follow, the sequelae of adolescent motherhood will be discussed.

The Abortion–Delivery Decision

Research suggests that a number of factors affect the decision to terminate pregnancy by abortion. First, younger adolescents are more likely than older adolescents to have abortions. In 1977, 53% of pregnant adolescents age 14 and younger chose to have abortions, whereas 37% of those age 15 and older chose to do so (Olson, 1980). Second, adolescents of high socioeconomic status choose abortion more often than did adolescents of lower socioeconomic status (Zelnick, Kantner, & Ford, 1981). Third, adolescents who choose to have abortions tend to be more academically oriented and show better school performance (Devaney & Hubley, 1981).

In a study designed to determine psychological and social factors that influence the abortion–delivery decision, Klerman, Bracken, Jekel, and Bracken (1982) controlled for demographic variables by matching adolescents on marital status, race, age, welfare status, and previous pregnancies. It was found that the psychosocial variables most likely to be associated with the decision to deliver were desire for the child, haphazard contraceptive use, longer delay before confirming the pregnancy, longer and more serious relationship with the male partner, presence of role models who are (or were) adolescent parents, and religiosity. Perhaps more important, of the adolescents who had been pregnant once before and had delivered, half had chosen to have abortions to end their current pregnancy. Similarly, half of the adolescents who had previously had abortions had chosen to deliver. These findings suggest that the decision about pregnancy outcome is largely related to factors surrounding the current pregnancy rather than to stable personality characteristics.

This interpretation is supported by the general inability of studies to find a consistent personality pattern distinguishing those adolescents who have abortions from those who deliver (Olson, 1980). What is consistently found is that about half of pregnant adolescents are very ambivalent and changeable about their decision to abort or deliver (Klerman, Bracken, Jekel, & Bracken, 1982; Rosen, 1980; Weinman, Robinson, Simmons, Schrieber, & Stafford, 1989). In Bracken and colleagues' (1982) study, about half the women who, at one point, had made a decision either to abort or to deliver had changed their minds before following through with the original decision. This ambivalence about the outcome of pregnancy may lead to delayed decisions and may help to explain the high rate of second-trimester abortions among adolescents (Burr & Schultz, 1980). Delay in obtaining abortion also may be due to the difficulty anticipated by those adolescents who are reluctant to discuss this issue with their parents in order to attain legal consent (Crosby & English, 1991; Greydanus, 1983).

To aid the decision-making process, most adolescents rely on their parents. Rosen (1980) surveyed 432 pregnant adolescents about their parents' contribution to the decision to have an abortion, deliver, or give up the infant for adoption. When they first found out they were pregnant, few adolescents sought advice from parents. When seeking medical confirmation of the pregnancy, 23% of the adolescents consulted their parents. After they were sure they were pregnant, 57% of the adolescents came to a decision about the pregnancy after consulting their parents, usually their mothers. Rosen found that young women who were certain about the "right" decision were unlikely to consult their parents, and if their parents did advise them, they were unlikely to consider their parents' advice if the proposed solution was not the same one they had chosen. Adolescents who felt undecided about the outcome of their pregnancy, or incompetent to do something about it, were more likely to ask their parents' advice and be influenced by them. These findings suggest that although all adolescents may benefit from objective information from a counselor, about half of them are very unsure about what to do and rely heavily on family members to help them make their decisions. In such cases, if both the young woman and her parents are willing, it may be of some benefit if the counselor would also provide the parents with objective information so that they may make a more informed decision along with their daughter.

Studies of psychological sequelae of abortion in adult women generally suggest that the most common reaction is one of relief, and that negative feelings of guilt or loss, if they occur, are transient (Olson, 1980). Although few studies of the psychological impact of abortion have been conducted with adolescents, these studies indicate that younger age is associated with more negative feelings after abortion (Adler & Dolcini, 1986; Campbell, Franco, & Jurs, 1988). However, the magnitude of this association is not very great (Adler & Dolcini, 1986). A factor that may contribute to adolescents' more negative response is that they are more likely than adult women to delay their decision and therefore must contend with second-trimester abortions (Adler & Dolcini, 1986; Hayes, 1987). Preabortion screening is necessary to identify adolescents who may be reluctant to make a timely decision, or who have psychiatric histories and may be more likely to experience extreme distress (Olson, 1980). Virtually all abortion clinics offer postabortion counseling in addition to standard preabortion counseling (Hayes, 1987).

Physiological Risks of Adolescent Pregnancy and Childbirth

In general, the less well developed an adolescent is gynecologically, the higher her risk of pregnancy complications and poor birth outcome (Hollingsworth,

Kotchen, & Felice, 1983). Adolescents further heighten their risk of pregnancy complications because they are more likely than adults to have poor eating habits (Jacobson & Heald, 1983), use substances that may harm the fetus (Hollingsworth, Kotchen, & Felice, 1983; Pletsch, 1988) and seek prenatal care late in pregnancy (Gunter & LaBarba, 1981; Young, McMahon, & Bowman, 1990). Several studies document that adolescents who are unaware of or are unconcerned about the risks associated with pregnancy are less likely to keep regular clinic appointments (Kinsman & Slap, 1992; Wells, McDiarmid, & Bayatpour, 1990; Young, McMahon, Bowman, & Thompson, 1989) and are also more likely to use alcohol and drugs (Lohr, Gillmore, Gilchrist, & Butler, 1992) during the prenatal period. If professionals working with pregnant adolescents carefully assess their patients' knowledge about the risks of pregnancy and attitudes toward prenantal care, they may then be able to identify those cases that may benefit from more extensive guidance, for example, involvement of social services, that may help increase compliance with health care regimens.

The Adoption–Motherhood Decision

In 1976 and in 1985, it was found that about 95% of adolescents who delivered kept their infants (Alan Guttmacher Institute, 1981; 1988). The rarity of adoption is striking when considering that, prior to the late 1960s, 90% of unwed adolescents relinquished their infants to adoption (Greer, 1982). It is likely that greater societal acceptance of single motherhood has influenced most adolescents who deliver to keep their infants. Adolescents who have no role models who are (or were) adolescent parents, and have mothers who oppose abortion, tend to relinquish their infants to adoption more often (Herr, 1989). Many adolescents who decide upon adoption early in their pregnancies change their minds shortly before or after delivery (Weinman et al., 1989). This finding underscores the ambivalence young women feel while making this decision.

Greer (1982) has stated that many who counsel pregnant adolescents assume that, unless an adolescent has an abortion, she will keep the child. Those who counsel pregnant adolescents should not make this assumption, and should present adoption as a realistic and responsible alternative to early parenthood.

Adolescent Marriage

Adolescent marriage is rare; approximately 8% of women younger than 19 are married, and only 2% of women marry between the ages of 15–17 (Alan Guttmacher Institute, 1981). Most adolescents who marry do so in order to legitimize a pregnancy (Hayes, 1987). Rates of adolescent marriage have declined since the late 1960s, when Furstenberg reported that 25% of a sample of 300 pregnant adolescents were married prior to delivery (Furstenberg, 1976). In general, these marriages did not last (Furstenberg, 1976; Lorenzi, Klerman, & Jekel, 1977). In Furstenberg's (1976) sample, 80% of couples who were married when the child was born were divorced just one year later. This finding suggests that marriage does little to increase, and may actually decrease, the stability in childbearing adolescents' lives.

PSYCHOSOCIAL SEQUELAE OF ADOLESCENT MOTHERHOOD

Socioeconomic sequelae

A substantial body of research documents lower socioeconomic attainment among young mothers (Card & Wise, 1978; Dryfoos, 1982; Furstenberg, 1976; Hayes, 1987; Moore, Hofferth, Caldwell, & Waite, 1979). In general, women who become mothers in adolescence complete fewer years of school, are less likely to earn high school diplomas, and are not likely to go on to college. In addition, adolescent mothers have fewer occupational opportunities, and often do not gain stable employment. Young mothers are frequently supported by welfare programs.

Although early childbearing is generally associated with lower socioeconomic attainment, it has been found that achieving an education, receiving parental support, and remaining primiparous positively affects outcome (Furstenberg, 1976). Regarding educational attainment, adolescents who demonstrate more academic ability and motivation to achieve are, of course, more likely to graduate from high school (Furstenberg, 1976). A less-expected finding is that those who give birth at age 16 or older are more likely to drop out of high school than those who give birth at younger ages (Furstenberg, 1976; Hofferth, 1987c). Furstenberg (1976) explains that those who give birth at younger ages are more likely to stay in their parents' home, and therefore, are more likely to have the child care and support they need in order to remain in school. Those who give birth at older ages are more likely to get a job and establish independent living arrangements. This responsibility makes it difficult for older adolescents to remain in school. In addition to completing an education, adolescent mothers who live with parents are also more likely to live without welfare assistance and be gainfully employed when they eventually do live on their own (Alan Guttmacher Institute, 1981; 1988). Those who do not return to school and those who choose to marry are more likely to have a second child shortly after the first (Darabi, Graham, & Philliber, 1982; Furstenberg, 1976). In general, approximately 25% of adolescent mothers have a second child within 30 months of their first (Darabi, Graham, & Philliber, 1982). In these families, socioeconomic problems associated with early pregnancy are obviously compounded.

Many factors considered to be sequelae of early childbearing are the same factors that often precede pregnancy (Chilman, 1989; Furstenberg, Brooks-Gunn, & Morgan, 1987; Hayes, 1987). For example, Hayes (1987) noted that although many pregnant adolescents drop out of high school after conceiving, a large number drop out even before they conceive. Therefore, it is difficult to implicate many factors as true sequelae. Nevertheless, childbearing does seem to have some direct impact on socioeconomic attainment that is not due to factors existing before pregnancy. Studies controlling for socioeconomic status, motivational factors, and academic ability continue to find that childbearing adolescents show lower educational and socioeconomic attainment (e.g., Card & Wise, 1978), which suggests that the responsibility of child care is specifically implicated as an obstacle to attaining economic stability.

Although virtually all adolescent mothers experience substantial economic setbacks, data from a 20-year longitudinal study of over 200 women who were adolescent mothers suggests that the socioeconomic problems of early motherhood sometimes attenuate in later years (Furstenberg, Brooks-Gunn, & Chase-Lansdale, 1989; Furstenberg, Brooks-Gunn, & Morgan, 1987). Young mothers who were able to complete high school, remain primiparous, and marry after the age of 20 were virtually indistinguishable from older childbearers. However, those who dropped out of school and became pregnant again shortly after their first child tended to experience the most poverty and had the fewest prospects of future betterment.

Psychiatric Sequelae

Despite the educational and economic setbacks of early motherhood, studies find that childbearing adolescents tend to experience the same levels of depression (Barth, Schinke, & Maxwell, 1983; Troutman, 1988; Troutman & Cutrona, 1990), and self-esteem (Barth, Schinke, & Maxwell, 1983; Ralph, Lochman, & Thomas, 1984; Troutman, 1988) as their nulliparous peers. Nevertheless, these studies also suggest that the level of psychological disturbance among adolescent mothers is higher than the level that would be expected among adult mothers. Although adolescent mothers usually are not psychologically disturbed, they may have more psychological difficulty than adults, which could present additional stress in their lives.

Impact on Offspring

Children of adolescent mothers, when compared with children of adult mothers, show more cognitive deficits and lower educational attainment (Belmont, Cohen, Dryfoos, Stein, & Zayac, 1981; Broman, 1981). The possible influence of factors that may lead to those outcomes, namely, the low socioeconomic status and educational attainment of adolescent mothers, makes it unclear that adolescent parenting per se leads to adverse outcomes in children (Belmont, Cohen, Dryfoos,

Stein, & Zayac, 1981; Broman, 1981; Furstenberg, Brooks-Gunn, & Chase-Lansdale, 1989; Hayes, 1987; Hofferth, 1987a). Furthermore, controlled studies comparing adolescent and adult mothers find virtually no differences in their parenting behaviors (Hofferth, 1987a) or in the likelihood that they will abuse or neglect their children (Kinard & Klerman, 1980). It is unlikely that interventions directed at improving the parenting skills of adolescent mothers will improve outcomes for their offspring. Nevertheless, adolescent mothers and their children could benefit from social and economic support that could ease the pressures associated with parenting. Adolescent mothers' need for support is especially salient if they do not live with their parents, because they are most often single or are in unstable marriages.

Implications for Intervention with Adolescent Mothers

A consistent finding in the literature is that parental support, both financial and emotional, is associated with adolescent mothers' well-being (Cutrona, 1989; Furstenberg, 1976; Furstenberg, Brooks-Gunn, & Morgan, 1987; Koniak-Griffin, 1988). Adolescents from supportive families are more likely to attain a high school education and stable employment, and are less likely to need support from the community. Programs designed to meet the financial needs of young mothers (e.g., Aid to Families with Dependent Children[AFDC]) typically provide assistance only to mothers who leave their parental homes (Ooms, 1984). Programs that provide education and psychological support are generally not as narrowly targeted. Some of these programs include high schools for adolescent mothers, life-skills training, and employment programs (Hayes, 1987; Hofferth, 1987b). Although it is clear that completing high school is associated with good outcome, there is a lack of research on the efficacy of programs designed to encourage education and otherwise enhance the well-being of adolescent mothers (Furstenberg, Brooks-Gunn, & Chase-Lansdale, 1989; Hayes, 1987).

SUMMARY OF CLINICAL IMPLICATIONS

The objective of this chapter was to familiarize professionals with research bearing on societal and psychological factors that influence young womens' decisions about preventing pregnancy, dealing with early pregnancy, and facing the task of early motherhood.

Most efforts to prevent adolescent pregnancy are community based. Professionals who work with adolescents should be familiar with family planning and school-based clinics, and with other agencies that provide sex education and contraception. Professionals should convey this infomation to adolescents in a way that makes these services seem accessible, for example, by giving phone numbers of free clinics and telling them that appointments are easy to make. The fear that sex education and contraceptive availability will encourage adolescent sexuality is clearly unfounded, and the possiblity that such interventions may prevent some young women from becoming pregnant cannot be overlooked. Community-based programs to prevent adolescent pregnancy are likely to be effective, but school-based programs may reach more adolescents, and thus be even more effective (Dryfoos, 1991).

A second role of the professional is to provide objective information about the options available to pregnant young women. One option is abortion. Approximately half of pregnant adolescents are sure that they either want or do not want an abortion, and half are ambivalent. For those who are ambivalent, it is likely that their parents will play a key role in determining the outcome of their pregnancy. If it is possible, professionals should involve parents in the counseling process so that they may make an informed decision along with their daughter. Young women should be given the names of clinics and physicians providing abortion services so that they may more easily avoid delay should they opt to have an abortion.

Another option for pregnant young women is, of course, continuation of the pregnancy and delivery. Adolescents choosing to deliver should be informed about the risks involved in pregnancy so that they may understand the importance of complying with a prenatal care regimen. Although most adolescents who deliver choose to keep their infants, this should not be assumed. Adoption should be presented as a realistic and responsible alternative. If possible, some counseling should be conducted to explore the means that adolescents have to care for a child and, if adoption is considered, discuss fears and concerns about relinquishing the infant. Counseling may prevent impulsive decision making that tends to occur close to the time of delivery. If possible, parents should be involved in this process.

Finally, professionals must be familiar with programs that provide adolescent mothers with financial and other forms of assistance. It should be kept in mind that if a young mother chooses to marry, this arrangement is likely to be unstable. Therefore, married adolescents should be provided with the same information about community support services as those who remain single. For all adolescents, the support that parents provide is a key predictor of good outcome, which includes staying in high school and delaying a second pregnancy until after age 20. In order to predict and optimize outcome, the degree of parental support should be assessed, along with the young mother's motivation to stay in school.

REFERENCES

Adler, J., Katz, S., & Jackson, D. (1985). A teen-pregnancy epidemic. *Newsweek, 105,* 90.

Adler, N. E., & Dolcini, P. (1986). Psychological issues in abortion for adolescents. In G. B. Melton (Ed.), *Adolescent abortion: Psychological and legal issues* (pp. 74–95). Lincoln: University of Nebraska Press.

Alan Guttmacher Institute (1981). *Teenage pregnancy: The problem that hasn't gone away.* New York: Author.

Alan Guttmacher Institute (1988). *Teenage pregnancy in the United States.* New York: Author.

Barth, R. P., Schinke, S. P., & Maxwell, J. S. (1983). Psychological correlates of teenage motherhood. *Journal of Youth and Adolescence, 12,* 471–487.

Belmont, L., Cohen, J., Dryfoos, J., Stein, Z., & Zayac, S. (1981). Maternal age and children's intelligence. In K. Scott, T. Field, & E. G. Robertson (Eds.), *Teenage parents and their offspring* (pp.177–194). New York: Grune & Stratton.

Broman, S. H. (1981). Long-term development of children born to teenagers. In K. Scott, T. Field, & E. G. Robertson (Eds.), *Teenage parents and their offspring* (pp.195–224). New York: Grune & Stratton.

Burr, W. A., & Schultz, K. F. (1980). Delayed abortion in an area of easy accessability. *Journal of the American Medical Association, 246,* 452–455.

Campbell, N. B., Franco, K., & Jurs, S. (1988). Abortion in adolescence. *Adolescence, 23,* 813–823.

Card, J. J., & Wise, L. L. (1978). Teenage mothers and teenage fathers: The impact of early childbearing on the parents' personal and professional lives. *Family Planning Perspectives, 10,* 199–205.

Chilman, C. S. (1989). Some major issues regarding adolescent sexuality and childbearing in the United States. *Journal of Social Work and Human Sexuality, 8,* 3–25.

Coddington, R. K. (1979). Life events associated with adolescent pregnancies. *Journal of Clincal Psychiatry, 40,* 180–185.

Crosby, M. C., & English, A. (1991). Mandatory parental involvement/judicial bypass laws: Do they promote adolescents' health? *Journal of Adolescent Health Care, 12,* 143–147.

Cutrona, C. E. (1989). Ratings of social support by adolescents and adult informants: Degree of correspondence and prediction of depressive symptoms. *Journal of Personality and Social Psychology, 57,* 723–730.

Darabi, K., Graham, E. H., & Philliber, S. G. (1982). The second time around: Birth spacing among teenage mothers. In I. R. Stuart & C. F. Wells (Eds.), *Pregnancy in adolescence* (pp. 427–438). New York: Van Nostrand Reinhold.

Dash, L. (1989). *When children want children.* New York: William Morrow.

Devaney, B. L., & Hubley, K. S. (1981). *The determinants of adolescent pregnancy and childbearing.* (Final report to the National Institute of Child Health and Human Development). Washington, DC: Mathematica Policy Research.

Dryfoos, J. G. (1982). The epidemiology of adolescent pregnancy: Incidence, outcomes, and interventions. In I. R. Stuart & C. F. Wells (Eds.), *Pregnancy in adolescence* (pp. 27–47). New York: Van Nostrand Reinhold.

Dryfoos, J. G. (1983). *Review of interventions in the field of prevention of adolescent pregnancy*. New York: Preliminary report to the Rockefeller Foundation.

Dryfoos, J. G. (1985). *Review of programs and services to foster responsible sexual behavior on the part of adolescent boys*. New York: Report to the Carnegie Corporation.

Dryfoos, J. G. (1991). Adolescents at risk: A summation of work in the field—programs and policies. *Journal of Adolescent Health, 12*, 630–637.

Furstenberg, F. F. (1976). *Unplanned parenthood*. New York: Free Press.

Furstenberg, F. F., & Brooks-Gunn, J. (1985). Adolescent fertility: Causes, consequences, and remedies. In L. Aiken & D. Mechanic (Eds.), *Applications of social science to clinical medicine and health policy* (pp. 29–45). New Brunswick, NJ: Rutgers University Press.

Furstenberg, F. F., Brooks-Gunn, J., & Chase-Lansdale, L. (1989). Teenaged pregnancy and childbearing. *American Psychologist, 44*, 313–320.

Furstenberg, F. F., Brooks-Gunn, J., & Morgan, S. P. (1987). *Adolescent mothers in later life*. New York: Cambridge University Press.

Greer, J. G. (1982). Adoptive placement: Developmental and psychotherapeutic issues. In I. R. Stuart & C. F. Wells (Eds.), *Pregnancy in adolescence* (pp. 386–406). New York: Van Nostrand Reinhold.

Greydanus, D. E. (1983). Abortion in adolescence. In E. R. McAnarney (Ed.), *Premature adolescent pregnancy and parenthood* (pp. 351–374). New York: Grune & Stratton.

Gunter, N. C., & LaBarba, R. C. (1981). Maternal and perinatal effects of adolescent childbearing. *International Journal of Behavioral Development, 4*, 333–357.

Hart, B., & Hilton, I. (1988). Dimensions of personality organization as predictors of teenage pregnancy risk. *Journal of Personality Assessment, 52*, 116–132.

Hayes, C. D. (1987). *Risking the future: Adolescent sexuality, pregnancy, and childbearing* (Vol. 1). Washington, DC: National Academy Press.

Herr, K. M. (1989). Adoption vs. parenting decisions among pregnant adolescents. *Adolescence, 27*, 795–799.

Hofferth, S. L. (1987a). The children of teen childbearers. In S. L. Hofferth & C. D. Hayes (Eds.), *Risking the future: Adolescent sexuality, pregnancy, and childbearing* (Vol. 2, pp. 174–206). Washington, DC: National Academy Press.

Hofferth, S. L. (1987b). The effects of programs and policies on adolescent pregnancy and childbearing. In S. L. Hofferth & C. D. Hayes (Eds.), *Risking the future: Adolescent sexuality, pregnancy, and childbearing* (Vol. 2, pp. 207–263). Washington, DC: National Academy Press.

Hofferth, S. L. (1987c). Social and economic consequences of teenage childbearing. In S. L. Hofferth & C. D. Hayes (Eds.), *Risking the future: Adolescent sexuality, pregnancy, and childbearing* (Vol. 2, pp. 123–144). Washington, DC: National Academy Press.

Hollingsworth, D. R., Kotchen, J. M., & Felice, M. E. (1983). Impact of gynecologic age on outcome of adolescent pregnancy. In E. R. McAnarney (Ed.), *Premature adolescent pregnancy and parenthood* (pp. 169–194). New York: Grune & Stratton.

Jacobson, M. S., & Heald, F. P. (1983). Nutritional risks of adolescent pregnancy and their management. In E. R. McAnarney (Ed.), *Premature adolescent pregnancy and parenthood* (pp. 119–136). New York: Grune & Stratton.

Jones, E. F. (1986). *Teenage pregnancy in industrialized countries*. New Haven, CT: Yale University Press.

Kinard, E. M., & Klerman, L. V. (1980). Teenage parenting and child abuse: Are they related? *American Journal of Orthopsychiatry, 50*, 481–488.

Kinsman, S. B., & Slap, G. B. (1992). Barriers to adolescent prenatal care. *Journal of Adolescent Health Care, 13*, 146–154.

Kirby, D. (1984). *Sexuality education: An evaluation of programs and their effect*. Santa Cruz, CA.: Network Publications.

Klerman, L. V., Bracken, M. B., Jekel, J. F., & Bracken, M. (1982). The delivery–abortion decision among adolescents. In I. R. Stuart & C. F. Wells (Eds.), *Pregnancy in adolescence* (pp. 219–235). New York: Van Nostrand Reinhold.

Koniak-Griffin, D. (1988). The relationship between social support, self-esteem and maternal–fetal attachment in adolescents. *Research in Nursing and Health, 11*, 269–278.

Kriepe, R. E. (1983). Prevention of adolescent pregnancy: A developmental approach. In E. R. McAnarney (Ed.), *Premature adolescent pregnancy and parenthood* (pp. 37–60). New York: Grune & Stratton.

Lohr, M. J., Gillmore, M. R., Gilchrist, L. D., & Butler, S. S. (1992). Factors related to substance abuse by pregnant, school-age adolescents. *Journal of Adolescent Health Care, 13*, 475–482.

Lorenzi, M. E., Klerman, L. V., & Jekel, J. F. (1977). School age parents: How permanent a relationship? *Adolescence, 12*, 13–22.

Meyerowitz, J. H., & Malev, J. S. (1973). Pubescent attitudinal correlates antecedent to adolescent illegitimate pregnancy. *Journal of Youth and Adolescence, 2*, 251–258.

Moore, D. S., & Erickson, P. I. (1985). Age, gender, and ethnic differences in sexual and contraceptive knowledge, attitudes, and behaviors. *Family and Community Health, 8*, 38–51.

Moore, K. A., Hofferth, S. L., Caldwell, S. B., & Waite, L. J. (1979). *Teenage motherhood: Social and economic consequences*. Washington, DC: Urban Institute.

Morrison, D. M. (1985). Adolescent contraceptive behavior: A review. *Psychological Bulletin, 98*, 538–568.

Olson, L. (1980). Social and psychological correlates of pregnancy resolution among adolescent women: A review. *American Journal of Orthopsychiatry, 50*, 432–445.

Ooms, T. (1984). The family context of adolescent parenting. In M. Sugar (Ed.), *Adolescent parenthood* (pp. 217–227). Jamaica, NY: Spectrum Publications.

Philliber, S., Namerow, P. B., Kaye, J. W., & Kunes, C. H. (1986). Pregnancy risk taking among adolescents. *Journal of Adolescent Research, 1*, 463–481.

Phoenix, A. (1989). Influences on previous contraceptive use/nonuse in pregnant 16–19 year olds. *Journal of Reproductive and Infant Psychology, 7*, 211–225.

Pletsch, P. K. (1988). Substance use and health activities of pregnant adolescents. *Journal of Adolescent Health Care, 9*, 38–43.

Quay, H. C. (1981). Psychological factors in teenage pregnancy. In K. G. Scott, T. Field, & E. G. Roberson (Eds.), *Teenage parents and their offspring* (pp. 73–90). New York: Grune & Stratton.

Ralph, N., Lochman, J., & Thomas, T. (1984). Psychosocial characteristics of pregnant and nulliparous adolescents. *Adolescence, 14*, 283–294.

Rosen, R. H. (1980). Adolescent pregnancy decision-making: Are parents important? *Adolescence, 15*, 43–54.

Rosen, E. J., Campbell, C., & Arima, L. (1961). A psychiatric, social and psychological study of illegitimate pregnancy in girls under the age of sixteen years. *Psychiatric Neurology, 142*, 44–60.

Semmens, J., & Lammers, W. (1968). *Teenage pregnancy*. Springfield, IL: Charles C Thomas.

Sirpa, U. (1989). Adolescent pregnancy: Standards and services in Finland. *Child Welfare, 68*, 167–182.

Troutman, B. R. (1988). *Living situation, social support and psychological adjustment among childbearing adolescents*. Unpublished doctoral dissertation, University of Iowa, Iowa City.

Troutman, B. R, & Cutrona, C. E. (1990). Nonpsychotic postpartum depression among adolescent mothers. *Journal of Abnormal Psychology, 99*, 69–78.

Wallace, H. M., & Vienonen, M. (1989). Teenage pregnancy in Sweden and Finland: Some implications for the United States. *Journal of Adolescent Health Care, 10*, 231–236.

Weinman, M. L., Robinson, M., Simmons, J. T., Schrieber, N. B., & Stafford, B. (1989). Pregnant teens: Differential pregnancy resolution and treatment implications. *Child Welfare, 68*, 45–55.

Wells, R. D., McDiarmid, J., & Bayatpour, M. (1990). Perinatal Health Belief Scales: A cost effective technique for predicting prenatal appointment keeping rates among pregnant teenagers. *Journal of Adolescent Health Care, 11*, 119–124.

Young, C. L., McMahon, J. E., & Bowman, V. M. (1990). Psychosocial concerns of women who delay prenatal care. *Families in Society, 71*, 408–414.

Zabin, L. S., Hirsch, M. B., Smith, E. A., Street, R., & Hardy, J. B. (1986). Evaluation of a pregnancy prevention program for urban teenagers. *Family Planning Perspectives, 18*, 119–126.

Zelnik, M. J., Kantner, J. F., & Ford, K. (1981). *Sex and pregnancy in adolescence*. Beverly Hills, CA: Sage Publications.

Zelnik, M. J., & Kim, Y. J. (1982). Sex education and its association with teenage sexual activity, pregnancy, and contraceptive use. *Family Planning Perspectives, 14*, 6–13.

PART IV
Decision Making

16

Medical Decision Making

Carol J. Hodne

Ethical principles and legal mandates have guided efforts to provide patients with information to allow informed consent to medical treatment (Faden, Beauchamp with King, 1986). Informed consent includes information regarding "the nature of the disorder and of the proposed intervention, the likely benefits, risks, and discomforts, and possible alternatives, including the option of no treatment, along with their risks and treatments" (Appelbaum & Grisso, 1988). Informed consent requires that the patient be able to: 1) understand the medical situation and its personal consequences; 2) use information rationally; 3) understand the information well enough to make a choice; 4) make and communicate a choice; and 5) be free from force, coercion, deceit, or duress (Appelbaum & Grisso, 1988; Wu & Pearlman, 1988).

Medical decision making and informed consent are becoming more oriented to patients' expectations, as they have been shaped by health consumerism (Haug & Lavin, 1983; Reiter, Lench, & Gambone, 1989), the health component of the women's movement (Rodin & Ickovics, 1990; Travis, 1988), and research on patient–physician communication (Anderson & Sharpe, 1991; Roter, Hall, & Katz, 1988).

This chapter describes models of informed consent which facilitate active patient participation in medical decision making. Social influences upon decision making are presented, along with the effects of judgment biases and cultural and gender differences between physicians and patients. Implications are suggested for clinical practice and assessment of competency to grant informed consent.

MODELS OF ACTIVE PATIENT PARTICIPATION IN DECISION MAKING

Informed consent information has often traditionally been presented in a complex-appearing document without dialogue or assessment of patients' abilities to understand the information (Tymchuk & Ouslander, 1991). In contrast, patient–centered models incorporate highly interactive patient–provider communication and decision making. For example, Gambone and Reiter's (1992) PREPARED™ informed-consent mnemonic model helps patients secure information regarding: 1) Procedure; 2) Reason for procedure; 3) Expectation for benefits; 4) Probability of benefits occurring; 5) Alternatives; 6) Risks; 7) Expense; and 8) Decision. Questions pertaining to these areas of information are noted in Table 16.1.

Ballard-Reisch (1990) proposed a compatible model of participative medical decision making with three phases: 1) diagnosis; 2) exploration of treatment alternatives; and 3) treatment decision, implementation, and evaluation. The phases are divided into 8 stages, which are noted in Table 16.2.

Wu and Pearlman (1988) found that the element of informed consent most often communicated by physicians was rationale for a procedure, followed, in order, by benefits, risks, and alternatives. Alternatives were communicated more often with more invasive procedures. The importance or risk of procedures did not affect communication in these four areas. Agreement in patients' and physicians' understanding was generally greater for rationale and benefits than it was for risks and alternatives. For invasive procedures, agreement regarding rationale and benefits improved, but worsened regarding risks. Agreement was not greater for important or risky procedures. The authors suggest that physicians' limited sharing of information is a barrier to informed consent and recommend greater patient participation in decision making.

Physicians' sharing of educational information, particularly regarding the prognosis, the cause of the problem, and prevention/future treatment, can increase their effectiveness in soliciting needed information from patients (Roter & Hall, 1987). Since physicians' sharing of information is related to patient disclosure and the extent of understanding between physicians and patients, it is likely that the use of the PREPARED™ mnemonic and the Ballard-Reisch (1990) model will improve communication and understanding. Ballard-Reisch (1990) suggests that her model allows patients and physicians to assess their progress through the stages of decision making; identify discrepancies between their perceptions,

TABLE 16.1   PREPARED™ for Health Care

P	Procedure. What is your understanding of the course of action which the doctor is recommending to you?
R	Reason. What is your medical diagnosis and what harm is it causing you?
E	Expectation. What benefits can you reasonably expect from the procedure?
P	Probability. What are the odds that you will get these benefits?
A	Alternatives. What other choices, including "watchful waiting," are available and what are their prospects for meeting your expectations?
R	Risks. What possible problems may be caused by the procedure?
E	Expense. What are all of the direct and indirect costs to you of having the procedure? (include insurance copayments, time lost from work, childcare costs, etc.)
D	Decision. Is this the best course of action for you at this time or not?

Note. From: *PREPARED for Health Care Patient Checklist*, by J. C. Gambone, R. C. Reiter, and M. R. DiMatteo, (1993), Los Angeles: HealthCare Works Foundation. Copyright 1993 by Health Care Works Foundation. Reprinted by permission.

needs, and values; negotiate their roles and relationships; and come to mutually agreeable treatment options.

METHODS OF AND ADVANTAGES TO ACTIVE PATIENT PARTICIPATION IN DECISION MAKING

Patients may gain more information from physicians by: 1) preparing questions to increase the number of questions they ask (Roter, 1984; Thompson, Nanni, & Schwanovsky, 1990); 2) learning how to read their medical records, ask questions, and negotiate decisions (Greenfield, Kaplan, & Ware, 1985); and 3) reading informative surgery preparation booklets (Wallace, 1986). Physicians may also increase patients' question asking by informing patients that they encourage questions (Thompson, Nanni, & Schwanovsky, 1990) and by being more explicit regarding instructions (Svarstad, 1976).

While patients may learn methods to increase the information they receive, situational and social factors also influence their participation in decision making. Only during interactions of at least 19 minutes did patients' desire for information correspond with their information-seeking behavior, particularly among older patients (Beisecker & Beisecker, 1990). Waitzkin (1985) found that greater information sharing was associated with longer acquaintance between physician and patient, uncertain or poor prognoses, fewer patients seen daily, as well as with patient characteristics of greater age, higher educational attainment, higher social class, and female sex.

Active information sharing and patient participation in decision making are associated with enhanced patients' perceptions of control and self-responsibility

TABLE 16.2   Participative Decision Making Model

Phase 1: Diagnostic
    Stage 1: Information gathering
    Stage 2: Information interpretation
Phase 2: Exploration of treatment alternatives
    Stage 3: Exploration of alternatives
    Stage 4: Criteria establishment for treatment
    Stage 5: Weighing of alternatives against criteria
Phase 3: Treatment decision, implementation, & evaluation
    Stage 6: Alternative selection
    Stage 7: Decision implementation
    Stage 8: Evaluation of implemented treatment

Note. From: A model of participative decision making for physician-patient interaction by D. S. Ballard-Reisch, (1990), *Health Communication, 2.*

regarding their health (Lerman, Brody, Caputo, Smith, Lazaro, & Wolfson, 1990; Thompson, Nanni, & Schwanovsky, 1990) and with improved health outcomes (Garrity & Lawson, 1989), such as faster recoveries (Wallace, 1986), improved treatment effectiveness (Brody, Miller, Lerman, Smith, & Caputo, 1989), and fewer limitations on patients' functional abilities (Greenfield, Kaplan, & Ware, 1985). Patients who were more active in decision making, compared with more passive patients, reported more control of and improvement in their health, more satisfaction with their physician, and less concern with their illness (Brody, Miller, Lerman, Smith, & Caputo, 1989).

Physicians may increase patients' adherence to treatment through the effective communication of information (DiMatteo, Hays, & Sherbourne, 1992), the willingness to answer all questions (DiMatteo, Sherbourne, Hays, Ordway, Kravitz, McGynn, Kaplan, & Rogers, 1993), the clarity of their instructions (Svarstad, 1976), and empathy with their patients (Squier, 1990).

Information sharing may also increase patients' satisfaction with their medical care (Ley, 1989; Thompson, Nanni, & Schwanovsky, 1990). Willingness to answer questions and a kind, caring attitude were considered the most helpful physician responses by women who had detected a lump in their breast (Hailey, Lavine, & Hogan, 1988). Physicians' humaneness, including their willingness to listen and inter-personal skill, was among the top predictors of patient satisfaction in Hall and Dornan's (1988) meta-analysis. However, training patients in more active participation (Greenfield, Kaplan, & Ware, 1985) and question-asking (Roter, 1984) did not lead to greater satisfaction with their visit. Thus, satisfaction is often, but not always, associated with greater information sharing.

COMPREHENSION AND RECALL OF
MEDICAL INFORMATION

In order to make informed decisions, patients need to comprehend as much medical information as possible. However, comprehension may be diminished by impairments of perceptual abilities associated with age, since by age sixty-five approximately 30% of women have experienced perceptual losses which impair social interaction (Garrity & Lawson, 1989). Tymchuk and Ouslander (1990) recommend that physicians assess the vision, hearing, decision-making capacity, and reading comprehension of some elderly patients, as well as conduct ongoing follow-up regarding their comprehension and maintenance of earlier decisions.

Certain medical problems may affect perceptual abilities and thus comprehension of medical information. Women with Premenstrual Syndrome (PMS) were less able to interpret nonverbal behavior, during the premenstrual phase, than were women without PMS (Giannini, Sorger, Martin, & Bates, 1989). This impairment parallels the decline in visual perception occurring at the premenstrual phase (Ward, Stone, & Sandman, 1977). Anorexia may also be associated with impaired visual perception, since anorexic female adolescents, compared with controls, gazed at psychologists with lower frequencies and lengths of individual and mutual gaze (Cipolli, Sancini, Tuozzi, Bolzani, Mutinelli, Flamigni, & Porcu, 1989).

Greater recall of medical information has been associated with: 1) a primacy effect, in which material presented first is better recalled; 2) statements perceived as more important; and 3) greater medical knowledge held by the patient (Ley, 1982, 1989). A recency effect also exists, in which material most recently presented is better recalled than intermediate material. Recency and primacy effects were found among nursing home residents for information regarding low-risk, but not high-risk, procedures (Tymchuk & Ouslander, 1991).

Physicians may improve patients' recall of information by varying the order of information presentation, routinely assessing patients' accuracy of recall and providing related feedback, and repeating the presentation of information not previously recalled (Bertakis, 1977; Tymchuk & Ouslander, 1991). Comprehension and recall of written information may be enhanced by use of easier words, shorter sentences (Folstein, Fostein, & McHugh, 1975), and storybook formats (Tymchuk, Ouslander, & Rader, 1986). Patients tend to recall for a considerable time what they recalled shortly after a medical visit (Ley, 1989). Therefore, efforts to increase their immediate recall may be especially effective. Patients may need more time during or shortly after an office visit to rehearse new information. Patients and those who accompany them may be encouraged to take notes during and/or after the visit.

When providing medical information to patients, it is important to consider their preferences for personal control over their health care and for information.

For example, individuals over 60 years of age, compared with younger adults, expressed more desire for health professionals to make decisions for them and lower perceived self-efficacy related to their health, which may contribute to their lower desire for control of their health care (Woodward & Wallston, 1987). For other ways in which aging affects informed consent, see Haug and Ory's (1987) review of research on medical interactions with elderly patients.

Miller and Mangan (1983) found that the levels of physiological arousal and tension for both patients desiring more information and those desiring less information were lower when the levels of preparatory information regarding colposcopy were consistent with their information preference. The authors recommend caution in using the traditional informed-consent model with its predetermined amounts and types of information.

The importance of physicians' sensitivity to both patients' and their own expressions of anxiety is suggested by findings that patients with low to moderate anxiety levels remember more information, recover more favorably, and are more satisfied with treatment quality (Sprecher, Thomas, Huebner, Norfleet, & Jacoby, 1983). For example, women viewed a videotaped presentation of ambiguous mammogram results portraying either worried or nonworried physician affect. Women viewing the worried physician recalled less information, perceived their medical condition as more severe, and reported more anxiety (Shapiro, Boggs, Melamed, & Graham-Pole, 1992).

Increased hand-to-body (but not hand-to-hand) self-touching was associated with patients' presentation of hidden agendas (i.e., issues involving anxiety or distress that were difficult to express directly; Shreve, Harrigan, Kues, & Kagas, 1988). Understanding of patients' concerns regarding high-anxiety issues may be increased through sensitivity to relevant self-touching cues and subsequent discussion of these issues. Physicians may encourage anxious patients' self-disclosure through greater vocal back-channels (i.e, noninterruptive simultaneous speech) to show attentiveness (e.g., "uh-huh") and briefer speaking turns (Street & Buller, 1987). Rapport with anxious patients (and other patients) may be increased by: 1) viewing them with moderate, rather than extended, eye contact; 2) sitting directly facing them, with uncrossed legs, and arms in symmetrical, side-by-side positions (Harrigan, Oxman, & Rosenthal, 1985); 3) leaning forward with open arm positions; and 4) nodding one's head (Harrigan & Rosenthal, 1983).

CAUSAL ATTRIBUTIONS AND JUDGMENT BIASES IN DECISION MAKING

Patients often report attributions for what caused their illness or injury. The frequency and content of these causal attributions are associated with illness variables (e.g., diagnosis, severity of illness). Reporting some type of attribution is associated with improved adjustment. However, the association between particular types of attributions and adjustment is less strong (Turnquist, Harvey, & Andersen, 1988).

Medical treatment is more likely to be effective when physicians and patients agree upon, or at least understand one another's view on causal attributions, as they influence the decision-making process. Attributions of responsibility for causes of problems may be distinguished from attributions of responsibility for solutions to problems. These separate attributions influence patients' and physicians' expectations for themselves and others, including their preferred forms of coping and helping (Brickman, Rabinowitz, Karuza, Coates, Cohn, & Kidder, 1982; Karuza, Zevon, Rabinowitz, & Brickman, 1982). Michela and Wood's (1986) review of literature on attributions and health includes therapeutic benefits of making explicit what may be implicit models of attributions of causality (e.g., providing a focus for intervention). Making explicit both physicians' and patients' views on both causes of and solutions to problems can enhance their mutual understanding, and can facilate the healing process.

Causal attributions and other aspects of medical decision making are often influenced by subjective judgment biases or "heuristics," which have been described as "intuitive rules that influence estimates of prevalence or likelihood, preferences among alternatives, and eventually affect policy" (decision making; Travis, Phillippi, & Tonn, 1989). Some types of medical decision making are influenced by heuristics due to high stress, uncertainty, and large amounts of information to be rapidly processed (Schaeffer, 1989). While heuristics often lead to appropriate decisions, they may also lead to less effective decisions, particularly if their potentially negative consequences are ignored (Redeimeier, Rozin, & Kahneman, 1993). This section focuses on definitions, examples, and implications of the following heuristics that were described by Travis, Phillippi, and Tonn (1989): *illusory correlations; availability bias; false consensus; representativeness heuristic; anchoring bias;* and *framing effects.*

Events that happen together, especially frequently, may inaccurately be considered causally related, creating *illusory correlations.* This bias may impede discrimination of relevant diagnostic information, particularly for problems for which specific causes are not well understood. *Illusory correlations* may falsely indicate treatment side effects, therefore lessening adherence to treatment. For example, if psychosexual problems began concurrently with a medication treatment, a patient may discontinue the medication, falsely believing it caused the psychosexual problem.

Evaluating the frequency or likelihood of an event on the basis of how readily instances or associations come to mind is called the *availability bias* (Tversky & Kahneman, 1973). Some diseases (e.g., Acquired Immune Deficiency Syndrome—AIDS) may be thought of more readily due to related media attention or public education, and may be considered a possible cause of symptoms to a greater extent than is appropriate (Travis et al., 1989). The *availability bias* may contribute to delay in seeking a diagnosis, leading to subsequent diminishment of treatment choices or effectiveness.

The tendency to view one's own behavior as typical, and to assume that others react similarly under the same circumstance is termed *false consensus*. Personal experiences influence one's estimates of the prevalence of behaviors or conditions in the population (Fiske & Taylor, 1991). *False consensus* may lead to interpreting symptoms in an inaccurate manner that fits one's perceptions of the general population or may lead to a lack of recognition that health care would be helpful. For example, the existence of eating disorders in some group settings (e.g., university housing or athletic teams; Crandall, 1988) may create distorted views of overall norms for healthy eating, and may, therefore, prevent women from recognizing their eating disorders as unhealthy.

The *representativeness heuristic* involves overreliance on small samples or special features of individual cases, while ignoring normative features or base rates of the population (Travis et al.,1989). This bias may lead to inaccurate estimates of the prevalence of a condition in the population, prolonged diagnostic processes, and incorrect diagnoses. For example, a physician whose residency at a Premenstrual Syndrome (PMS) Clinic involved mostly treatment of older patients is now working with a younger population. A young patient presenting the symptoms of tension, depression, and irritability may be misdiagnosed with PMS unless the social context of the symptoms are discussed (Riessman, 1983), allowing the identification of a situational stressor (e.g., stressful employment) that may be alleviated through psychotherapy and/or group advocacy.

Anchoring bias may occur when physicians view new cases against initial or extreme evaluations (Travis et al., 1989) or experiences or when they too slowly adapt their initial diagnoses to consider changes in symptoms or health status. Guarding against this form of *anchoring bias* is especially important since physicians tend to generate a set of tentative diagnostic hypotheses based on initial signs and symptoms (Schiffmann, Cohen, Nowik, & Selinger, 1978). For example, a physician's disinclination to prescribe birth control pills may be due to one of their patients experiencing a rare complication of stroke while on the birth control pill.

Framing effects (i.e., the way in which information is presented) may influence decision making. For example, health behaviors may be framed with an emphasis on risks or benefits. Undergraduates who read a pamphlet framed in terms of the negative consequences of not performing breast self-examination (BSE), compared with those who read a pamphlet framed in terms of the positive benefits of performing BSE, had more positive attitudes toward performing BSE and the greatest increase in performing BSE at 4-month follow-up (Meyerowitz & Chaiken, 1987).

Another example of framing effects is that delayed gains are often viewed as less beneficial, while the consequences of future risks are discounted (Travis et al., 1989). Such biases make it difficult to utilize expectancy management (wait and see) which may often be the most effective, least risky option. For example, patients with abnormal bleeding may choose hysterectomy, while discounting its risks, in order to stop the bleeding, while viewing the delayed gains achieved through hormonal treatment or nonsurgical management as less beneficial.

Travis (1985) analyzed how the aggregate benefits for elective hysterectomies (i.e., life expectancy, avoiding costs of gynecologic surgery and cancer treatment, quality of life) are small relative to risks (i.e., morbidity, mortality, psychological sequelae), and suggested that *framing effects* contribute to distorted perceptions of risks. When two options are negative, individuals often select the riskier option, choosing to risk a possible large loss to avert certain moderate losses. Choosing a hysterectomy entails the possibility of larger losses, while choosing not to have one may be associated with the continuation of symptoms.

Negative consequences of *framing effects* may be lessened by considering the issue from multiple perspectives and discussing it with others with different opinions (Reideimeier, Rozin, & Kahneman, 1993). Discussion between patients and physicians of elements of informed consent (Travis, 1985) and of whether any risk and benefit distortions or heuristics are operating in their decision making may prevent the potentially negative influences of distortions and judgment biases.

SOCIAL SUPPORT, COPING, AND SOCIAL INFLUENCES ON DECISION MAKING

Consideration of patients' social support is an important part of decision making because social support: 1) has direct or mediating effects on illness; 2) influences patients' perceptions of aspects of informed consent; and 3) is linked to personal relationships (Duck with Silver, 1990). In their meta-analysis of research on social support and health, Schwarzer and Leppin (1991) distinguish three categories of social support: 1) social integration—the quantity, structure, and nature of social relationships and important roles; 2) cognitive social support—perceived available support; and 3) behavioral social support—the actual receipt of support, which is of the emotional, instrumental, or material type, and the evaluation of the received support. They found that reports of physical symptoms were inversely related to satisfaction with support, instrumental support, emotional support, cognitive support, and social integration, in descending order of the size of the (negative) correlations.

Cohen and Wills' (1985) literature review reveals empirical support for two central models of how social support affects health: 1) the main-effect model (i.e., social support has beneficial effects whether or not individuals are under stress, primarily through integration in social networks); and 2) the buffering model (i.e., when stress occurs, social support prevents behavioral and biological responses to stress which have adverse effects on health and increases beneficial responses). Cohen (1988) describes how main-effect models operate through four types of social support:

1. Information-provision—a wide range of network relationships provides multiple sources of information regarding preventive medical care, health promotion, or avoidance of stress;
2. Identity and self-esteem—social support increases feelings of self-esteem, self-identity, and control over one's environment, which lessen despair, increase motivation for self-care, and enhance immune functioning;
3. Social influence—social controls and peer pressure influence normative health behaviors;
4. Tangible resources—network members provide aid and tangible and economic services that promote better health and health care.

Cohen (1988) similarly describes how buffering models may operate through these four types of social support. His focus on perceived availability of support centers on individuals' appraisal of the relative potential harm of stressors, assessment of their coping capacities, and their emotional effects.

While high levels of social support are generally associated with improved physical health among men, the relationship between social support and health is more complex and weak among women. This is possibly due to women's greater responsibilities for providing support to network members, including children and parents, resulting in increased stress and exposure to negative social outcomes (Shumaker & Hill, 1991). Although research on social support and health has focused on males, therefore leaving its generalizability to females in question, the main-effect and buffering models provide a framework for describing various social influences upon medical decision making.

Patients' different ways of coping with their illness affect their expectations for treatment and the decision-making process. Coping, including assessment of the potential consequences of a stressor and of one's options and resources, is a mediator of various stressful events and subsequent physical and mental health outcomes (Folkman, Lazarus, Dunkel-Schetter, DeLongis, & Gruen, 1986). In general, avoidant coping, which diverts attention from the stressor, is more adaptive in the short term, while attentional coping, which focuses on the stressor, is more adaptive in the long term (Suls & Fletcher, 1985). For example, recent-onset pain patients using primarily avoidant coping, compared with those using attentional coping, were less depressed and anxious and had more social activity, while chronic pain patients using mostly attentional coping, compared with those using avoidant coping, experienced similar benefits (Holmes & Stevenson, 1990).

Similar benefits of coping strategies focused on minimizing worry were found in a study that exemplified the information-provision type of support within the buffering model of social support (Cohen, 1988). Ridgeway and Mathews (1982) presented three types of hysterectomy preparation manuals: 1) an information manual regarding the surgery and its effects; 2) a cognitive coping manual on how to think positively regarding worrisome aspects of the surgery; and 3) an attention control booklet. Patients receiving the cognitive coping manual had fewer worries and used fewer analgesics, while those receiving the information manual knew the most about the surgery. Another study of hysterectomy patients similarly revealed that subjective distress was predicted less by medical variables than by social psychological variables, including cognitive coping (e.g., negative attitudes toward the consequences of hysterectomy, low internal control, low dependence on powerful others, and low social support; Schulze, Florin, Matschin, Sougioullzi, & Schulze, 1988).

Severe, chronic, or trauma-induced medical conditions may require more elaborate or phase-oriented cognitive coping. Taylor (1983) proposed three cognitive processes in adjusting to threatening events, including illness and stress: 1) a search for meaning; 2) an attempt to regain mastery over the event and one's life; and 3) restoration of self-esteem through positive self-evaluations. The social aspects of this process may be viewed as an example of the identity and self-esteem type of support within the buffering model of social support. Horowitz (1976, 1987) described an ongoing, sometimes cyclical, process of cognitive adaptation to severe trauma and stress that includes stages of crying out and stunned reactions, avoidance, oscillation between avoidance and intrusive thoughts, and transition to an integrated processing of the information, including new long-term cognitions, including of self-concept.

Patients coping with severe conditions (e.g., cancer), chronic conditions (e.g., physical disability), or the consequences of traumatic stressors (e.g., war, sexual abuse, or assault; Bachmann, Moeller, & Benett, 1988) may exhibit: 1) fluctuations in avoidant and attentional coping; 2) shifts in perceptions of meaning, mastery, and self-esteem (Taylor, 1983); and 3) changes in their value preferences or treatment expectations relative to their stage in coping. Such patients may particularly benefit from the open and flexible discussion promoted by patient-centered models of informed consent. Physician collaboration with psychologists also fosters patients' ongoing coping, healing, and stage-appropriate decision making (Hunter, 1989; Roth & Newman, 1991).

Patients' preferences for treatment may also change over time due to changes in their health status. Christensen-Szalanski (1984) found that women preferred to avoid using anesthesia during childbirth when they were asked one month before labor and during early labor. During labor, preferences shifted toward using anesthesia and then, one month postpartum, shifted back toward avoiding anesthesia. The author suggests that physicians grant patients a choice between stating their anesthesia preference prior to labor or allowing them to change their preference. In order to ethically provide informed consent, physicians need to discuss and be tolerant of how patients' value preferences may change over the course of treatment, including due to changes in their health (Llewellyn-Thomas, Sutherland, Tritchler, Lockwood, Till, Ciampi, Scott, Lickley, & Fish, 1991) or changes in their social support (e.g., tangible resources).

While models of informed consent often focus on decision making by autonomous individuals, it is crucial to consider the influence of patients' social context, including their close relationships. Ewart (1991) emphasizes how patients' efforts to regulate their health (including cognitive schemas, self-goals, and problem-solving activities) are influenced by various social mechanisms, including interdependence within personal relationships. An example of how social interdependence affects patients' treatment preference is that women's childbirth preferences were more influenced by social factors than by their physician's advice (McClain, 1987). Only 3 of the 28 respondents choosing repeat cesarean section and 1 of 65 choosing vaginal birth after a cesarean section described their physician's advice as the only influence on their choice. Social motives for their choice were most common, particularly husband's needs, child care, return to work, and future childbearing.

Women's social situations were more influential than their physician's medical diagnosis in women's constructions of meaning for their illnesses (Hunt, Jordan, & Irwin, 1989). Women adapted their views of their illness to the changing requirements of their everyday lives. Part of this meaning-construction process was the sharing of their accounts with others, particularly family members, friends, and those with similar problems. Account-making (i.e., the development of stories including explanations, memories, and emotions) facilitates healing from illness and stress (Harvey, Orbuch, & Weber, 1990) and contributes to feelings of control, clearer understanding, higher self-esteem, emotional purging, closure, enlightenment, and enhanced will and hope (Harvey, Weber, & Orbuch, 1990).

Cultural differences exist in the relative emphasis on decision making by autonomous individuals or by individuals within the context of their personal relationships. Although Japanese physicians generally supported granting of informed consent by individual patients, they preferred to involve patients' family members, sometimes as a substitute for patients' informed consent, in order to minimize patients' emotional upheaval in cases of high-risk diagnostic procedures, cancer, or patients' unwillingness to undergo treatment (Hattori, Salzberg, Kiang, Fujimiya, Tejima, & Furuno, 1991). This practice was partially explained by selfhood in Japan being more defined in relationship to others, including family members, than in the autonomous sense prevalent in Western societies.

Jecker and Berg (1992) similarly suggest that rural primary-care physicians often make medical resource allocation decisions that incorporate views of justice that go beyond patients' individual needs to include the maintenance of social relationships.

The above findings suggest advantages to the interactive, patient-centered informed-consent models which allow an open process to accommodate the amount and type of information preferred by patients (Ballard-Reisch, 1990). These preferences vary with patients' appraisals of illness severity and chronicity, their stage in coping, and relative emphasis on attentional or avoidant coping. As these factors change over time, patients' preferences for information may shift. Discussion regarding these preferences may help patients gain the benefits of more appropriate information, while minimizing inappropriate information.

The benefits of a patient's social support network may be further enhanced by discussing the following issues during medical decision making:

1. Type, amount, and effectiveness of available social support from particular individuals;
2. Identification of individuals that the patient considers part of the decision-making process and with whom the patient shares social responsibilities;
3. Ways in which social support influences the patient's perspectives on elements of informed consent (e.g., perceptions of risks and benefits of proposed treatments, expectations for treatment); and
4. How social support may influence the patient's adherence to treatment.

SEXUAL AND RELATED PSYCHOSOCIAL ISSUES

Concurrent discussion of related sexual and psychosocial issues is often helpful. Stellman and colleagues (1984) recommend information sharing and ongoing psychosexual counseling, for patients undergoing vulvectomies and their partners, to address common problems of depression, sexual guilt, and difficulties in reality testing. Cairns and Valentich (1986) similarly recommend that informed consent regarding vaginal reconstruction include discussion of psychosocial and sexual adjustment issues with both partners and that ongoing counseling be made available. Their review of research on vaginal reconstruction suggests that its sexual and psychosocial consequences have been underemphasized and that definitions of the need for and success of vaginal reconstruction often reflect male stereotypes of women's health that are narrowly focused upon capacity for heterosexual intercourse.

Even though breast reconstruction may reduce the feelings of diminished femininity and attractiveness that follow mastectomy, and may improve behaviors related to body image (Wellisch et al., 1989), it has been chosen by less than 1% of the more than half million women in the United States who have had mastectomies, according to Winder and Winder (1985). They recommend that counseling and education designed to overcome barriers to choosing breast reconstruction should address: 1) psychological responses to mastectomy, including acceptance of loss; 2) motivation for reconstruction; and 3) possible guilt, shame, or fear regarding body image. They propose that counselors help women take an active role in medical decision making and help them prepare questions for physicians.

Women commonly want to discuss sexual health issues with their physicians. Metz and Seifert's (1988) survey of female patients of primary-care physicians revealed that: 1) 84% of patients wanted physician initiative in sexual health discussions; 2) 32% wanted more physician initiative; 3) 41% would not discuss sexual issues without physician initiative; and 4) physicians were the main professional with whom 68% had discussed sexual issues. Empathy, warmth, professional competence, and confidentiality were the most desired qualities and were especially important for the 20% of the sample who had been sexually abused. Successful coping with sexual assault or abuse is associated with receiving helpful reactions when confiding about the assault or abuse (Harvey, Orbuch, Chwalisz, & Garwood, 1990).

COMPETENCY TO GRANT INFORMED CONSENT

When patients' competency to give informed consent is in question, Appelbaum and Grisso (1988) recommend that physicians ask patients to: 1) state their preferences regarding a proposed procedure more than once to check for relative consistency; 2) paraphrase and interpret information; 3) express their perceptions of the meaning of their illness, treatment needs, and likely outcomes; and 4) state the main reasons for their decisions and the weight attached to each reason. In order to enhance the accuracy and fairness of the competency assessment, they encourage physicians to: 1) conduct more than one examination; 2) talk with knowledgeable family members or care givers; and 3) minimize cultural and class barriers to understanding. Treatments to enhance mental functioning may restore patients' abilities to fully participate in decision making.

An example of assessing and enhancing competency to give informed consent is contraceptive use among women with chronic mental illness. McCullough, Coverdale, Bayer, and Chervenak (1992) describe how these pregnancies may involve particular risks to mothers and children. In order to balance protection against these risks with the protection of women's decision-making autonomy, the authors propose guidelines for informed consent to obstetric and gynecologic care, including contraception. Depending on the degree to which their autonomy is chronically and variably imparied, the women are divided into groups of those who: 1) can achieve thresholds of autonomy; 2) are irreversibly near thresholds of autonomy; and 3) are irreversibly below thresholds of autonomy.

Guidelines for Group 1 focus on interventions to improve autonomous decision making (e.g., repeated provision of information and removal of psychosocial stressors). Group 2 guidelines focus on presenting options for care that are consistent with a patient's values to which the patient may meaningfully agree. Guidelines for Group 3 include evaluation of the social costs of pregnancy, avoidance of forced sterilization, and usage of highly effective contraception.

CULTURAL DIFFERENCES

Medical training and practice are set within larger cultural and subcultural contexts and are influenced by dominant cultural values and ideologies (Waitzkin, 1989). Payer (1988) documents how aspects of medical care (e.g., diagnoses, treatment preferences, physician–patient relationships) differ significantly among the United States, England, West Germany, and France, parallel to differences in overall national philosophies and cultural values.

Cultural differences between patients and physicians may create divergent expectations of treatment processes and goals and decrease adherence to treatment (Garrity & Lawson, 1989). Communication problems associated with differences in patients' and physicians' language, worldviews, and conceptions of illness have been identified with patients from Appalachian (Tripp-Reimer, 1982) and North American Indian (Kaplan, 1989) backgrounds. Fox and Stein (1991) identified language differences between physicians and patients to be one cause of Hispanic women's lower utilization of mammograms than that of black and white women. Hispanic women were least likely to receive mammogram information, the main predictor of utilization.

Since most physicians come from and maintain upper-middle class status (Waitzkin, 1989), sensitivity is encouraged regarding how social and economic aspects of lower-income patients' lives may affect decision making. While exposed to high levels of health-endangering occupational and social stressors, the poor often have minimal access to health resources. Poor women in rural areas face particular problems in maintaining their health (e.g., high incidence of chronic disorders, environmental hazards, and low occupational status). They also experience problems in receiving medical services due to limited access to specialists, related human services, health insurance, and transportation (Bushy, 1990; Richardson, 1988) and exhibit a traditional reliance upon informal social networks (Bushy, 1990).

While decision making must incorporate the realities of such poverty-induced constraints, it is important to utilize existing resources (e.g., effective self-help remedies, social support networks) and to expand choices when possible. Curbow (1986) found that low-income women expressed more negative evaluations of hypothetical Medicaid health plans when they were offered less choice of providers. Since the women did not derogate the quality of care and interpersonal relations of the restricted services, the use of patient-centered decision-making models to enhance choices regarding aspects of treatment may lessen the derogation of other aspects of the restricted services.

Garrity and Lawson (1989) warn physicians against holding negative stereotypes of low-income patients (e.g., minimal understanding of disease, limited vocabulary, passive orientation to health and prevention). Waitzkin (1985) found that physicians gave more time, explanations, and nondiscrepant responses to upper-class patients than to lower-class patients, despite the lack of difference in patients' desires for information. This may be due to lower-class patients' greater use of nonverbal communication to express intent, relative to physicians' greater use of and expectation of related verbal communication. In addition, lower-income patients are often reluctant to ask questions of physicians due to social distance, their lack of familiarity with technical terms, and their belief that physicians don't expect questions (Waitzkin, 1985).

Physicians who work in settings that are different than their own cultural background are encouraged to increase their understanding of: 1) their own cultural perspectives (Moffic, 1983; Tripp-Reimer, 1982); 2) the socioeconomic context of their patients' health concerns (Ewart, 1991; Riessman, 1983); 3) differences in nonverbal communication; and 4) ways to utilize indigenous resources (e.g., community-based patient advocates; Kaplan, 1989). Physicians may develop culturally appropriate roles and treatments by asking patients to communicate in their most comfortable language; using paraphrasing; and assessing patients' cultural histories, folk beliefs, and perspectives on the problem, prior remedies, and treatment conceptions (Moffic, 1983). Participatory models of decision making provide a process to help implement the above recommendations and provide safeguards against the potentially negative effects of cultural differences by creating ways to: (1) identify potential differences in perceptions and expectations, including those which are beneficial to the treatment process; (2) minimize negative stereotypes; and (3) encourage question asking. The provision of culturally-appropriate health education through self-help groups may help address low-income, rural, or minority patients' needs for more access to medical care, including preventive care. Stewart's (1990) review of research on self-help groups suggests that professionals who interact with self-help groups through indirect, non-authoritarian roles as collaborative partners are often effective.

GENDER DIFFERENCES

Female physicians, compared with male physicians, have been found to: 1) conduct longer medical visits; 2) discuss psychosocial factors more; and 3) engage in more positive talk, partnership building, question asking, information giving, and acknowledgements (Maheaux, Dufort, Beland, Jacques, & Levesque, 1990; Meeurwesen, Schaap, & Van Der Staak, 1991; Roter, Lipkin, & Korsgaard, 1991).

Physicians' gender may affect their interactions with patients (e.g., information content, affective tone, and negotiatory quality) through: 1) sex-role attitudes; 2) increased similarity of status between physicians and patients of the same gender; and 3) patients' different expectations of male and female physicians (Weisman & Teitelbaum, 1985). For example, patients have different gender-based expectations for how physicians are to gain their adherence to treatment. Patients, regardless of sex, expected female and male physicians to use nonaggressive (nondirective) and mid-level aggressive persuasion strategies, respectively. Patients' satisfaction with and adherence to treatment was related to physicians behaving consistently with patients' expectations, with the additional allowance of nonaggressive strategies for male physicians (Burgoon, Birk, & Hall, 1991). Since patient-centered models of decision making encourage negotiation of patient and physician roles (Ballard-Reisch, 1990), these models may facilitate negotiation of effective boundaries of directiveness by physicians, enhancement of patients' satisfaction with and adherence to treatment, and discussion of sex-role expectations (Fennema, Meyer, & Owen, 1990).

SUMMARY OF CLINICAL IMPLICATIONS

Patients are most likely to communicate choices that are consistent with their goals when they receive appropriate informed-consent information (i.e., nature of the illness and treatment, probabilities of treatment effectiveness, risks, costs, and alternatives). Patients' knowledge and participation in decision making are increased through physicians' sharing of information, encouragement of questions, and use of educational materials. Patients' active role in decision making is associated with improvements in their knowledge, control, health status, adherence to treatment, and satisfaction with medical care.

Two overall suggestions for clinical practice are offered. First, agreement in physicians' and patients' understanding of the elements of informed consent can be facilitated by joint decision-making tools (e.g., the PREPARED™ protocol) and can improve ultimate health outcomes. Second, provision of informed-consent information and medical decision-making are most effective when done with sensitivity to individual differences among patients. General guidelines for

TABLE 16.3   Differences in Patients to Consider while Sharing Information

Preferences for information depending on previous similar experiences and existing
    medical knowledge
Needs for alternative formats, or orders, of information presentation, information
    rehearsal, and feedback regarding accuracy of understanding
Expectations for health outcomes, self-responsibility, and self-efficacy
Stages and styles of coping with illness and stress
Severity and chronicity of the evident disorder or of other disorders having an impact on
    capacities to grant informed consent
General perceptual, cognitive, and reading capacities
Needs and support capacities of family and friends
Cultural and gender differences, including those between patients and physicians

Note. From: "Decision-making in women's health care" by C. J. Hodne and R. C. Reiter (1994),
Clinical Obstetrics and Gynecology, 37 (1). The table was originally published by the J.B. Lippincott
Company, Philadelphia, PA, and is reprinted with permission.

providing information in a manner consistent with patients' preferences for
information (Hodne & Reiter, 1994) are summarized in Table 16.3.

Patients' preferences and expectations for treatment may change over time,
reflecting changes in their health status and various social influences (e.g., needs
and support of social network members). Therefore, flexibility in decision making is helpful. Patient-centered models of decision making offer ways to match
information provision with patients' preferences by allowing patients and physicians to: 1) identify individual differences and preferences in an early and ongoing manner; 2) assess the extent of agreement of understanding and readily
remedy any misunderstandings; 3) anticipate and communicate any changes in
preferences and expectations as they occur; and 4) negotiate adjustment of
treatment as needed.

Finally, patient-centered models of decision making provide ways to prevent
and remedy the potentially negative consequences of judgment biases, cultural
differences, and gender differences by creating opportunities to compare perspectives, gain from the benefits of different perspectives, and enhance agreement.

REFERENCES

Anderson, L. A., & Sharpe, P. A. (1991). Improving patient and provider communica-
    tion: A synthesis and review of communication interventions. *Patient Education and
    Counseling, 17,* 99–134.
Appelbaum, P. S., & Grisso, T. (1988). Assessing patients' capacities to consent to treat-
    ment. *New England Journal of Medicine, 319,* 1635–1638.
Bachmann, G. A., Moeller, T. P., & Benett, J. (1988). Childhood sexual abuse and the
    consequences in adult women. *Obstetrics and Gynecology, 71,* 631–642.

Ballard-Reisch, D. S. (1990). A model of participative decision making for physician–patient interaction. *Health Communication, 2,* 91–104.

Beisecker, A. E., & Beisecker, T. D. (1990). Patient information-seeking behaviors when communicating with doctors. *Medical Care, 28,* 19–28.

Bertakis, K. D. (1977). The communication of information from physician to patient: A method of increasing patient retention and satisfaction. *Journal of Family Practice, 5,* 217–222.

Brickman, P., Rabinowitz, V. C., Karuza, J., Jr., Coates, D., Cohn, E., & Kidder, L. (1982). Models of helping and coping. *American Psychologist, 37,* 368–384.

Brody, D. S., Miller, S. M., Lerman, C. E., Smith, D. G., & Caputo, G. C. (1989). Patient perception of involvement in medical care: Relationship to illness attitudes and outcomes. *Journal of General Internal Medicine, 4,* 506–511.

Burgoon, M., Birk, T. S., & Hall, J. R. (1991). Compliance and satisfaction with physician–patient communication: An expectancy theory interpretation of gender differences. *Human Communication Research, 18,* 177–208.

Bushy, A. (1990). Rural U.S. women: Traditions and transitions affecting health care. *Health Care for Women International, 11,* 503–513.

Cairns, K. V., & Valentich, M. (1986). Vaginal reconstruction in gynecologic cancer: A feminist perspective. *Journal of Sex Research, 22,* 333–346.

Christensen-Szalanski, J.J.J. (1984). Discount functions and the measurement of patients' values: Women's decisions during childbirth. *Medical Decision Making, 4,* 47–58.

Cipolli, C., Sancini, M., Tuozzi, G., Bolanzi, R., Mutinelli, P., Flamigni, C., & Porcu, E. (1989). Gaze and eye-contact with anorexic adolescents. *British Journal of Medical Psychology, 62,* 365–369.

Cohen, S. (1988). Psychosocial models of the role of social support in the etiology of physical disease. *Health Psychology, 7,* 269–297.

Cohen, S., & Wills, T. A. (1985). Stress, social support, and the buffering hypothesis. *Psychological Bulletin, 98,* 310–357.

Crandall, C. S. (1988). Social contagion of binge eating. *Journal of Personality and Social Psychology, 55,* 588–598.

Curbow, B. (1986). Health care and the poor: Psychological implications of restrictive policies. *Health Psychology, 5,* 375–391.

DiMatteo, M. R., Hays, R. D., & Sherbourne, C. D. (1992). Adherence to cancer regimens: Implications for treating the older patient. *Oncology, 6,* 50–57.

DiMatteo, M. R., Sherbourne, C. D., Hays, R. D., Ordway, L., Kravitz, R. L., McGlynn, E. A., Kaplan, S., & Rogers, W. H. (1993). Physicians' characteristics influence patients' adherence to medical treatment: Results from the medical outcomes study. *Health Psychology, 12,* 93–103.

Duck, S., (with R. C. Silver) (1990). *Personal relationships and social support.* London: Sage.

Ewart, C. K. (1991). Social action theory for a public health psychology. *American Psychologist, 46,* 931–946.

Faden, R. R., & Beauchamp, T. L. (with N.M.P. King) (1986). *A history and theory of informed consent.* New York: Oxford University Press.

Fennema, K., Meyer, D. L., & Owen, N. (1990). Sex of physician: Patients' preferences and stereotypes. *Journal of Family Practice, 30,* 441–446.

Fiske, S. T., & Taylor, S. E. (1991). *Social cognition.* (2nd ed.) New York: Random House.

Folkman, S., Lazarus, R. S., Dunkel-Schetter, C., DeLongis, A., & Gruen, R. J. (1986). Dynamics of a stressful encounter: Cognitive appraisal, coping, and encounter outcomes. *Journal of Personality and Social Psychology, 50,* 992–1003.

Folstein, J., Fostein, S., & McHugh, P. (1975). Mini-mental state. *Journal of Psychiatric Research, 12,* 189–198.

Fox, S. A., & Stein, J. A. (1991). The effect of physician–patient communication on mammography utilization by different ethnic groups. *Medical Care, 29,* 1065–1081.

Gambone, J. C., & Reiter, R. C. (1992). *Prepared for health care: A consumer's guide to better medical decisions.* Beaverton, OR: Great Performance.

Garrity, T. F., & Lawson, E. J. (1989). Patient–physician communication as a determinant of medication misuse in older, minority women. *Journal of Drug Issues, 19,* 245–259.

Giannini, A. J., Sorger, L. G., Martin, D. M., & Bates, L. (1988). Impaired reception of nonverbal cues in women with premenstrual tension syndrome. *Journal of Psychology, 122,* 591–596.

Greenfield, S., Kaplan, S., & Ware, J. E. (1985). Expanding patient involvement in care. *Annals of Internal Medicine, 102,* 520–528.

Hailey, B. J., Lavine, B., & Hogan, B. (1988). The mastectomy experience: Patients' perspectives. Women *and Health, 14,* 75–88.

Hall, J. A., & Dornan, M. C. (1988). Meta-analysis of satisfaction with medical care: Description of research domain and analysis of overall satisfaction levels. *Social Science and Medicine, 27,* 637–644.

Harrigan, J. A., & Rosenthal, R. (1983). Physicians' head and body positions as determinants of perceived rapport. *Journal of Applied Social Psychology, 13,* 496–509.

Harrigan, J. A., Oxman, T. E., & Rosenthal, R. (1985). Rapport expressed through nonverbal behavior. *Journal of Nonverbal Behavior, 9,* 95–110.

Harvey, J. H., Orbuch, T. L., Chwalisz, K. D., & Garwood, G. (1990). Coping with sexual assault: The role of account-making and confiding. *Journal of Traumatic Stress, 4,* 515–531.

Harvey, J. H., Orbuch, T. L., & Weber, A. L. (1990). A social psychological model of account-making in response to severe stress. *Journal of Language and Social Psychology, 9,* 191–207.

Harvey, J. H., Weber, A. L., & Orbuch, T. L. (1990). *Interpersonal accounts: A social psychological perspective.* Cambridge, MA: Basil Blackwell.

Hattori, H., Salzberg, S. M., Kiang, W. P., Fujimiya, T., Tejima, Y., & Furuno, J. (1991). The patient's right to information in Japan—Legal rules and doctor's opinions. *Social Science and Medicine, 32,* 1007–1016.

Haug, M., & Lavin, B. (1983). *Consumerism in medicine: Challenging physician authority.* Beverly Hills, CA: Sage Publications.

Haug, M. R., & Ory, M. G. (1987). Issues in elderly patient–provider interactions. *Research on Aging, 9,* 3–44.

Hodne, C. J., & Reiter, R. C. (1994). Decision-making in women's health care. *Clinical Obstetrics and Gynecology, 37,* 162–179.

Holmes, J. A., & Stevenson, C.A.Z. (1990). Differential effects of avoidant and attentional coping strategies on adaptation to chronic and recent-onset pain. *Health Psychology, 9,* 577–584.

Horowitz, M. J. (1976). *Stress response syndromes.* New York: Jason Aronson.

Horowitz, M. J. (1987). *States of mind.* New York: Plenum.

Hunt, L. M., Jordan, B., & Irwin, S. (1989). Views of what's wrong: Diagnosis and patients' concepts of illness. *Social Science and Medicine, 28,* 945–956.

Hunter, M. (1989). Gynaecology. In A. K. Broome (Ed.), *Health psychology: Processes and applications* (pp. 312–343). London: Chapman and Hall.

Jecker, N. S., & Berg, A. O. (1992). Allocating medical resources in rural America: Alternative perceptions of justice. *Social Science and Medicine, 34,* 467–474.

Kaplan, T. (1989). An intercultural communication gap: North American Indians vs. the mainstream medical profession. In W. von Raffler-Engel (Ed.), *Doctor–patient interaction* (pp. 45–59). Amsterdam: John Benjamins Publishing.

Karuza, J., Jr., Zevon, M. A., Rabinowitz, V. C., & Brickman, P. (1982). Attribution of responsibility by helpers and recipients. In T. A. Wills (Ed.), *Basic processes in helping relationships* (pp. 107–129). New York: Academic Press.

Lerman, C. E., Brody, D. S., Caputo, G. C., Smith, D. G., Lazaro, C. G., & Wolfson, H. G. (1990). Patients' perceived involvement in care scale: Relationship to attitudes about illness and medical care. *Journal of General Internal Medicine, 5,* 29–33.

Ley, P. (1982). Giving information to patients. In J. R. Eiser (Ed.), *Social psychology and behavioral science* (pp. 339–373). London: John Wiley.

Ley, P. (1989). Improving patients' understanding, recall, satisfaction and compliance. In A. K. Broome (Ed.), *Health psychology: Processes and applications* (pp. 74–102). London: Chapman and Hall.

Llewellyn-Thomas, H. A., Sutherland, H. J., Tritchler, D. L., Lockwood, G. A., Till, J. E., Ciampi, A., Scott, J. F., Lickley, L. A., & Fish, E. B. (1991). Benign and malignant breast disease: The relationship between women's health status and health values. *Medical Decision Making, 11,* 180–188.

Maheaux, B., Dufort, F., Beland, F., Jacques, A., & Levesque, A. (1990). Female medical practitioners: More preventive and patient oriented? *Medical Care, 28,* 87–92.

McClain, C. S. (1987). Patient decision making: The case of delivery method after a previous cesarean section. *Culture, Medicine, and Psychiatry, 11,* 495–508.

McCullough, L. B., Coverdale, J., Bayer, T., & Chervenak, F. A. (1992). Ethically justified guidelines for family planning interventions to prevent pregnancy in female patients with chronic mental illness. *American Journal of Obstetrics and Gynecology, 167,* 19–25.

Meeurwesen, L., Schaap, C., & Van Der Staak, C. (1991). Verbal analysis of doctor–patient communication. *Social Science and Medicine, 32,* 1143–1150.

Metz, M. E., & Seifert, M. H. (1988). Women's expectations of physicians in sexual health concerns. *Family Practice Research Journal, 7,* 141–152.

Meyerowitz, B. E., & Chaiken, S. (1987). The effect of message framing on breast self-examination attitudes, intentions, and behavior. *Journal of Personality and Social Psychology, 52,* 500–510.

Michela, J. L., & Wood, J. V. (1986). Causal attributions in health and illness. In P. C. Kendall (Ed.), *Advances in cognitive–behavioral research and therapy, Vol. 5* (pp. 179–235). New York: Academic Press.

Miller, S. M., & Mangan, C. E. (1983). Interacting effects of information and coping style in adapting to gynecologic stress: Should the doctor tell all? *Journal of Personality and Social Psychology, 45,* 223–236.

Moffic, H. S. (1983). Sociocultural guidelines for clinicians in multicultural settings. *Psychiatric Quarterly, 55,* 47–54.

Payer, L. (1988). *Medicine and culture: Varieties of treatment in the United States, England, West Germany, and France.* New York: Penguin Books.

Redeimeier, D. A., Rozin, P., & Kahneman, D. (1993). Understanding patients' decisions: Cognitive and emotional perspectives. *Journal of the American Medical Association, 270,* 72–76.

Reiter, R. C., Lench, J. B., & Gambone, J. C. (1989). Consumer advocacy, elective surgery, and the "golden era of medicine." *Obstetrics and Gynecology, 74,* 815–817.

Richardson, H. (1988). The health plight of rural women. *Women & Health, 12,* 41–54.

Ridgeway, V., & Mathews, A. (1982). Psychological preparation for surgery: A comparison of methods. *British Journal of Clinical Psychology, 21,* 271–280.

Riessman, C. K. (1983). Women and medicalization: A new perspective. *Social Policy, 14,* 3–18.

Rodin, J., & Ickovics, J. R. (1990). Women's health: Review and research agenda as we approach the 21st century. *American Psychologist, 45,* 1018–1034.

Roter, D. L. (1984). Patient question asking in physician–patient interaction. *Health Psychology, 3,* 395–409.

Roter, D. L., & Hall, J. A. (1987). Physicians' interviewing styles and medical information obtained from patients. *Journal of General Internal Medicine, 2,* 325–328.

Roter, D. L., Hall, A., & Katz, N. R. (1988). Patient-physician communication: A descriptive summary of the literature. *Patient Education and Counseling, 12,* 99–119.

Roter, D., Lipkin, M., & Korsgaard, A. (1991). Sex differences in patients' and physicians' communication during primary care medical visits. *Medical Care, 29,* 1083–1093.

Roth, S., & Newman, E. (1991). The process of coping with sexual trauma. *Journal of Traumatic Stress, 4,* 279–297.

Schaeffer, M. H. (1989). Environmental stress and individual decision-making: Implications for the patient. *Patient Education and Counseling, 13,* 221–235.

Schiffmann, A., Cohen, S., Nowik, R., & Selinger, D. (1978). Initial diagnostic hypotheses: Factors which may distort physicians' judgment. *Organizational Behavior and Human Performance, 21,* 305–315.

Schulze, C., Florin, I., Matschin, E., Sougioultzi, C., & Schulze, H. (1988). Psychological distress after hysterectomy—A predictive study. *Psychology and Health, 2,* 1–12.

Schwarzer, R., & Leppin, A. (1991). Social support and health: A theoretical and empirical overview. *Journal of Social and Personal Relationships, 8,* 99–127.

Shapiro, D. E., Boggs, S. R., Melamed, B. G., & Graham-Pole, J. (1992). The effect of varied physician affect on recall, anxiety, and perceptions in women at risk for breast cancer: An analogue study. *Health Psychology, 11,* 61–66.

Shreve, E. G., Harrigan, J. A., Kues, J. R., & Kagas, D. K. (1988). Nonverbal expressions of anxiety in physician–patient interactions. *Psychiatry, 51,* 378–384.

Shumaker, S. A., & Hill, D. R. (1991). Gender differences in social support and physical health. *Health Psychology, 10,* 102–111.

Sprecher, P. L., Thomas, E. R., Huebner, L. A., Norfleet, B. E., & Jacoby, K. E. (1983).

Effects of increased physician–patient communication on patient anxiety. *Professional Psychology: Research and Practice, 14,* 251–255.

Squier, R. W. (1990). A model of empathic understanding and adherence to treatment regimens in practitioner–patient relationships. *Social Science and Medicine, 30,* 325–339.

Stellman, R. E., Goodwin, J. M., Robinson, J., Dansak, D., Hilgers, R. D. (1984). Psychological effects of vulvectomy. *Psychosomatics, 25,* 779–783.

Stewart, M. J. (1990). Professional interface with mutual-aid self-help groups: A review. *Social Science and Medicine, 31,* 1143–1158.

Street, R. L., & Buller, D. B. (1987). Nonverbal response patterns in physician–patient interactions: A functional analysis. *Journal of Nonverbal Behavior, 11,* 234–253.

Suls, J., & Fletcher, B. (1985). The relative efficacy of avoidant and nonavoidant coping strategies: A meta-analysis. *Health Psychology, 4,* 249–288.

Svarstad, B. S. (1976). Physician–patient communication and patient conformity with medical advice. In D. Mechanic (Ed.), *The growth of bureaucratic medicine* (pp. 220–238). New York: John Wiley.

Taylor, S. E. (1983). Adjustment to threatening events: A theory of cognitive adaptation. *American Psychologist, 38,* 1161–1173.

Thompson, S. C., Nanni, C., & Schwankovsky, L. (1990). Patient-oriented interventions to improve communication in a medical office visit. *Health Psychology, 9,* 390–404.

Travis, C. B. (1985). Medical decision making and elective surgery: The case of hysterectomy. *Risk Analysis, 5,* 241–251.

Travis, C. B. (1988). *Women and health psychology: Biomedical issues.* Hillsdale, NJ: Lawrence Erlbaum.

Travis, C. B., Phillippi, R. H., & Tonn, B. E. (1989). Judgment heuristics and medical decisions. *Patient Education and Counseling, 13,* 211–220.

Tripp-Reimer, T. (1982). Barriers to health care: Variation in interpretation of Appalachian client behavior by Appalachian and non-Appalachian health professionals. *Western Journal of Nursing Research, 4,* 179–191.

Turnquist, D. C., Harvey, J. H., & Andersen, B. L. (1988). Attributions and adjustment to life-threatening illness. *British Journal of Clinical Psychology, 27,* 55–65.

Tversky, A., & Kahneman, D. (1973). Availability: A heuristic for judging frequency and probability. *Cognitive Psychology, 5,* 207–232.

Tymchuk, A. J., & Ouslander, J. G. (1990). Optimizing the informed consent process with elderly people. *Educational Gerontology, 16,* 245–257.

Tymchuk, A. J., & Ouslander, J. G. (1991). Informed consent: Does position of information have an effect upon what elderly people in long-term care remember? *Educational Gerontology, 17,* 11–19.

Tymchuk, A. J., Ouslander, J. G., & Rader, N. (1986). Informing the elderly: A comparison of four methods. *Journal of the American Geriatrics Society, 34,* 818–822.

Waitzkin, H. (1985). Information giving in medical care. *Journal of Health and Social Behavior, 26,* 81–101.

Waitzkin, H. (1989). A critical theory of medical discourse: Ideology, social control, and the processing of social context in medical encounters. *Journal of Health and Social Behavior, 30,* 220–239.

Wallace, L. M. (1986). Communication variables in the design of presurgical preparatory information. *British Journal of Clinical Psychology, 25,* 111–118.

Ward, M. M., Stone, S. C., & Sandman, C. A. (1977). Visual perception in women during the menstrual cycle. *Physiology and Behavior, 20,* 239–243.

Weisman, C. S., & Teitelbaum, M. A. (1985). Physician gender and the physician–patient relationship: Recent evidence and relevant questions. *Social Science and Medicine, 20,* 1119–1127.

Wellisch, D. K., DiMatteo, R., Silverstein, M., Landsverk, J., Hoffman, R., Waisman, J., Handel, N., Waisman-Smith, E., & Schain, W. (1989). Psychosocial outcomes of breast cancer therapies. *Psychosomatics, 30,* 365–373.

Winder, A. E., & Winder, B. D. (1985). Patient counseling: Clarifying a woman's choice for breast reconstruction. *Patient Education and Counseling, 7,* 65–75.

Woodward, N. J., & Wallston, B. S. (1987). Age and health care beliefs: Self-efficacy as a mediator of low desire for control. *Psychology and Aging, 2,* 3–8.

Wu, W. C., & Pearlman, R. A. (1988). Consent in medical decision making: The role of communication. *Journal of General Internal Medicine, 3,* 9–14.

Index

SP *Springer Publishing Company*

TREATING ABUSE IN FAMILIES
A Feminist and Community Approach

Elaine Leeder, MSW, CSW, MPH, PhD

The author presents a practical, alternative model of treatment for psychologists and other therapists who deal with abuse in families. Based on her own clinical experiences, Dr. Leeder proposes treating the perpetrator and the victim as part of a community or family system. Unlike traditional approaches that favor removing the victim from the abusive environment, the author advocates family and community interventions to stabilize the violent behavior and keep the family together.

Contents:

Springer Series: Focus on Women

1994   232pp   0-8261-8530-4   hardcover

536 Broadway, New York, NY 10012-3955 • (212) 431-4370 • Fax (212) 941-7842

Ⓢ *Springer Publishing Company*

WOMEN AND SUICIDAL BEHAVIOR

Silvia Sara Canetto, PhD, and **David Lester,** PhD, Editors

A comprehensive and definitive work on women and suicide is long overdue, especially because women in most countries are more likely than men to exhibit suicidal behavior. This book fills a major gap in the suicide literature and contrasts with previous works that have tended to address suicidal behavior on women from a male perspective. This volume considers the social and cultural factors involved and also provides useful intervention strategies.

Partial Contents:

I: INTRODUCTION. Women and Suicidal Behavior: Issues and Dilemmas, *S. S. Canetto & D. Lester*

II: EPIDEMIOLOGY. Women and Suicidal Behavior: Epidemiology, Gender, and Lethality in Historical Perspective, *H. I. Kushner* • The Epidemiology of Women's Suicidal Behavior, *S. S. Canetto & D. Lester*

III: THEORIES. Gender Socialization and Women's Suicidal Behaviors, *A. Kay Clifton & D. E. Lee* • Through a Glass Darkly: Women and Attitudes Toward Suicidal Behavior, *J. M. Stillion* • The Pseudosuicidal Female: A Cautionary Tale, *B. Joyce Stephens*

IV: DIVERSE EXPERIENCES OF SUICIDAL WOMEN. Suicidal Behavior and Employment, *B. Yang & D. Lester* • Suicidal Adolescent Latinas: Culture, Female Development, and Restoring the Mother-Daughter Relationship, *J. K. Zimmerman & L. H. Zayas* • Suicidal Behavior in African-American Women, *M. H. Alston & S. Eylar Anderson* • Suicidal Behavior in Asian-American Women, *F. A. Ibrahim* • American Indian Female Adolescent Suicide, *T. LaFromboise & B. Howard-Pitney* • Elderly Women and Suicidal Behavior, *S. S. Canetto*

V: INTERVENTION. Suicidal Women: Intervention and Prevention Strategies, *S. S. Canetto* • Women as Survivors of Suicide: An Experience of Integration, *L. Sapsford*

Springer Series: Focus on Women

1994   288pp   0-8261-8630-0   hardcover

536 Broadway, New York, NY 10012-3955 • (212) 431-4370 • Fax (212) 941-7842

§P *Springer Publishing Company*

WOMEN AND ANGER

Sandra P. Thomas, PhD, RN, Editor

"The study, the first large-scale detailed look at anger in the lives of average middle-class american women, puts the lie to many long-standing beliefs about the role of this emotion in women's lives."
— **New York Times**

"Thomas and her colleagues make sense out of why anger is a special health problem for women, and why anger is an excellent example of a 'dis-ease' in need of study when considering the evolution of a new health paradigm focusing on the fit between person and environment. It has made me think that how a person handles anger should be a part of every health professional's assessment of a new patient."
— **Angela Barron McBride,** PhD

Contents:

Emotions and How They Develop, *S. P. Thomas* • Anger and Its Manifestations in Women, *S. P. Thomas* • Anger: Targets and Triggers, *G. Denham and K. Bultemeier* • Women's Anger and Self-Esteem, *M. Saylor and G. Denham* • Stress, Role Responsibilities, Social Support, and Anger, *S.P. Thomas and M. M. Donnellan* • Values and Anger, *C. Smucker, J. Martin, and D. Wilt* • Unhealthy, Unfit, and Too Angry to Care? *M.A. Modrcin-McCarthy and J. Tollett* • Women's Anger and Eating, *S.S. Russell and B. Shirk* • Women's Anger and Substance Use, *E.G. Seabrook* • Women, Depression, and Anger, *P.G. Droppleman and D. Wilt* • Treatment of Anger, *D. Wilt*

Springer Series : Focus on Women
1993   332pp   0-8261-8100-7   hardcover

536 Broadway, New York, NY 10012-3955 • (212) 431-4370 • Fax (212) 941-7842

SP *Springer Publishing Company*

BREAST CANCER
A Psychological Treatment Manual

Sandra Haber, PhD, Editor

This volume, originally published by the Division of Independent Practice of the American Psychological Association, was designed to educate and involve therapists and counselors in the psychological treatment of patients and their families. This manual represents a collaborative venture of 10 women psychologists who address the emotional responses of breast cancer patients, families, and caretakers, as well as the psychological, social, and behavioral factors that may influence cancer morbidity and mortality.

Contents:

I: Medical Aspects of Breast Cancer. Medical Treatment of Breast Cancer • The Relationships Among Patient, Physician and Psychologist

II: Stages of Breast Cancer: Patient's Experience and Treatment. Psychological Reactions to Diagnosis and Treatment • Psychological Reactions to Posttreatment • Recurrence and Terminal Illness

III: Psychotherapy with the Breast Cancer Patient. The Patient-Psychologist Relationship • Support Groups/Group Therapy • Special Populations: High Risk Women, Lesbian Women, Women of Poverty and Ethnicity, and Older Women • Countertransference

IV: Psychological Interventions with the Family. Husbands and Significant Others • Helping the Children

V: Interventions and Resources. Specific Interventions • Research on the Effectiveness of Psychological Interventions • Resources • Selected Medical Glossary

1994   144pp (est.)   0-8261-8790-0   hardcover

536 Broadway, New York, NY 10012-3955 • (212) 431-4370 • Fax (212) 941-7842